876.47

The Role of Emotions in Preventative Health Communication

The Role of Emotions in Preventative Health Communication

Jessica Gall Myrick

LEXINGTON BOOKS
Lanham • Boulder • New York • London

Published by Lexington Books
An imprint of The Rowman & Littlefield Publishing Group, Inc.
4501 Forbes Boulevard, Suite 200, Lanham, Maryland 20706
www.rowman.com

Unit A, Whitacre Mews, 26-34 Stannary Street, London SE11 4AB

British Library Cataloguing in Publication Information Available

Library of Congress Cataloging-in-Publication Data

Myrick, Jessica Gall, 1984- , author.
The role of emotions in preventative health communication / Jessica Gall Myrick.
p. cm.
Includes bibliographical references and index.
ISBN 978-0-7391-9147-7 (cloth : alk. paper) -- ISBN 978-0-7391-9148-4 (ebook)
I. Title. [DNLM: 1. Emotions. 2. Health Communication. 3. Health Behavior. 4. Health Knowledge,
Attitudes, Practice. 5. Preventive Medicine. WA 590]
RA427.8
613--dc23
2015024055

Printed in the United States of America

To Scott, with love.

Contents

Acknowledgments

As I reflect on my early academic career, I can't help but notice that the people I have most leaned on during this time have been strong, intelligent, inspiring, and caring women. Without these women, I am pretty sure I wouldn't be where I am now or publishing a book about scholarly research.

Margie Hershey first exposed me to media research when I was an undergraduate political science student at Indiana University. And when I started wandering naively toward graduate school, she also made sure I ended up where I needed to be.

Once I was enrolled in the journalism master's program at Indiana University, Amy Reynolds, Bonnie Brownlee, Lesa Major, Radhika Parameswaran, and Betsi Grabe planted the seed in my head that being a professor was a meaningful and interesting career path. I am extremely humbled and grateful to now be working as a faculty member at the same place and with many of the same wonderful people who gave me my start down this academic path.

Once I started the doctoral program at the University of North Carolina at Chapel Hill, Rhonda Gibson kept me on track, despite many off-the-rails moments. Her service on behalf of graduate students was unmatched.

While writing a literature review for a paper in Rhonda's class, I happened upon one of Robin Nabi's articles. I proceeded to read every one of Robin's papers I could find and then hunted her down at communication conferences to ask questions. She always took the time to answer my inquiries and chat with me. This book would be quite thin without Robin's influential scholarship.

One of the most fortuitous events that happened to me while I was at UNC was to meet Mary Beth Oliver. She not only taught me how to construct and test a structural equation model but also has provided constant support and encouragement. I feel so lucky to have her as a mentor and friend.

Merely saying "thanks" to these women feels quite insufficient considering all they've done for me. Nonetheless, I do thank them and hope they know how much I appreciate them.

There are many others I want to thank for helping to make this book possible. Faculty and staff at the Indiana University Media School have been supportive of all of my research activities. My graduate research assistant, Rachelle Pavelko, helped gather background research for many of the chapters and was a lifesaver when it came to creating the index. I can't wait to see what she does in her own academic career.

Francie Hill and George Thompson read over the initial contract that came from the publisher and also offered encouragement throughout the writing process. Everyone I've encountered at Lexington Books has been extremely helpful, too. A special thanks goes to Alison Pavan for guiding me through this book-writing gig for the first time.

Brian Murer and Jona Kerr helped me restore my physical health after I spent too much time sitting hunched over a laptop. Their ELDOA classes (and the classmates) provided much needed respites between writing and revising.

Scott Myrick kept me focused when I tried to procrastinate and listened patiently when I would ramble on about various aspects of the book. Biscuit Myrick was—literally—by my side throughout this project. I love them both.

I must also thank my dad, sister, and other family members for their support and encouragement in all of my endeavors.

Introduction

Emotions and Preventative Health Communication

There can be no knowledge without emotion. We may be aware of a truth, yet until we have felt its force, it is not ours. To the cognition of the brain must be added the experience of the soul. —Arnold Bennett, *The Journals of Arnold Bennett*, entry for March 18, 1897

PREVENTION AND HEALTH

In 1992, Congress appended the words "and Prevention" to the formal title of the Centers for Disease Control (Centers for Disease Control 1992). This change recognized and emphasized the CDC's role in preventing disease, injury, and disability, not just controlling them. More than 20 years later, prevention has become a common topic in health behavior and health communication circles. More than half of all Americans live with at least one serious but preventable health condition (Trust for America's Health and Robert Wood Johnson Foundation 2014). Between 20 and 40 percent of annual deaths from the five leading causes of death in the United States (heart disease, cancer, chronic lower respiratory diseases, stroke, and unintentional injuries) are preventable (Yoon, Bastian, Anderson, Collins, and Jaffe 2014). These preventable conditions are even more common in minority communities in the United States (Centers for Disease Control 2009; 2011). Given these statistics, the increasing interest in prevention is no surprise.

Despite the high number of preventable conditions, more than three-quarters of health care dollars in the United States are spent on treating disease instead of preventing it (Anderson 2004; Sensenig 2007; Trust for America's

Health 2006). Meanwhile, the growing costs of disease treatment are helping drive health care spending rates higher and higher (Thorpe 2013). In a paper tellingly titled "Greater use of preventive services in U.S. health care could save lives at little or no cost," Maciosek, Coffield, Flottemesch, Edwards, and Solberg (2010) analyzed the costs and the benefits of adopting doctor-recommended clinical health services. The researchers found that use of these 20 prevention services could save more than 2 million years of life (called "life-years") each year. What is more, the data indicate that the greater use of preventive services would also save the country money.

The three most cost-effective of these preventive services include a daily aspirin for men over age 40 and women over age 50, childhood immunizations, and smoking cessation advice/help to quit (Maciosek et al. 2006). Maciosek et al.'s data also suggest that greater use of services such as alcohol screening and counseling, colorectal cancer screening, hypertension screening and treatment, influenza immunization, and vision screening would be cost-effective ways to ease the burden of disease on individuals and on society. Public policy has attempted to address these burdens. For example, the Patient Protection and Affordable Care Act of 2010 established the National Prevention Strategy and Prevention Fund with the goal of expanding insurance coverage for preventive services and helping communities improve health through prevention-focused initiatives (Trust for America's Health and Robert Wood Johnson Foundation 2014).

Beyond government agencies and public health advocates, the public itself is increasingly aware of the need to undertake prevention and not just depend on treatment. In fact, 84 percent of Americans support the provision of public funding for prevention programs and are even willing to pay higher taxes to fund such programs (Centers for Disease Control 2009). But this type of funding is hard to come by during times of economic and political constraints.

Greater accessibility of clinical services, along with behavioral changes in the modifiable risk factors at the root of the preventable diseases (e.g., tobacco use, second hand smoke, indoor and outdoor air pollutants, high blood pressure, high cholesterol, type 2 diabetes, poor diet, overweight, lack of physical activity, exposure to ultraviolet radiation, occupational hazards, exposure to certain chemicals, drug and alcohol use, as well as unsafe home and community environments, see Yoon et al. 2014), would go a long way toward improving quality of life. Many of the modifiable risk factors mentioned above are behaviors that most people can change on their own *if* they have the necessary knowledge, motivation, resources, and support to do so. Other illness-preventing measures, as well as widespread implementation of the aforementioned clinical services, would likely require collective action and policy change to occur.

The importance of prevention takes on additional meaning in the context of health communication. That is because it is a challenge to communicate the importance of prevention to individuals who often feel invincible to health threats or who want to avoid thinking about health threats at all. It is much easier to convince an individual to pay attention *after* symptoms or a diagnosis are present. Moreover, there is no guarantee that the effort required by preventative actions, such as maintaining an exercise routine and healthy diet, will ensure perfect health. Since even the most healthy and mindful individuals can still get cancer or have a heart attack, countless individuals remain dissuaded from engaging in preventative health actions.

The obstacles to effectively focusing the public's attention on prevention-oriented messages and then motivating people to take action based on those messages are many. Because it is more difficult to gain and keep the public's attention on prevention messages and their target behaviors, this realm of health communication differs qualitatively from research on messages directed at diagnosed patients and/or their family members. The emotional reactions associated with those messaging contexts can be quite different, too. For example, humor may seem inappropriate for communicating with someone with a recent stage four cancer diagnosis. However, in a prevention-focused environment, humor may be an effective tool for getting the attention of individuals who would otherwise ignore such health information.

Effective prevention-focused health messages are vital if society is to find a way to improve individual and public health. How can researchers and health message creators overcome the hurdles presented by the public's apathy and avoidance of prevention behaviors? One answer to this question is to more closely examine the role of emotions in shaping public reactions to prevention-focused health messages. By analyzing the psychology of message-relevant emotions within the context of preventative health communication, researchers can better understand the ability of these messages to improve health outcomes. This vein of research can also improve understanding of the effects of particular forms of health messages on audiences, from public service announcements to news stories and even video games.

By "emotions," this book adopts Nabi's (2009; 2010) definition of the concept: Internal mental states of various intensities that denote evaluative and valenced reactions to events, agents, or objects (Ortony, Clore, and Collins 1988). Emotions differ from the more general concept of affect, which is an umbrella term to describe evaluative reactions to one's environment. Discrete emotions (e.g., fear, anger, hope, joy) also differ from moods, which are more diffuse and longer-lasting states that individuals typically cannot associate with particular events (see chapter 1 on theoretical foundations for a more detailed discussion of the conceptual definitions used in this book).

This book is focused on message-relevant, or integral, emotions that arise from consuming prevention-oriented health messages. Various features (e.g., visuals versus text, choice of colors, etc.) and components (e.g., framing of the message, inclusion of threat and efficacy information, etc.) of messages may elicit different emotions in different audiences. For instance, a story about an insect-borne illness like Lyme disease may frighten the average news consumer, but the same story may result in feelings of interest and curiosity in an entomologist. It is the effects of these message-relevant emotional reactions to health messages on subsequent health-related attitudes and behaviors that are the focus of this book. This is not to say that the relationship between prevention messages, emotions, and health behaviors is entirely linear, one causing the other in lock step. The process can be reciprocal and nuanced with many intermediate steps (e.g., Baumeister, Vohs, Nathan De-Wall, and Zhang 2007).

This book makes the argument that if prevention-focused health messages are to be effective in motivating behavior, they need to tug at the heartstrings, and researchers need to understand more precisely how different discrete emotional reactions influence health message effects. In making this case, this book takes a quantitative, social science–based approach to understanding the role of emotions in shaping individual-level effects to preventative health messages disseminated (primarily) through mass media channels.

EMOTIONS AND MEDIATED HEALTH MESSAGES

As the twenty-first century advances, mass media continue to be a fundamental part of the human experience. Health-related media permeate our modern experience, from using an online search engine to reading a pamphlet about vaccinations at the doctor's office or watching a television news report on the dangers of sitting too much. Media of all types and about all topics have one aspect in common: They make people feel *something*, be it frightened, elated, intrigued, depressed, inspired, or some mix of emotions (Döveling, von Scheve, and Konijn 2011). Döveling, von Scheve, and Konijn argue that the emotional ramifications of media consumption are important areas of scholarly inquiry: "[H]ow we feel in and about our society, or indeed about the world in which we live, is affected by our experiencing this world through the mass media" (2).

Evidence from the field of social psychology also provides an impetus for studying the role of emotions in media effects, particularly as they relate to preventative health behaviors. Emotions help form the primary motivational system for human beings, prompting people to take action to either change or maintain their surroundings (Izard 1977). Emotions assist individuals in determining what events, people, or objects are relevant to well-being and which are not (Frijda 1986). Emotions help people navigate society and foster social connections that can benefit us down the road (Fredrickson

1998; Keltner and Haidt 1999). Evolutionary perspectives argue that emotions evolved to help individuals adapt and learn how best to handle situations in order to ensure their welfare (Darwin 2009). And work in neurology has demonstrated that when individuals have brain damage to the parts of the brain that regulate emotions, they often act irrationally and alienate those around them (Damasio 2006).

Moreover, research also suggests that emotion is tied directly to health and well-being (Consedine and Moskowitz 2007; Williams and Evans 2014). This literature indicates that emotions like anger or anxiety can negatively impact physiological processes, but also shows that anticipated emotions may spur health-related behavior (e.g., anticipating regret for not exercising can motivate people to exercise). Research acknowledging the centrality of emotions to human life, understanding how prevention-focused health messages evoke emotions, and how these emotional reactions shape subsequent thoughts and behavior are crucial activities for developing more substantive theories of health communication effects and more effective health messages.

Along these lines, in an article titled "Rethinking communication in the e-health era," Neuhauser and Kreps (2003) provide guidance for advancing the field of health communication in the digital age. First on their list of axioms for moving the field forward is the following: "Health communication is more effective when it reaches people on an emotional as well as rational level" (10). They point out that knowledge alone, though necessary, is not enough to motivate people to engage in positive health behavior changes. This type of behavior change is difficult to sustain without some form of emotional involvement to provide motivation and foster perseverance. Yet, as Nabi (2015) notes, only limited research to date, on only a limited subset of discrete emotions, has dug deeply into the role of discrete emotions in health communication.

This lack of work on media processes and effects related to discrete emotional reaction to media messages is not unique to the field of health communication. Communication research as a whole has largely focused on cognitive aspects of message processes and effects. It wasn't until the 1980s and 1990s that emotion gained a foothold as a worthwhile topic of study in mainstream media effects research (Nabi 2009). And even then, emotion remains underexplored. By overlooking one of the most important determinants of human behavior, health messages that do not take into account the role of discrete emotional states often fall short of fostering long-term behavior change. Likewise, health communication research often fails to explain a large portion of the variance in health communication processes and effects, perhaps due to the lack of a detailed analysis of the role of emotions.

The good news is that a growing body of research is beginning to recognize and analyze the role of emotions in the realm of communication. Origi-

nally, research on media effects modeled on the behaviorist tradition of social psychology treated emotions as noise or interference (Konijn and ten
Holt 2011). Ultimately, though, communication scholars came to recognize
emotion as a central component in understanding the complex ways in which
the media may (or may not) impact audiences. For instance, Zillmann and his
colleagues led a movement to study the role of emotion in entertainment
media selection and entertainment effects (e.g., Bryant, Roskos-Ewoldsen,
and Cantor 2003; Cantor 2009; Zillmann 1971; 1988; 2006; Zillmann and
Bryant 1985).

Eventually communication researchers studying health-related messages
effects likewise developed the groundwork to better understand the important
role of emotion in their outcomes of interest (e.g., Dillard 1994; Dillard and
Peck 2000; 2001; Lang 2006; Nabi 1999; 2002; 2003; Shen and Dillard
2007; Turner, Rimal, Morrison, and Kim 2006; Witte 1992). Standing on
their shoulders, more and more health communication scholars are beginning
to include emotional components in their own research designs and measures. Yet there is still much work to be done to more widely instill the notion
that emotions are central to an adequate understanding of health communication processes and effects.

In applying emotion theories to the analysis of health message effects, it
is also important to consider what features of messages evoke which type and
intensity of emotion. Communication researchers have developed a plethora
of literature in this area. One body of research looks at how the packaging
and editing of content can influence emotional reactions. Media features such
as color (e.g., Detenber, Simons, and Reiss 2000; Detenber and Winch
2001), pacing of cuts and edits (e.g., Lang, Bolls, Potter, and Kawahara
1999), screen size (e.g., Reeves, Lang, Kim, and Tatar 1999), and many
others can influence audience reactions to media content without necessarily
changing the core message.

Even the order of emotional elicitation in a message can impact audience
reactions and behavior. For instance, research has found that individuals tend
to best recall the peak emotional experience and the final emotional experience for a given event (Kahneman, Fredrickson, Schreiber, and Redelmeier
1993). Nabi (2015) posits that the emotional flow, or "the evolution of the
emotional experience during exposure to a health message, marked by one or
more emotional shifts" (117), may increase or decrease the persuasiveness of
health messages, particularly narrative health messages. According to Nabi,
information describing a health threat that is likely to evoke fear in audiences
may be best placed at the beginning of a health message in order to attract
attention, but then a more positive approach-oriented emotion, like hope,
should be evoked by later parts of the message so that audiences finish the
message consumption inspired to take action.

Another body of literature examines the ways in which differences in the core message or style of the content impacts audience reactions to media. Framing a health issue as angering, frightening, or even saddening has been shown to result in different emotional reactions in audience members—the differences arising due to the different patterns of appraisals and action tendencies associated with those respective emotions (e.g., Kim and Cameron 2011; Kühne and Schemer 2013; Major 2011; Nabi 2003). In the health communication literature, framing content as either a *gain* (e.g., "You will have healthy skin if you avoid ultra violet rays" or "You will decrease your chances of getting skin cancer if you avoid ultra violet rays") or a *loss* (e.g., "You won't have healthy skin if you do not avoid ultra violet rays" or "You will increase your chances of getting skin cancer if you do not avoid ultra violet rays") is a common strategic messaging tactic. In their seminal piece, Rothman and Salovey (1997) argued that gain frames, which promote the benefits of a behavior, are more effective for promoting prevention behaviors that are perceived as low risk by audiences. Conversely, detection behaviors, which the authors argued carry greater perceptions of risk, may be best advocated for via the use of loss-framed messages. Meta-analyses have not found this argument to hold true across domains (O'Keefe and Jensen 2007; 2009); therefore, more work is needed to understand the relationship between message framing, affective responses to frames, and health behaviors (O'Keefe 2012).

Beyond framing, narrative (versus non-narrative) presentations of information has been shown to have an impact on emotional reactions of audiences, with narratives typically evoking stronger emotions than the drier, information-focused message (e.g., Murphy, Frank, Chatterjee, and Baezconde-Garbanati 2013; Oliver, Dillard, Bae, and Tamul 2012; Yoo, Kreuter, Lai, and Fu 2014). Given that many health messages are embedded in narratives such as plots in television dramas or blogs detailing personal experiences with health conditions, differences in narrative format is another important consideration for scholars studying the role of emotions in prevention-focused health messages (see the appendix for more on narratives).

The aforementioned pieces are just a few of the many studies examining the impact of form, style, and content on emotional reactions and other message outcomes. What this area of research demonstrates is that there are multiple aspects of a message that may evoke and/or regulate emotions in audiences. However, another important consideration when studying the connection between health media and emotional reactions is that different audience members are frequently impacted in different ways by each of these various message features or themes. People react differently to the same stimuli because emotions are highly dependent on one's relationship with his or her environment. As stated by Cacioppo and Gardner (1999), "relativity governs the province of emotion" (196). For one person, a popular song on the radio might be reason to smile and sing along in joy, while for another that same song may remind the listener of a lost relationship and instead provoke sadness.

OVERVIEW AND ORGANIZATION OF THIS BOOK

This book aims to provide an in-depth discussion of the relationships between prevention-focused health messages and discrete emotions. This is but one step in a larger effort to more fully integrate the study of emotions into the study of health communication. Specifically, the book focuses on the many ways in which *discrete emotions evoked by preventative health media messages influence how audiences respond to those messages.* Are they persuaded to change their behavior? Will they seek more information? Will they share the information with others? Will they support or oppose certain health-related policies? While a rich literature exists on the effects of health-related fear appeals on audiences, researchers have yet to fully explore the role that other discrete emotions play in health communication processes and outcomes. This book aims to start filling that gap by providing an overview of the role of nine different emotions in various prevention-focused health communication settings.

This book is not a full treatise on every type of emotion that may be evoked by a health message. Nor is it an attempt to cover every single conceptualization of emotion discussed in the communication literature. Instead, the book introduces readers to commonly employed emotional theories and concepts and then dives into how various discrete emotions have been studied in a relation to prevention-focused health messages.

This book also takes a very broad approach to what counts as a prevention-focused health message. Some health communication researchers differentiate between the prevention of negative behaviors, like smoking or overeating, and the promotion of positive behaviors, like eating vegetables and exercising (Rice and Atkin 2013). However, the present work looks at any message that promotes or discusses any behavior that may prevent disease—from quitting smoking to practicing mindfulness—as a prevention-focused health message. Furthermore, some early detection and screening behaviors (also known as secondary prevention behaviors) are also considered preventative in nature since they can help prevent more advanced disease states (e.g., Hesse, Beckjord, Rutten, Fagerlin, and Cameron 2015). This applied "big umbrella" definition of preventative health messages can provide researchers with a more inclusive view of how media help or hurt efforts to prevent illness (at all of its stages) as well as promote health and wellness.

Within the myriad of ways in which individuals encounter preventative health messages—from other people, from health care providers, from medical websites, from social media, from the news, and many combinations of those sources—emotional responses are a common thread in predicting an individual's reactions to such messages. This book provides an overview of the psychology of discrete emotions alongside the study of health-related media effects. In addition to its conceptual basis in appraisal theories of emotions (Lazarus 1991), this book also provides numerous empirical examples of the ways in which emotions have had a profound impact on our reactions to and the effectiveness of preventative health messages.

The emphasis of this book is on health-related communication processes and effects that take place in a mediated environment. As such, this book largely focuses on processes and effects related to mass communication and mass media. However, it is impossible to fully separate mass and interpersonal communication as the two often intersect and co-occur, particularly in an era of social media. Therefore, this book also touches occasionally on interpersonal communication processes (e.g., sharing health information with or seeking health information from others) where existing literature links these practices together.

It is also important to note that this book focuses on micro-level media processes and effects on individuals. Micro-level effects are those studied by assessing how individuals respond to media (Chaffee and Berger 1987). As such, most of the work featured in this book is quantitative in nature and examines the effects of health messages on individuals. However, it is also important to understand that individual effects do not take place in a vacuum. Social-ecological models of behavior note that one's relationships, community, and society also influence individual behavior (Stokols 1996). This book acknowledges the influence of these macro-level processes. Because of the importance of environmental and societal factors in shaping individual behaviors, the nine chapters about discrete emotions in this book also include a brief discussion of how the various emotions may influence public support and advocacy for health-related public policies.

Policy changes are one of the most effective ways to improve health for a large number of people. As the Centers for Disease Control and Prevention stated in its report "The Power of Prevention," "adopting healthy behaviors is much easier if we establish supportive community norms and adopt a philosophy that embraces health in all policies and settings" (2009). Such policies include land-use and design strategies that promote physical activity, healthier menu selections at restaurants, schools, and workplaces, requirements for physical education in schools, smoking bans, and other measures to collectively improve health. Investigating the role of message-relevant emotions in motivating civic engagement with such policies can help researchers better understand the relationship between preventative health messages and public health.

This book begins with a chapter on theoretical foundations. The main conceptual framework used throughout the book to analyze the role of emotions in prevention-focused health messages is that of appraisal theory. While many researchers contributed to the development of this paradigm (see Scherer, Schorr, and Johnstone 2001), the one whose work is most influential to the present volume is Lazarus (1991). In short, Lazarus argues that emotions are shaped by how people (largely subconsciously) appraise, or evaluate, their situations. These appraisals include assessments of if the situation is relevant to one's goals or not, if it is helping or hurting one's goals, amount of individual control, certainty of the situation, and coping potential. While many theoretical traditions provide valuable insights for studying the role of emotions in media effects, the appraisal, or functional, approach is particularly fruitful for health communication scholars given its nuance and ability to predict behavioral responses to messages (Nabi 2010; 2015). The appendix of this book offers descriptions of additional theoretical perspectives on emotions as well as discussions of related concepts, such as empathy, narratives, meta-emotions, and identification.

While this book approaches the study of emotional reactions to prevention messages from a discrete, appraisal theory paradigm, it does not ignore the valence-based view of emotion (e.g., positive versus negative emotions). In fact, according to appraisal theory, valence is akin to appraisals of goal-congruence—one of the primary appraisals that determines the nature of an emotional experience (Lazarus 1991; Smith and Lazarus 1993). Therefore, the first two sections of this book describe groups of negative and positive emotions, respectively.

Negative emotions are those emotions that an individual appraises as contrary to one's goals. Frijda (1988) argued that negative emotions are so impactful on human behavior because they alert people to a threat that demands action and they motivate people to avoid that threat in order to survive. Humans are more sensitive to and tend to react more strongly to negative events than positive ones, a propensity labeled the negative bias (Cacioppo and Berntson 1994). Negative emotions focus an organism's attention on a threat and motivate avoidance of that threat (Cacioppo and Berntson 1999; Cacioppo and Gardner 1999). Although an overabundance of sustained negative emotion can cause physiological harm (Consedine and Moskowitz 2007), these negative feelings serve evolutionary functions and can enhance functioning and even well-being in appropriate situations. For instance, anger can motivate individuals to overcome obstacles and to demonstrate strength and optimism in the face of adversity (Hess 2014; Lerner and Tiedens 2006), while reasonable levels of anxiety are associated with improved performance and greater conscious awareness of one's situation (Perkins and Corr 2014).

Media content that is likely to evoke negative emotions is common in health messages, from campaigns to health news articles. In fact, fear is the most frequently utilized emotional overtone in strategic health messages (Hale and Dillard 1995; Rice and Atkin 2013), although audiences may experience many emotions other than fear as the result of consuming fear appeals (Dillard, Plotnick, Godblod, Freimuth, and Edgar 1996). Anger and guilt are two other commonly used negative emotional tones for health messages, although their efficacy also depends on a number of contextual factors (Turner 2012). Moreover, feelings of sadness may result from consuming media stories about people struggling and succumbing to illness. Each of these negatively valenced emotional outcomes of health media consumption may impact audiences' health-related cognitions and behaviors.

The second section of the book includes five chapters dedicated to *positive emotions*, or emotions that signal that the current situation benefits well-being and goal pursuit (i.e., humor, pride, interest, hope, and elevation). While positive emotions serve different adaptive functions than negative emotions, they are more common in everyday life. The *positivity offset* is the notion that people typically experience a slightly positive state (Cacioppo and Gardner 1999). This tendency to have a (weakly) positive status quo likely encourages individuals to explore and learn. The broaden-and-build theory (Fredrickson 1998; 2001) also argues that positive emotions serve useful functions in that they, unlike negative emotions, broaden one's scope of attention, cognition, and action, while also encouraging people to build skills for the future.

There are advantages to utilizing content that is likely to evoke positive emotions in health messages. For one, health messages laced with positive emotion can gain the audiences' attention, lead to greater receptiveness, prompt reconsideration of an issue, facilitate recall, and lead to more positive attitudes toward the message (Monahan 1995). Moreover, people have an inclination to avoid threatening information about themselves in order to maintain a positive self-image (Baumeister 2010), implying that positively toned messages might prevent message avoidance for certain individuals. Indeed, positive emotions have been shown to motivate people to attend to self-relevant threats—information that will help them improve and benefit in the long run (Das and Fennis 2008; Raghunathan and Trope 2002; Trope and Neter 1994; Trope and Pomerantz 1998). In a prevention context, Dillard, Meyer, Solomon, and Manni (2015) found that healthy women who decided to enroll in a clinical trial aimed at reducing biomarkers of breast cancer risk experienced more positive emotions and fewer negative emotions than did those who chose not to participate. The authors note that placing a greater emphasis on practical and psychosocial benefits (i.e., positive emotions) in messages used to recruit participants may improve participation in such prevention-related health activities.

Research also indicates that news stories (Berger and Milkman 2012) and advertisements (Eckler and Bolls 2011) with positive emotional overtones are more likely to be shared with others than are negatively toned or neutral messages. So if one goal of a health message is for it to improve audience receptiveness or to be disseminated via grassroots channels, then messages that elicit positive emotions are a promising option for health advocates. However, as is demonstrated in the individual chapters on positive emotions, much research remains to be done to delineate the processes by which positive emotions evoked by preventative health messages are (or are not) beneficial in motivating prevention behaviors.

After the section of the book dedicated to positive emotions, four chapters discuss the role of emotions in specific health communication contexts: campaigns, journalism, information seeking, and eHealth. Each of these domains is a sub-field of health communication with its own research traditions and varying areas of conceptual emphasis. The purpose of these four chapters is to illustrate how multiple emotions can influence aspects of audience responses to prevention-oriented health messages in these contexts. For instance, whereas the chapter on fear discusses how audiences are likely to respond to fear appeals, the chapter on campaigns discusses not only fear responses to such appeals but also other emotions that may be evoked by campaign messages, ranging from anger to hope. These context-based chapters aim to provide a more holistic view of the role of emotions in common types of health messages. The chapters also may provide insight to content-area experts who have yet to consider the role of emotion in their particular research domain.

CONCLUSION

Predicting how people will *think* and *act* regarding health issues is often a direct consequence of how people *feel*. For example, young adult females are acutely aware that indoor tanning is bad for them (Noar, Myrick, Morales-Pico, and Thomas 2014). They have the knowledge that ultraviolet radiation is strongly linked to skin cancer, and they rationally understand the danger. Yet, they tan anyway. Why? Research tells us they continue to tan because it feels good and they expect it to give them feelings of pride and social acceptance (Noar et al. 2014). As this anecdote indicates, health education alone will not solve the many public health crises facing the globe.

No matter how often health communicators attempt to educate the public about preventative measures necessary to decrease health risks, and no matter how often such well-meaning messages ask the public to rationally calculate the risks, the public must be motivated to take action if any of these messages are to be effective. If individuals do not *feel* like they can change their behavior for the better, or if they do not *feel* they can make a difference for the health of others, then little change will come in this era of global preventable health crises, from obesity to cancer. The power of message-relevant emotions to motivate individuals to take preventative health actions is the core theme of this book.

Flashback to the 1990s, the same year that the CDC appended the word "prevention" to its title: A book called "The Strategy of Preventive Medicine" argued that the medical and health care community needed to tactfully, but swiftly, turn its attention toward prevention efforts (Rose 1992). Rose pointed out that there are many economic motivations for trying to prevent illness. However, he contended that the humanitarian reason to pursue prevention is more persuasive than the economic one: "It is better to be healthy than ill or dead. That is the beginning of the end of the only real argument for preventive medicine. It is sufficient" (4).

REFERENCES

Anderson, G. 2004. *Chronic conditions: Making the case for ongoing care.* Baltimore, MD: Johns Hopkins University.

Baumeister, R. F. 2010. The self. In R. F. Baumeister and E. J. Finkel (Eds.), *Advanced social psychology: The state of the science* (pp. 139–75). Oxford: Oxford University Press.

Baumeister, R. F., K. D. Vohs, C. Nathan DeWall, and L. Zhang. 2007. How emotion shapes behavior: Feedback, anticipation, and reflection, rather than direct causation. *Personality and Social Psychology Review* 11(2):167–203. doi: 10.1177/1088868307301033.

Berger, J., and K. L. Milkman. 2012. What makes online content viral? *Journal of Marketing Research* 49(2):192–205. doi: 10.1509/jmr.10.0353.

Bryant, J., D. Roskos-Ewoldsen, and J. R. Cantor. 2003. *Communication and emotion: Essays in honor of Dolf Zillmann.* Mahway, NJ: Lawrence Erlbaum.

Cacioppo, J. T., and G. G. Berntson. 1994. Relationship between attitudes and evaluative space: A critical review, with emphasis on the separability of positive and negative substrates. *Psychological Bulletin* 115(3):401–23. doi: 10.1037/0033-2909.115.3.401.

———. 1999. The affect system: Architecture and operating characteristics. *Current Directions in Psychological Science* 8(5):133–37. doi: 10.1111/1467-8721.00031.

Cacioppo, J. T., and W. L. Gardner. 1999. Emotion. *Annual Review of Psychology,* 50(1):191–214. doi: 10.1146/annurev.psych.50.1.191.

Cantor, J. R. 2009. Fright reactions to mass media. In J. Bryant and M. B. Oliver (Eds.), *Media effects: Advances in theory and research* (Third ed., pp. 287–303). New York: Routledge.

Centers for Disease Control. 1992. CDC: The nation's prevention agency. *MMWR Morbidity and Mortality Weekly Report* 41(44):833.

———. 2009. *The power of prevention: Chronic disease . . . the public health challenge of the 21st century.* Retrieved from http://www.cdc.gov/chronicdisease/pdf/2009-power-of-prevention.pdf.

———. 2011. CDC health disparities and inequalities report—United States 2011. *MMWR Morbidity and Mortality Weekly Report.*

Chaffee, S. H., and C. R. Berger. 1987. Levels of analysis: An introduction. In C. R. Berger and S. H. Chaffee (Eds.), *Handbook of communication science* (pp. 143–45). Newbury Park, CA: Sage.

Consedine, N. S., and J. T. Moskowitz. 2007. The role of discrete emotions in health outcomes: A critical review. *Applied and Preventive Psychology* 12(2):59–75. doi: 10.1016/j.appsy.2007.09.001.

Damasio, A. R. 2006. *Descartes' error: Emotion, reason and the human brain.* London: Vintage.

Darwin, C. 2009. *The expression of the emotions in man and animals*. London; New York: Penguin.

Das, E., and B. M. Fennis. 2008. In the mood to face the facts: When a positive mood promotes systematic processing of self-threatening information. *Motivation and Emotion* 32(3):221–30.

Detenber, B. H., R. F. Simons, and J. E. Reiss. 2000. The emotional significance of color in television presentations. *Media Psychology* 2(4):331–55. doi: 10.1207/S1532785XMEP0204_02.

Detenber, B. H., and S. P. Winch. 2001. The impact of color on emotional responses to newspaper photographs. *Visual Communication Quarterly* 8(3):4–14. doi: 10.1080/15551390109363461.

Dillard, J. P. 1994. Rethinking the study of fear appeals: An emotional perspective. *Communication Theory* 4(4):295–323. doi: 10.1111/j.1468-2885.1994.tb00094.x.

Dillard, J. P., B. J. F. Meyer, D. H. Solomon, and A. Manni. 2015. Factors associated with participation in a prevention trial aimed at reducing biomarkers of breast cancer risk. *Patient Education and Counseling*. doi: 10.1016/j.pec.2015.01.007.

Dillard, J. P., and E. Peck. 2000. Affect and persuasion: Emotional responses to public service announcements. *Communication Research* 27(4):461–95. doi: 10.1177/009365000027004003.

———. 2001. Persuasion and the structure of affect: Dual systems and discrete emotions as complementary models. *Human Communication Research* 27(1):38–68. doi: 10.1111/j.1468-2958.2001.tb00775.x.

Dillard, J. P., C. A. Plotnick, L. C. Godblod, V. S. Freimuth, and T. Edgar. 1996. The multiple affective outcomes of AIDS PSAs: Fear appeals do more than scare people. *Communication Research* 23(1):44–72. doi: 10.1177/009365096023001002.

Döveling, K., C. von Scheve, and E. A. Konijn. 2011. Emotions and mass media. In K. Döveling, C. von Scheve, and E. A. Konijn (Eds.), *The Routledge handbook of emotions and mass media* (pp. 1–12). New York: Routledge.

Eckler, P., and P. Bolls. 2011. Spreading the virus: Emotional tone of viral advertising and its effect on forwarding intentions and attitudes. *Journal of Interactive Advertising* 11(2):1–11. doi: 10.1080/15252019.2011.10722180.

Fredrickson, B. L. 1998. What good are positive emotions? *Review of General Psychology* 2(3):300–319. doi: 10.1037/1089-2680.2.3.300.

———. 2001. The role of positive emotions in positive psychology: The broaden-and-build theory of positive emotions. *American Psychologist* 56(3):218–26. doi: 10.1037/0003-066X.56.3.218.

Frijda, N. H. 1986. *The emotions*. Cambridge, England: Cambridge University Press.

———. 1988. The laws of emotion. *American Psychologist* 43(5):349–58. doi: 10.1037/0003-066X.43.5.349.

Hale, J. L., and J. P. Dillard. 1995. Fear appeals in health promotion campaigns: Too much, too little, or just right? In E. W. Maibach and R. Parrott (Eds.), *Designing health messages: Approaches from communication theory and public health practice* (pp. 65–80). Thousand Oaks, CA: Sage.

Hess, U. 2014. Anger is a positive emotion. In W. G. Parrott (Ed.), *The positive side of negative emotions* (pp. 55–76). New York: Guilford Press.

Hesse, B. W., E. Beckjord, L. J. F. Rutten, A. Fagerlin, and L. D. Cameron. 2015. Cancer communication and informatics research across the cancer continuum. *American Psychologist* 70(2):198–210. doi: 10.1037/a0036852.

Izard, C. E. 1977. *Human emotions*. New York: Plenum.

Kahneman, D., B. L. Fredrickson, C. A. Schreiber, and D. A. Redelmeier. 1993. When more pain is preferred to less: Adding a better end. *Psychological Science* 4(6):401–5. doi: 10.1111/j.1467-9280.1993.tb00589.x.

Keltner, D., and J. Haidt. 1999. Social functions of emotions at four levels of analysis. *Cognition and Emotion* 13(5):505–21. doi: 10.1080/026999399379168.

Kim, H. J., and G. T. Cameron. 2011. Emotions matter in crisis: The role of anger and sadness in the publics' response to crisis news framing and corporate crisis response. *Communication Research* 38(6):826–55. doi: 10.1177/0093650210385813.

Konijn, E. A., and J. M. ten Holt. 2011. From noise to nucleus: Emotion as key construct in processing media messages. In K. Döveling, C. von Scheve, and E. A. Konijn (Eds.), *The Routledge handbook of emotions and mass media* (pp. 37–59). New York: Routledge.

Kühne, R., and C. Schemer. 2013. The emotional effects of news frames on information processing and opinion formation. *Communication Research*. doi: 10.1177/0093650213514599.

Lang, A. 2006. Using the Limited Capacity Model of Motivated Mediated Message Processing to design effective cancer communication messages. *Journal of Communication* 56:S57–S80. doi: 10.1111/j.1460-2466.2006.00283.x.

Lang, A., P. Bolls, R. F. Potter, and K. Kawahara. 1999. The effects of production pacing and arousing content on the information processing of television messages. *Journal of Broadcasting and Electronic Media* 43(4):451–75. doi: 10.1080/08838159909364504.

Lazarus, R. S. 1991. *Emotion and adaptation*. New York: Oxford University Press.

Lerner, J. S., and L. Z. Tiedens. 2006. Portrait of the angry decision maker: How appraisal tendencies shape anger's influence on cognition. *Journal of Behavioral Decision Making* 19:115–37.

Maciosek, M. V., A. B. Coffield, N. M. Edwards, T. J. Flottemesch, M. J. Goodman, and L. I. Solberg. 2006. Priorities among effective clinical preventive services. *American Journal of Preventive Medicine* 31(1):52–61. doi: 10.1016/j.amepre.2006.03.012.

Maciosek, M. V., A. B. Coffield, T. J. Flottemesch, N. M. Edwards, and L. I. Solberg. 2010. Greater use of preventive services in U.S. health care could save lives at little or no cost. *Health Affairs* 29(9):1656–60. doi: 10.1377/hlthaff.2008.0701.

Major, L. H. 2011. The mediating role of emotions in the relationship between frames and attribution of responsibility for health problems. *Journalism and Mass Communication Quarterly* 88(3):502–22. doi: 10.1177/107769901108800303.

Monahan, J. L. 1995. Thinking positively: Using positive affect when designing health messags. In E. W. Maibach and R. Parrott (Eds.), *Designing health messages: Approaches from communication theory and public health practice* (pp. 81–98). Thousand Oaks, CA: SAGE.

Murphy, S. T., L. B. Frank, J. S. Chatterjee, and L. Baezconde-Garbanati. 2013. Narrative versus nonnarrative: The role of identification, transportation, and emotion in reducing health disparities. *Journal of Communication* 63(1):116–37. doi: 10.1111/jcom.12007.

Nabi, R. L. 1999. A cognitive-functional model for the effects of discrete negative emotions on information processing, attitude change, and recall. *Communication Theory* 9(3):292–320. doi: 10.1111/j.1468-2885.1999.tb00172.x.

———. 2002. Anger, fear, uncertainty, and attitudes: A test of the cognitive-functional model. *Communication Monographs* 69(3):204–16.

———. 2003. Exploring the framing effects of emotion. *Communication Research* 30(2):224–47. doi: 10.1177/0093650202250881.

———. 2009. Emotion and media effects. In R. L. Nabi and M. B. Oliver (Eds.), *The SAGE handbook of media processes and effects* (pp. 205–21). Thousand Oaks, CA: Sage.

———. 2010. The case for emphasizing discrete emotions in communication research. *Communication Monographs* 77(2):153–59. doi: 10.1080/03637751003790444.

———. 2015. Emotional flow in persuasive health messages. *Health Communication* 30(2):114–24. doi: 10.1080/10410236.2014.974129.

Neuhauser, L., and G. L. Kreps. 2003. Rethinking communication in the ehealth era. *Journal of Health Psychology* 8(1):7–23. doi: 10.1177/1359105303008001426.

Noar, S. M., J. G. Myrick, B. Morales-Pico, and N. E. Thomas. 2014. Development and validation of the comprehensive indoor tanning expectations scale. *JAMA Dermatology* 150(5):512–21. doi: 10.1001/jamadermatol.2013.9086.

O'Keefe, D. J. 2012. From psychological theory to message design: Lessons from the story of gain-framed and loss-framed persuasive messages. In H. Cho (Ed.), *Health communication message design: Theory and practice* (pp. 3–20). Los Angeles: SAGE.

O'Keefe, D. J., and J. D. Jensen. 2007. The relative persuasiveness of gain-framed loss-framed messages for encouraging disease prevention behaviors: A meta-analytic review. *Journal of Health Communication* 12(7):623–44. doi: 10.1080/10810730701615198.

———. 2009. The relative persuasiveness of gain-framed and loss-framed messages for encouraging disease detection behaviors: A meta-analytic review. *Journal of Communication* 59(2):296–316. doi: 10.1111/j.1460-2466.2009.01417.x.

Oliver, M. B., J. P. Dillard, K. Bae, and D. J. Tamul. 2012. The effect of narrative news format on empathy for stigmatized groups. *Journalism and Mass Communication Quarterly* 89(2):205–24. doi: 10.1177/1077699012439020.

Ortony, A., G. L. Clore, and A. Collins. 1988. *The cognitive structure of emotions.* New York: Cambridge University Press.

Perkins, A. M., and P. J. Corr. 2014. Anxiety as an adaptive emotion. In W. G. Parrott (Ed.), *The positive side of negative emotions* (p. 2). New York: Guilford Press.

Raghunathan, R., and Y. Trope. 2002. Walking the tightrope between feeling good and being accurate: Mood as a resource in processing persuasive messages. *Journal of Personality and Social Psychology* 83(3):510–25. doi: 10.1037/0022-3514.83.3.510.

Reeves, B., A. Lang, E. Y. Kim, and D. Tatar. 1999. The effects of screen size and message content on attention and arousal. *Media Psychology* 1(1):49–67. doi: 10.1207/s1532785xmep0101_4.

Rice, R. E., and C. K. Atkin (Eds.). 2013. *Public communication campaigns* (Fourth ed.). Los Angeles, CA: SAGE.

Rose, G. 1992. *The strategy of preventive medicine.* New York, NY: Oxford University Press.

Rothman, A. J., and P. Salovey. 1997. Shaping perceptions to motivate healthy behavior: The role of message framing. *Psychological Bulletin* 121(1):3–19. doi: 10.1037/0033-2909.121.1.3.

Scherer, K. R., A. Schorr, and T. Johnstone. 2001. *Appraisal processes in emotion: Theory, methods, research.* Oxford: Oxford University Press.

Sensenig, A. L. 2007. Refining estimates of public health spending as measured in national health expenditures accounts: The United States experience. *Journal of Public Health Management and Practice* 13(2):103–14.

Shen, L., and J. P. Dillard. 2007. The influence of behavioral inhibition/approach systems and message framing on the processing of persuasive health messages. *Communication Research* 34(4):433–67. doi: 10.1177/0093650207302787.

Smith, C. A., and R. S. Lazarus. 1993. Appraisal components, core relational themes, and the emotions. *Cognition and Emotion* 7(3–4):233–69.

Stokols, D. 1996. Translating social ecological theory into guidelines for community health promotion. *American Journal of Health Promotion* 10(4):282–98. doi: 10.4278/0890-1171-10.4.282.

Thorpe, K. E. 2013. Treated disease prevalence and spending per treated case drove most of the growth in health care spending in 1987–2009. *Health Affairs* 32(5):851–58. doi: 10.1377/hlthaff.2012.0391.

Trope, Y., and E. Neter. 1994. Reconciling competing motives in self-evaluation: The role of self-control in feedback seeking. *Journal of Personality and Social Psychology* 66(4):646–57. doi: 10.1037/0022-3514.66.4.646.

Trope, Y., and E. M. Pomerantz. 1998. Resolving conflicts among self-evaluative motives: Positive experiences as a resource for overcoming defensiveness. *Motivation and Emotion* 22(1):53–72. doi: 10.1023/a:1023044625309.

Trust for America's Health. 2006. Shortchanging America's health 2006: A state-by-state look at how federal public health dollars are spent. Washington, DC.

Trust for America's Health and Robert Wood Johnson Foundation. 2014. Investing in America's health: A state-by-state look at public health funding and key health facts. Washington, DC.

Turner, M. M. 2012. Using emotional appeals in health messages. In H. Cho (Ed.), *Health communication message design: Theory and practice* (pp. 59–72). Thousand Oaks, CA: SAGE.

Turner, M. M., R. N. Rimal, D. Morrison, and H. Kim. 2006. The role of anxiety in seeking and retaining risk information: Testing the risk perception attitude framework in two studies. *Human Communication Research* 32(2):130–56. doi: 10.1111/j.1468-2958.2006.00006.x.

Williams, D. M., and D. R. Evans. 2014. Current emotion research in health behavior science. *Emotion Review* 6(3):277–87. doi: 10.1177/1754073914523052.

Witte, K. 1992. Putting the fear back into fear appeals: The extended parallel process model. *Communication Monographs* 12(4):329–49. doi: 10.1080/03637759209376276.

Yoo, J. H., M. W. Kreuter, C. Lai, and Q. Fu. 2014. Understanding narrative effects: The role of discrete negative emotions on message processing and attitudes among low-income African American women. *Health Communication*, 29(5):494–504. doi: 10.1080/10410236.2013.776001.

Yoon, P. W., B. Bastian, R. N. Anderson, J. L. Collins, and H. W. Jaffe. 2014. Potentially preventable deaths from the five leading causes of death—United States, 2008–2010. *MMWR Morbidity and Mortality Weekly Report* 63(17).

Zillmann, D. 1971. Excitation transfer in communication-mediated aggressive behavior. *Journal of Experimental Social Psychology* 7(4):419–34. doi: 10.1016/0022-1031(71)90075-8.

———. 1988. Mood management through communication choices. *American Behavioral Scientist* 31(3):327–40. doi: 10.1177/000276488031003005.

———. 2006. Exemplification effects in the promotion of safety and health. *Journal of Communication* 56, S221–S237. doi: 10.1111/j.1460-2466.2006.00291.x.

Zillmann, D., and J. Bryant. 1985. *Selective exposure to communication.* Hillsdale, NJ: Erlbaum Associates.

Chapter One

Theoretical Foundations

Emotions guide and organize human behavior, pointing individuals toward salient goals. For researchers, theories provide a similar sort of guidance toward the goal of advancing knowledge about a particular domain and improving predictive power. The aim of this chapter is to outline the conceptual foundations that will form the groundwork for later discussions of discrete emotions and health media effects. After providing a general definition of the nature and structure of emotions, this chapter focuses on the tenets of appraisal theory. Appraisal theory is the overarching theoretical framework from which this book approaches the study of message-relevant emotions in prevention-focused health messages. This chapter also discusses ways in which mediated messages are likely to impact audience member's emotional reactions.

WHAT IS AN EMOTION, EXACTLY?

People experience emotion on a nearly constant basis. Sometimes they notice it, as tears stream down the cheeks or when one jumps for joy. Other times, emotional states may be muted or masked and barely, if at all, register in our consciousness. Despite any lack of awareness, emotions still shape neural firing patterns, heart rate, and facial expressions, among other automatic reactions that give away their presence (Ekman and Rosenberg 1998; Lang et al. 1998; LeDoux 1996).

While they are omnipresent in our lives, researchers have struggled to agree upon a precise definition of the concept of emotion. Many feisty debates exist in the literature about the exact nature of emotion as multitudes of psychologists and philosophers have attempted to answer William James's (1884) question, "What is an emotion?" One proposed answer is that an

1

emotion is a multifaceted experience that includes phenomenological, expressive, behavioral, and motivational components (see Roseman 2011). Researchers have also described emotions as mental states of varying intensity that occur as reactions to events, agents, or objects in the environment and that characterize evaluative, valenced reactions to those events, agents, or objects (Nabi 2009; Ortony, Clore, and Collins 1988).

Beyond defining an emotion, it is also helpful to describe the precursors of emotional states. Nabi (1999) outlines five components necessary for emotional arousal: (1) cognitive appraisal of a situation; (2) physiological arousal; (3) motor expression (e.g., facial expressions, goose bumps); (4) motivation (e.g., behavioral intentions or readiness); and (5) a subjective feeling state. The last component, a subjective feeling state, is the emotional component most frequently discussed and measured in communication research.

Emotions are part of the broader umbrella concept of affect. Researchers have conceptualized affect as the embodiment of evaluative reactions (Batson, Shaw, and Oleson 1992). That is, affect is the way a person feels about an event, object, or agent, whereas the way a person thinks about an event, object, or agent is typically labeled cognition. While affect differs from cognition, the two concepts are interrelated, and there is overlap in some (but not all) of the areas of the brain that deal with affect and cognition (LeDoux 1996).

Affect is the overarching psychological concept that encompasses both moods and emotions. Moods are more general than emotions and are typically defined by valence alone (e.g., a person is in a good mood or a bad mood). Moods cannot be attributed to a single cause; that is, people often have difficulty explaining why they are in a good or bad mood (Schwarz and Clore 1988). Moods also can last for many hours and are not very intense. Emotions, on the other hand, can take on many discrete forms within and between valences (e.g., anger, fear, happiness, surprise, etc.) and have a clear cause associated with them, yet they are often shorter in duration—lasting from a few seconds to many minutes—than are moods that can last for hours (Gross 1998). Furthermore, emotions are expressed automatically in the face through different facial muscle reactions, whereas moods are not usually signaled to others in this way (Ekman and Rosenberg 1998). In sum, emotions are more temporally bound, more intense, and more specific than the general affective state of moods (Frijda 1986; Lazarus 1991a; Plutchik 1980; Schwarz and Clore 1988). Emotions are, therefore, very important for understanding reactions to messages as they are more likely to be evoked by a specific message-related stimulus than are diffuse mood states (Nabi 1999).

Notably, emotions are not static states. They are dynamic and part of an ever-changing relationship between an organism and its environment. As soon as the person-environment relationship changes—be it through emotion regulation or external variation in the environment—individuals will automatically reappraise the situation and recalibrate their emotional reactions (Gross 1998; Lazarus 1991b). Combined with their short duration, the changing nature of emotions may make them appear too ephemeral to be of use to researchers hoping to gain insights into human behavior. However, emotions are one of the best predictors of human attitudes *and* behavior because of their inherent action tendencies, motivational components, and influence on subsequent cognitions (Frijda, Manstead, and Bem 2000; Izard 1977; Roseman 2011).

As dynamic processes, emotional reactions can be somewhat difficult for researchers to measure and analyze. However, scholars have a number of tools at their disposal for gauging emotional reactions, from self-report measures (Bradley and Lang 1994; Dillard and Shen 2007) to psychophysiological indicators like facial muscle movements, heart rate, and/or skin conductance (Ekman and Rosenberg 1998; Lang, Greenwald, Bradley, and Hamm 1993). Additionally, brain-scanning techniques such as fMRI are increasingly used to study media-provoked changes in parts of the brain dealing with emotional reactions (Anders, Lotze, Erb, Grodd, and Birbaumer 2004; Davidson and Irwin 1999; Lang et al. 1998).

While various emotions (e.g., fear, anger, joy) differ in their psychological and physiological markers, emotions can also differ in their relationship to the current situation. Integral emotions are those feeling states central to the context at hand (Keltner and Lerner 2010). That is, an integral emotion is sparked by the current person-environment relationship. This is the type of emotion most likely to be evoked by messages or a specific communication. For instance, while watching a fear appeal public service announcement about smoking on television, feelings of fear and anxiety would be integral emotions. In the communication context, integral emotions are often referred to as message-relevant emotions (Nabi 2009).

Besides integral emotions, people may experience emotions that are incidental to the present context. An incidental emotion is one that happens to be experienced at the same time but was not evoked by the situation at hand (Bodenhausen 1993). Basically, these are carryover emotions elicited by a previous situation but still not dissipated and therefore influencing subsequent events. Returning to the fear appeal example, if the viewer had just ended an adversarial phone call with a cable company customer service representative and was irate about the rise in her monthly cable bill, then those feelings of anger will still be present when the fear-evoking message appears on television, making her anger incidental to the public service announcement, yet still acutely present. While this book focuses on message-relevant integral emotions, an awareness of incidental emotions is helpful for appreciating the role of emotions in health media effects because it is unlikely that audiences come to a health message as affective blank slates completely devoid of emotion.

DISCRETE VERSUS DIMENSIONAL APPROACHES

Given that researchers continue to debate about the precise definition of emotion, it should come as no surprise that views on the structure of affect and emotions also differ. The dimensional view of emotion posits that there are only a limited number of dimensions that differentiate affective states from each other. According to this paradigm, the most basic distinction that can be made between two types of affect is that they differ on the dimension of valence: positive versus negative (Green, Salovey, and Truax 1999).

Beyond a single dimension of valence, other proponents of the dimensional view propose two dimensions upon which all emotions fall. Early in the line of modern psychological research on emotion, Schachter and Singer (1962) argued that individuals experience physiological arousal first, which then gives rise to a cognitive evaluation of the valence of a situation as good or bad. This work established arousal and valence as two important dimensions in emotion research. Additionally, Watson and Tellegen (1985) argued for a two-factor structure where all types of affect vary along the axes of negative and positive activation. With a two-factor structure, variations on the poles of activation and valence (positive or negative) can be mapped onto a circumplex model of affect that includes the following emotional states, each positioned 45 degrees apart from each other on a circle: pleasure, excitement, arousal, distress, displeasure, depression, sleepiness, and relaxation (Russell 1980). Later, Russell and Barrett (1999) argued that "core affect" is the psychological state based only on arousal and valence.

There is an alluring parsimony in limiting the dimensions upon which affect is studied. And a meaningful amount of variance between different affective states can be determined based on the two dimensions of arousal and valence alone. However, evidence from multiple research paradigms indicates that emotion is a more complex phenomenon than the dimensional view encapsulates. For instance, Ekman and colleagues' work on basic emotions displayed in facial expressions demonstrates that people from different cultures across the world exhibit similar automatic physiological reactions representing at least six, if not more, qualitatively different emotional states (Ekman 1992; Ekman et al. 1987; Ekman and Rosenberg 1998). Animal studies also indicate that the brain is likely wired to experience multiple discrete emotions that differ by more than valence and arousal alone (Panksepp 2007). While there is disagreement as to which emotions are basic (i.e., inherent and not learned), research has established a greater number of basic discrete emotions (anger, disgust, fear, happiness, sadness, and surprise) than there are poles in bivalent approaches to emotion (Ekman 1992).

In short, the discrete perspective allows for a more intricate analysis of emotion that also reflects some of the body's own nuanced reactions to emotional situations. When comparing discrete versus dimensional approaches, DeSteno, Petty, Rucker, Wegener, and Braverman (2004) make the following arugment: "Indeed, the bifurcation of emotional phenomena into positive versus negative states stands in direct opposition to the view espoused by many classical practitioners of persuasion. It also represents a gross oversimplification of emotional experience; distinctions among negative emotions (e.g., sadness, anger, disgust) and among positive emotions (e.g., gratitude, joy) are lost" (43).

In another study, Dillard and Peck (2001) tested dual systems (i.e., dimensional) and discrete approaches to emotion in the context of health-related public service announcements. Consistent with the dimensional approach, self-report scales of motivational inhibition predicted arousal of negative emotions, while scales of motivational activation predicted the arousal of positive emotions. However, perceived effectiveness of the health PSAs was better predicted by discrete emotional reactions than by approach or avoidance motivation. As the authors argue, the two approaches to understanding the structure of affect may be more appropriate for different domains, but discrete models are rather useful for studying message effects.

Given its ability to embrace nuance and its applicability for analyzing and understanding media effects, the discrete emotional approach is a good fit for the study of how emotions shape reactions to health messages discussing prevention behaviors. The finer-grained distinctions provided by the view of emotions as qualitatively different and discrete entities fits well with the study of the general field of communication, particularly given that communication is itself a complex and multifaceted process (Nabi 2010). Below, a theoretical foundation based in the discrete view, one that forms the basis of this book's perspective on the role of emotions in health-related media effects, is described.

APPRAISAL THEORY

The discrete view of emotion posits that various emotions are categorically different from each other. But what determines these differences between types of emotions, between fear and anger, between hope and happiness, and how do those differences impact subsequent behaviors? These are the questions appraisal theory aims to answer. Appraisal theories of emotion postulate that emotions arise from people's automatic cognitive appraisals of a situation such that each emotion is differentiated from another by its specific pattern of cognitive appraisals (Lazarus 1991a; Roseman 1984; Scherer 1984; Scherer, Schorr, and Johnstone 2001; C. A. Smith and Ellsworth 1985). As mentioned above, the concepts of emotion and cognition are tangled together and rather inseparable. Affect and cognition work in concert, one shaping the other and vice versa (Frijda et al. 2000). In fact, Clore and Ortony (2008) define emotions as "cognitively elaborated affective states" (629). Appraisal theory relies on the closeness of these two central concepts to explain why we feel afraid in one situation yet sad in another.

Although research camps differ slightly in their views on the number and exact nature of appraisals that determine unique emotional reactions, they tend to agree that the most important initial appraisal involves a person's evaluation of how personally relevant the present situation is (Lazarus 1991a; C. A. Smith and Ellsworth 1985; 1987; C. A. Smith and Lazarus 1993). Once an individual appraises the situation as personally relevant, then an emotional reaction is possible. In short, people have a difficult time emoting unless they make some sort of personal connection to the situation.

Beyond an initial appraisal of personal relevance, C. A. Smith and Ellsworth (1985) delineated eight appraisal dimensions important for determining subjective feeling states: attention, certainty, control (i.e., ability to cope with a situation), pleasantness (i.e., hedonic valence), perceived obstacle, responsibility, legitimacy (i.e., deservedness of the outcome), and anticipated effort. Lazarus (1991a) argues for a slightly shorter list of appraisals (six) that are separated into two groups—primary and secondary appraisals. Primary appraisals include goal relevance, goal congruency, and ego-involvement (i.e., an impact on some aspect of the self such as self-esteem or self-efficacy). Secondary appraisals include blame/credit, coping potential, and future expectations.

To give an example of Lazarus's (1991a) alignment of appraisal patterns, an individual who experiences fear when put in a room with a large snake would first make automatic primary appraisals related goal relevance (e.g., I have a goal to avoid snake bites), goal incongruence (e.g., this snake may bite me), and a lack of ego involvement (e.g., this situation is unrelated to my sense of self). Then, the individual would evaluate the secondary appraisal dimensions of the situation as uncertain (e.g., I don't know if this snake will bite me or not), as unclear as to who deserves blame (e.g., I don't know how this snake got here), and as there being questionable coping potential (e.g., I'm not sure I could handle it if the snake did bite me) (Lazarus 1991a).

Another example is the emotion of sadness, which shares the first two appraisals with fear (goal relevance and goal incongruity). However, the ego is often involved in feelings of sadness such that there may be a negative impact on esteem or other parts of the self. As for secondary appraisals, sadness involves an appraisal that there is nobody to blame (if there is an external agent to blame, then anger would be felt instead, whereas if an individual blamed oneself then guilt would ensue instead of sadness or anger). The appraisal of the coping potential associated with sadness is low potential, and appraisals of the future outlook for this emotion are appraised as bleak. Lazarus (1991a) further contends that, when taken as a whole, the patterns of appraisal associated with each emotion point to a core relational theme, a key defining essence. For example, the core relational theme of fear is imminent harm, while the core relational theme of hope is fearing the worst but yearning for better.

In addition to differing by appraisal components and core relational themes, discrete emotions vary based on their associations with unique action tendencies, which are motivations to take on a specific type of action in response to the emotional state (Frijda 1987; Frijda, Kuipers, and ter Schure 1989; Lazarus 1991a; Roseman, Wiest, and Swartz 1994). For example, the action tendency associated with feelings of fear is to seek protection from an imminent threat, while the action tendency associated with hope is to approach a yearned-for goal (Lazarus). It is this connection between discrete emotions and their associated action tendencies that makes appraisal theory useful for predicting potential behavioral outcomes associated with media exposure. Although a number of contextual factors and individual differences may prevent a tendency toward a certain action from translating into actual behavior, these tendencies are nonetheless powerful motivators of behavior and aid theorists in predicting behavior (Roseman 2011).

Because action tendencies differentiate discrete emotions from each other, appraisal theories are sometimes referred to as functional because they help humans function in their environments. Darwin (2009) argued in his seminal studies on emotional expressions in humans and other animals that actions that occur in response to an emotion serve adaptive functions, and these functions have been honed through thousands of centuries of evolution. Keltner and Gross (1999) argue that emotions are human adaptations to problems and opportunities related to survival, be it survival of the physical or social kind.

As mentioned above, appraisal theorists posit that the process of experiencing an emotion takes place in phases, many or even all of which occur below the level of consciousness. First, individuals perceive an event/object and make an appraisal as to its relevance. Then, additional appraisals are made (e.g., certainty, coping potential, etc.), and the patterns of these appraisals determine states of action readiness. Finally, "[t]hese action tendencies are associated with physiological changes that, together with the action tendency, influence future perceptions, cognitions, and even behaviors in accordance with the goal set by the action tendency" (Nabi 1999, 296). These outcomes of the emotional process serve adaptive functions for individuals as they try to navigate their relationships with their environment and with other social beings.

There are a number of reasons as to why a discrete approach to emotion, particularly one that includes appraisals and action tendencies, can be useful to communication researchers. For instance, Lerner and Keltner (2000; 2001) demonstrated that feelings of anger or fear, although both negative in their valence, result in different patterns of risk assessment. Across a series of experiments the researchers found that fear is associated with pessimistic risk judgments and anger with optimistic judgments, outcomes that comport with each emotion's unique appraisal patterns. Fear is associated with appraisals of low certainty and low control, whereas anger is associated with appraisals of high certainty and high control. Simply measuring arousal (likely to be high for both fear and anger) and valence (negative for both) would have missed the differences in risk evaluations fostered by these two emotional states. Given the use of risk information in many forms of preventative health communication, this research is a prime example of how the discrete approach to emotion can provide insight into the role of emotional experiences in shaping audience reactions to health messages.

Furthermore, a discrete approach to emotion is particularly useful in predicting what type of messages will elicit which emotions in audiences. As described by Nabi (2010), "Not only would we use different words to calm a person in an angry, sad, or fearful state, but the underlying appraisals resulting in those affects suggest how we might accomplish this task. For example, as blame is central to anger, addressing issues of fault may be useful. If lack of control is central to fear, conversation around this issue might help calm one who is frightened" (155). Based on knowledge of emotional appraisals and action tendencies, message designers and researchers can better include components that mimic those features of emotional states, or at least take them into account. Appraisal theory has been applied in research studies by many health communication and media effects scholars (e.g., Afifi and Morse 2009; Nabi 1999; 2015; S. W. Smith et al. 2010).

Yet much additional work is needed in this area to better grasp the relationships between messages, emotional reactions, and preventative behaviors. Given that discrete emotions are typically short lasting, little is known as to how these intense responses to health media impact audiences weeks, months, or years down the line. The answers likely deal with the link between memory and emotion (e.g., Levine and Burgess 1997; Newhagen and Reeves 1992) as well as with variables such as amount or repetitions of exposure, previous life experiences, health literacy, cognitive abilities, and also post-message consumption behaviors (i.e., did the individual share the information, do an online search for more information, and/or deliberate on it, or keep it to oneself and move on to the next flashy message?). While emotions are temporally short in duration, their strong impact on subsequent cognitions and behaviors makes them more than worthwhile for studying in the context of preventative health messages and behavior change. Moreover, while discrete emotions may be qualitatively different from each other, that does not mean they cannot occur simultaneously (e.g., Dillard, Plotnick, Godblod, Freimuth, and Edgar 1996; Du, Tao, and Martinez 2014; Ersner-Hershfield, Mikels, Sullivan, and Carstensen 2008; Larsen, McGraw, and Cacioppo 2001). Additional work into the ways that various combinations of emotions shape subsequent short- and long-term behavior will be useful in advancing our understanding of how messages impact health prevention behaviors.

CONCLUSION

Emotions are key to the human experience, and as such, they help guide human behavior. However, psychology and communication scholars differ in their view of the definition and structure of this concept that is so central to understanding how audiences react to health messages. Multiple theoretical perspectives on emotion, and affect more generally, can help guide research on the effects of health media on audiences. Yet given the predictive power afforded by the discrete approach, it and the tenets of appraisal theories are the dominant conceptualization of emotion used throughout this book.

REFERENCES

Afifi, W. A., and C. R. Morse. 2009. Expanding the role of emotion in the theory of motivated information management. In T. D. Afifi and W. A. Afifi (Eds.), *Uncertainty, information management, and disclosure decisions: Theories and applications* (pp. 87–105). New York: Routledge.

Anders, S., M. Lotze, M. Erb, W. Grodd, and N. Birbaumer. 2004. Brain activity underlying emotional valence and arousal: A response-related fMRI study. *Human Brain Mapping* 23(4):200–209. doi: 10.1002/hbm.20048.

Batson, C. D., L. L. Shaw, and K. C. Oleson. 1992. Differentiating affect, mood, and emotion: Toward functionally based conceptual distinctions. In M. S. Clark (Ed.), *Emotion. Review of personality and social psychology* (Vol. 13, pp. 294–326). Thousand Oaks, CA: Sage Publications, Inc.

Bodenhausen, G. V. 1993. Emotion, arousal, and stereotypic judgment: A heuristic model of affect and stereotyping. In D. Mackie and D. Hamilton (Eds.), *Affect, cognition, and stereotyping: Interactive processes in intergroup perception* (pp. 13–27). San Diego, CA: Academic Press.

Bradley, M. M., and P. J. Lang. 1994. Measuring emotion: the Self-Assessment Manikin and the semantic differential. *J Behav Ther Exp Psychiatry* 25(1):49–59. doi: 10.1016/0005-7916(94)90063-9.

Clore, G. L., and A. Ortony. 2008. Appraisal theories: How cognition shapes affect into emotion. In M. Lewis, J. M. Haviland-Jones, and L. F. Barrett (Eds.), *Handbook of emotions* (Third ed., pp. 628–42). New York: Guilford.

Darwin, C. 2009. *The expression of the emotions in man and animals*. London; New York: Penguin.

Davidson, R. J., and W. Irwin. 1999. The functional neuroanatomy of emotion and affective style. *Trends in Cognitive Sciences* 3(1):11–21. doi: 10.1016/S1364-6613(98)01265-0.

DeSteno, D., R. E. Petty, D. D. Rucker, D. T. Wegener, and J. Braverman. 2004. Discrete emotions and persuasion: The role of emotion-induced expectancies. *Journal of Personality and Social Psychology* 86(1):43–56. doi: 10.1037/0022-3514.86.1.43.

Dillard, J. P., and E. Peck. 2001. Persuasion and the structure of affect: Dual systems and discrete emotions as complementary models. *Human Communication Research* 27(1):38–68. doi: 10.1111/j.1468-2958.2001.tb00775.x.

Dillard, J. P., C. A. Plotnick, L. C. Godblod, V. S. Freimuth, and T. Edgar. 1996. The multiple affective outcomes of AIDS PSAs: Fear appeals do more than scare people. *Communication Research* 23(1):44–72. doi: 10.1177/009365096023001002.

Dillard, J. P., and L. Shen. 2007. Self-report measures of discrete emotions. In R. A. Reynolds, R. Woods, and J. D. Baker (Eds.), *Handbook of research on electronic surveys and measurements* (pp. 330–33). Hershey, PA: Idea Group Reference.

Du, S., Y. Tao, and A. M. Martinez. 2014. Compound facial expressions of emotion. *Proceedings of the National Academy of Sciences* 111(15):E1454–E1462. doi: 10.1073/pnas.1322355111.

Ekman, P. 1992. An argument for basic emotions. *Cognition & Emotion* 6(3-4):169–200. doi: 10.1080/02699939208411068.

Ekman, P., W. V. Friesen, M. O'Sullivan, A. Chan, I. Diacoyanni-Tarlatzis, K. Heider, . . . A. Tzavaras. 1987. Universals and cultural differences in the judgments of facial expressions of emotion. *Journal of Personality and Social Psychology* 53(4):712–17. doi: 10.1037/0022-3514.53.4.712.

Ekman, P., and E. L. Rosenberg. 1998. *What the face reveals: Basic and applied studies of spontaneous expression using the Facial Action Coding System (FACS)*. Oxford University Press, USA.

Ersner-Hershfield, H., J. A. Mikels, S. J. Sullivan, and L. L. Carstensen. 2008. Poignancy: Mixed emotional experience in the face of meaningful endings. *Journal of Personality and Social Psychology* 94(1):158–67.

Frijda, N. H. 1986. *The emotions*. Cambridge, England: Cambridge University Press.

Frijda, N. H. 1987. Emotion, cognitive structure, and action tendency. *Cognition and Emotion* 1(2):115–43. doi: 10.1080/02699938708408043.

Frijda, N. H., P. Kuipers, and E. ter Schure. 1989. Relations among emotion, appraisal, and emotional action readiness. *Journal of Personality and Social Psychology* 57(2):212–28. doi: 10.1037/0022-3514.57.2.212.

Frijda, N. H., A. S. R. Manstead, and S. Bem. 2000. *Emotions and beliefs: How feelings influence thoughts*. Cambridge: Cambridge University Press.

Green, D. P., P. Salovey, and K. M. Truax. 1999. Static, dynamic, and causative bipolarity of affect. *Journal of Personality and Social Psychology* 76(5):856–67. doi: 10.1037/0022-3514.76.5.856.

Gross, J. J. 1998. The emerging field of emotion regulation: An integrative review. *Review of General Psychology* 2(3):271–99.

Izard, C. E. 1977. *Human emotions*. New York: Plenum.

James, W. 1884. What is an emotion? *Mind* 9(34):188–205. doi: 10.2307/2246769.

Keltner, D., and J. J. Gross. 1999. Functional accounts of emotions. *Cognition and Emotion* 13(5):467–80. doi: 10.1080/026999399379140.

Keltner, D., and J. S. Lerner. 2010. Emotion. In D. T. Gilbert, S. T. Fiske, & G. Lindzey (Eds.), *The handbook of social psychology* (pp. 317–52). New York: Wiley.

Lang, P. J., M. M. Bradley, J. R. Fitzsimmons, B. N. Cuthbert, J. D. Scott, B. Moulder, and V. Nangia. 1998. Emotional arousal and activation of the visual cortex: An fMRI analysis. *Psychophysiology* 35(2):199–210. doi: 10.1111/1469-8986.3520199.

Lang, P. J., M. K. Greenwald, M. M. Bradley, and A. O. Hamm. 1993. Looking at pictures: Affective, facial, visceral, and behavioral reactions. *Psychophysiology* 30(3):261–73. doi: 10.1111/j.1469-8986.1993.tb03352.x.

Larsen, J. T., A. P. McGraw, and J. T. Cacioppo. 2001. Can people feel happy and sad at the same time? *Journal of Personality and Social Psychology* 81(4):684–96. doi: 10.1037/0022-3514.81.4.684.

Lazarus, R. S. 1991a. *Emotion and adaptation*. New York: Oxford University Press.

————. 1991b. Progress on a cognitive-motivational-relational theory of emotion. *American Psychologist* 46(8):819–34.

LeDoux, J. E. 1996. *The emotional brain: The mysterious underpinnings of emotional life.* New York: Simon & Schuster.

Lerner, J. S., and D. Keltner. 2000. Beyond valence: Toward a model of emotion-specific influences on judgment and choice. *Cognition & Emotion* 14(4):473–93. doi: 10.1080/026999300402763.

Lerner, J. S., and D. Keltner. 2001. Fear, anger, and risk. *Journal of Personality and Social Psychology* 81(1):146–59. doi: 10.1037/0022-3514.81.1.146.

Levine, L. J., and S. L. Burgess. 1997. Beyond general arousal: Effects of specific emotions on memory. *Social Cognition* 15(3):157–81. doi: 10.1521/soco.1997.15.3.157.

Nabi, R. L. 1999. A cognitive-functional model for the effects of discrete negative emotions on information processing, attitude change, and recall. *Communication Theory* 9(3):292–320. doi: 10.1111/j.1468-2885.1999.tb00172.x.

————. 2009. Emotion and media effects. In R. L. Nabi & M. B. Oliver (Eds.), *The SAGE handbook of media processes and effects* (pp. 205–21). Thousand Oaks, CA: Sage.

————. 2010. The case for emphasizing discrete emotions in communication research. *Communication Monographs* 77(2):153–59. doi: 10.1080/03637751003790444.

————. 2015. Emotional flow in persuasive health messages. *Health Communication* 30(2):114–24. doi: 10.1080/10410236.2014.974129.

Newhagen, J. E., & Reeves, B. 1992. The evening's bad news: Effects of compelling negative television news images on memory. *Journal of Communication* 42(2):25–41. doi: 10.1111/j.1460-2466.1992.tb00776.x.

Ortony, A., G. L. Clore, and A. Collins. 1988. *The cognitive structure of emotions.* New York: Cambridge University Press.

Panksepp, J. 2007. Neurologizing the psychology of affects: How appraisal-based constructivism and basic emotion theory can coexist. *Perspectives on Psychological Science* 2(3):281–96. doi: 10.1111/j.1745-6916.2007.00045.x.

Plutchik, R. 1980. *Emotion: A psychoevolutionary synthesis.* New York: Harper & Row.

Roseman, I. J. 1984. Cognitive determinants of emotion: A structural theory. *Review of Personality & Social Psychology* 5:11–36.

Roseman, I. J. 2011. Emotional behaviors, emotivational goals, emotion strategies: Multiple levels of organization integrate variable and consistent responses. *Emotion Review* 3(4):434–43. doi: 10.1177/1754073911410744.

Roseman, I. J., C. Wiest, and T. S. Swartz. 1994. Phenomenology, behaviors, and goals differentiate discrete emotions. *Journal of Personality and Social Psychology* 67(2):206–21. doi: 10.1037/0022-3514.67.2.206.

Russell, J. A. 1980. A circumplex model of affect. *Journal of Personality and Social Psychology* 39(6):1161–78. doi: 10.1037/h0077714.

Russell, J. A., and L. F. Barrett. 1999. Core affect, prototypical emotional episodes, and other things called emotion: Dissecting the elephant. *Journal of Personality and Social Psychology* 76(5):805–19. doi: 10.1037/0022-3514.76.5.805.

Schachter, S., and J. Singer. 1962. Cognitive, social, and physiological determinants of emotional state. *Psychological Review* 69(5):379–99. doi: 10.1037/h0046234.

Scherer, K. R. 1984. On the nature and function of emotion: A component process approach. In K. R. Scherer and P. Ekman (Eds.), *Approaches to emotions* (pp. 293–318). Hillsdale, NJ: Lawrence Erlbaum.

Scherer, K. R., A. Schorr, and T. Johnstone. 2001. *Appraisal processes in emotion: Theory, methods, research.* Oxford: Oxford University Press.

Schwarz, N., and G. L. Clore. 1988. How do I feel about it? The informative function of mood. In K. Fiedler & J. P. Forgas (Eds.), *Affect, cognition and social behavior* (pp. 44–62). Toronto: C. J. Hogrefe.

Smith, C. A., and P. C. Ellsworth. 1985. Patterns of cognitive appraisal in emotion. *Journal of Personality and Social Psychology* 48(4):813–38. doi: 10.1037/0022-3514.48.4.813.

Smith, C. A., and P. C. Ellsworth. 1987. Patterns of appraisal and emotion related to taking an exam. *Journal of Personality and Social Psychology* 52(3):475–88. doi: 10.1037/0022-3514.52.3.475.

Smith, C. A., and R. S. Lazarus. 1993. Appraisal components, core relational themes, and the emotions. *Cognition & Emotion* 7(3–4):233–69.

Smith, S. W., L. M. Hamel, M. R. Kotowski, S. Nazione, C. LaPlante, and C. K. Atkin. 2010. Action tendency emotions evoked by memorable breast cancer messages and their association with prevention and detection behaviors. *Health Communication* 25:737–46.

Watson, D., and A. Tellegen. 1985. Toward a consensual structure of mood. *Psychological Bulletin* 98(2):219–35. doi: 10.1037/0033-2909.98.2.219.

Chapter Two

Fear

Of the emotions studied in the context of prevention-focused health messages, fear is by far the most commonly examined. Health message creators frequently use fear-evoking imagery and phrasing in hopes of scaring audiences into taking action to improve their health. Beyond these persuasive fear appeals, fear is a common audience reaction to any message featuring a health threat, from health news reports to online discussion board exchanges about these threats. As such, it is nearly impossible to avoid feelings of fear in the context of preventative health messages.

It is beyond the scope of this chapter to examine the entire corpus of work on fear in preventative health message effects. Instead, the goal of this chapter is to provide the necessary background to understand the role of this emotion in shaping audience reactions to health messages. To begin, this chapter outlines the psychological qualities of fear before then discussing existing work on fear and communication. This discussion involves an overview of the evolution of research on fear appeals as well as the application of these theories to preventative health contexts. This chapter then examines the role of fear in motivating civic engagement with health issues before describing ethical concerns that come with using fear in health messages.

PSYCHOLOGICAL QUALITIES OF FEAR

The core relational theme of fear is the existence of an imminent threat (Lazarus 1991). According to Lazarus, fear is associated with appraisals of uncertainty, negative future expectancies, and low coping potential. The experience of fear is accompanied by multiple physical reactions including a pounding heart, raised eyebrows, and wide eyes (Roseman, Wiest, and Swartz 1994). The action tendency of fear is to move away from and avoid whatever individuals perceive to be the source of fear (Roseman 2011; Roseman et al. 1994).

Fear is an evolutionarily important emotion. Feelings of fright likely helped protect early humans from nearby predators and adverse weather, while they also likely aided in the establishment of social order within groups of humans (Öhman 2009). Fear reactions often occur automatically and swiftly in response to a relevant threat because there are strong neural connections between fear responses and the evolutionarily older part of the brain called the amygdala (Öhman 2009). Fear can be easily primed by threatening stimuli because of these strong associative connections in the brain's neural networks (Esteves, Parra, Dimberg, and Öhman 1994). Moreover, fear can be the result of unconscious associative learning processes whereby past experiences or juxtapositions of stimuli with fear can easily spark fright reactions in individuals (Esteves, Parra, Dimberg, and Öhman 1994).

Fear differs slightly from the emotion of anxiety because fear is tied to an imminent physical threat whereas anxiety is associated with an existential threat (Lazarus 1991). The emotions have biological differences, too, as they are related to the activation of different brain systems (Lang, Davis, and Öhman 2000). Both fear and anxiety, though, can arise from a specific stimulus or become chronic. Fear becomes chronic when individuals develop a phobia of a specific object, situation, or behavior. For example, while most humans display an innate fear of snakes, certain individuals are severely afraid of the slithering creatures to the point where they develop a phobia (Öhman 2009). Individuals also differ in their trait levels of anxiety (Spielberger, Gorsuch, and Lushene 1970a). Multiple experiences of anxiety can develop into psychological conditions associated with chronic anxiety, known as anxiety disorders (MacLeod 1999). Despite their differences, fear and anxiety are part of the ame family of emotions (Lazarus 1991), and, overall, are similar in their appraisal components and action tendencies. While many researchers group the two emotions into one category, deeper insight into the role of each would be beneficial for future work in this area (see So 2013).

FEAR AND COMMUNICATION

Fear has long garnered the attention of communication scholars, particularly in the area of persuasion (see Janis and Feshbach 1953; Rogers 1975; Witte 1992). Witte, Meyer, and Martell (2000) define a fear appeal as "a persuasive message that arouses fear by outlining the negative consequences that occur if a certain action is not taken" (2). The "certain action" referred to in that definition has also been called a coping component, which has been defined as information about how audiences can avoid the threat outlined in the message (Rogers 1975).

Communication scholars have been studying fear appeals since the 1950s when Janis and Feshbach (1953) used the drive model to examine the connection between fear and the persuasiveness of dental hygiene messages. The drive model posits that fear is a state of tension, and people experience a drive to reduce this tension-filled state by whatever means are most effective (Hovland, Janis, and Kelly 1953). Therefore, if a particular method for reducing fear is effective (e.g., distraction), even if that method does not entirely dissipate the actual threat that initially evoked feelings of fear, then the individual will prefer to employ that same fear-reducing behavior in future frightening situations.

In the 1970s, multiple researchers proposed alternatives to the drive model. Leventhal's (1970) parallel process model posited that individuals worked to control their fear as well as simultaneously control the danger presented in the message. As the name indicates, individuals would experience one of these processes or the other, not both. Rogers's (1975) protection motivation theory (PMT) took an expectancy-value approach to predicting the effects of fear appeals on audiences. He theorized that appraisals of the magnitude of a threat (i.e., severity), the likelihood it would occur (i.e., susceptibility), and appraisals of response efficacy (i.e., the effectiveness of the suggested remedy) and self-efficacy (i.e., confidence in one's ability to enact the suggested remedy) would interact to determine if and how individuals would respond to fear appeals. Appraisals of a threat as severe and likely to occur, when accompanied by adequate coping information in the form of self- and response-efficacy, should result in protection motivation, which Rogers defined as a cognitive response akin to a behavioral intention. While useful for its clear definition of the components of threat and efficacy, PMT practically discarded the role of fear in fear appeals, leaving a noticeable void in the theory related to affective routes to persuasion (Dillard 1994; Mongeau 2013; Witte 1992).

The Extended Parallel Process Model

As the aforementioned theories of fear appeals evolved, theoretical explanations for fear appeal effects gradually lost their emphasis on the emotion that motivated their creation. Instead, these theories focused heavily on cognitive reactions as the driving mechanisms behind message effects (Dillard 1994). Dillard argued that this cognitive focus left fear appeal theories wanting and unable to accurately explain the effects of fear on audiences. In an effort to put "the fear back into fear appeals" (329), Witte (1992) introduced the extended parallel process model (EPPM). This model reincorporated fear as a causal mechanism in fear appeal effects while retaining the cognitive appraisals related to threat and efficacy that were proposed by previous theorists.

The EPPM provides scholars with a framework for understanding how psychological reactions to messages that contain a threat and evoke fear may encourage or prevent adaptive *as well as* maladaptive behaviors (Witte 1992). The EPPM suggests that in response to fear appeals, individuals appraise the threat in terms of its severity and their own susceptibility. Fear arises in response to these threat appraisals, as postulated in the EPPM. According to Witte, a minimum level of perceived threat is necessary for a fear appeal to have an effect on audience members. If they do not perceive any threat, the EPPM states that audiences will not attend to the message because it will not be perceived as relevant to their well-being.

After appraising the threatening aspect of a message, individuals then appraise the efficacy of the response advocated by the message. Those efficacy appraisals are conceptualized as response and self-efficacy, respectively. Response efficacy is the perception that the response suggested by a fear appeal message (e.g., get a vaccine in order to avoid the threat of influenza) is effective and will actually prevent the threatening outcome. Self-efficacy, as the name implies, is the perception tied not to the response but to the self. It is how confident an individual feels in her ability to perform the recommended behavior (Bandura 1993).

Together, cognitive appraisals of threat (i.e., severity and susceptibility) and efficacy (i.e., response-efficacy and self-efficacy) are the mechanisms behind fear appeal effects in the EPPM (Witte 1992; 1994). These mechanisms interact to determine message effects. If appraisals of threat are stronger than appraisals of efficacy, then individuals will seek to diminish the fear through maladaptive behaviors, such as denigrating the source of information or rationalizing behaviors. These reactions are labeled fear control processes in the EPPM. An example of maladaptive reactions would be avoiding additional information about the threat or rejecting the message altogether (Goodall and Reed 2013; Lewis, Watson, and White 2013; Witte 1992; Witte and Allen 2000; Witte et al. 2000).

However, if efficacy appraisals are as strong or stronger than threat appraisals, then the EPPM predicts that individuals will feel capable of addressing the threat and will then enact adaptive, danger control behaviors (Witte 1992; Witte et al. 2000). One such adaptive reaction to a threat-containing message is information seeking (Goodall and Reed 2013; Turner, Rimal, Morrison, and Kim 2006), but others include taking direct behavior to prevent or ameliorate a threat. Witte's model suggests that fear-arousing messages must be high in both threat and efficacy if they are to persuade audiences to take adaptive actions (Witte and Allen 2000).

Some of the predictions put forth in the EPPM have received empirical support. For instance, higher levels of threat and higher levels of efficacy related to persuasion and meta-analysis indicates there is a positive linear relationship between message-induced fear and persuasion (Witte and Allen 2000). However, there are also notable shortcomings of the model and the ways in which various researchers have applied it. While fear is conceptualized as an important component of the EPPM, research has yet to explicitly connect fear reactions to each of the steps in the fear control process (Mongeau 2013). Likewise, fear reactions may also impact danger control processes such that fear may motivate some individuals to take action to reduce the threat, regardless of efficacy levels. For example, an individual may be afraid of the flu after seeing a PSA about the virus, but he still has no idea which type of vaccine is best (nasal or injection) or where he can get the vaccine and which locations will accept his insurance. In this situation, self-efficacy is low. However, the fear of the threat—influenza—could motivate the individual to search online for more information and take action, both behaviors typically described as danger control processes in the EPPM.

Yzer, Southwell, and Stephenson (2013) also note that while strong perceptions of threat and efficacy are typically correlated with message acceptance, the interactions between these appraisals predicted by the EPPM have not received strong empirical support (de Hoog, Stroebe, and de Wit 2007; Witte and Allen 2000). Furthermore, Popova (2012) analyzed twenty-nine studies that tested at least one of the EPPM's twelve propositions. She found that only seven of the twelve constructs received any empirical support; however, none of those seven constructs received a majority of support from the studies in the sample. That is, many studies have found mixed or contradictory results for those seven constructs. Meanwhile, the other five constructs of the EPPM have been mostly untested and require empirical evidence before researchers can rely on their accuracy. Clearly, more work is needed to understand if or how the constructs in the EPPM hold up to empirical scrutiny and to refine the model.

Some more recent work has taken up that call to find concepts that may supplement or supplant the EPPM. Rintamaki and Yang (2014) found that including response cost (i.e., drawbacks associated with a proposed response to a health threat) measures improved the ability of the model that also included EPPM-related variables to predict condom use. Additionally, So (2013) proposed an extended EPPM (E-EPPM) where emotional appraisals and dispositional coping style (i.e., monitoring versus blunting) are included in the model. So argues that the E-EPPM advances the literature by considering both cognitive and affective components of risk perceptions that undergird reactions to fear appeals. Uncertainty and severity (cognitive components) and anxiety and fear (affective components) combine organically in the E-EPPM, and both of these sets of components can impact whether an individual engages in fear or danger control. Central to the E-EPPM is the idea that it is the emotional arousal (fear and/or anxiety) that sparks coping appraisals. The E-EPPM, though, has yet to be tested empirically.

The Cognitive-Functional Model

Nabi (1999; 2002) proposed the cognitive-functional model (CFM) as a way to advance the literature on negative emotional appeals, in general. However, her model speaks directly to fear appeal effects, too. The CFM combines aspects of cognitive response models of persuasion with appraisal theory with a particular focus on two concepts: motivated attention and motivated processing. The model predicts that fear, because of its nature as an emotion that motivates individuals to avoid a threatening situation, can lead audiences to avoid processing a message.

However, if an individual experiencing message-relevant fear is also feeling uncertain as to whether the remainder of the message will contain personally relevant or useful information, then the CFM predicts that a fearful individual would become motivated to more deeply process the message. This deeper processing in the face of uncertainty occurs, according to the CFM, because the audience member is trying to find any information that might satisfy the fear-induced goal to prevent a danger. Nabi readily admits that the CFM is complex. However, she points to the complexity of communication processes and emotions as justification for more thorough explanations for potential message effects.

In a preliminary test of the CFM, Nabi (2002) established some empirical support for the prediction that avoidance negative emotions, like fear, would promote more shallow information processing than approach negative emotions, like anger, or than being in a neutral emotional state. She also found support for the position that a lack of certainty about the information in the rest of the message would lead to deeper information processing. However, there was not a significant interaction between type of emotion (approach or avoidance) and expectation of reassurance (certain or uncertain), as was predicted by the CFM. Nabi suggests that this lack of an interaction could possibly be due to the context of the study (attitudes toward domestic terrorism legislation) or on participants' perceived or actual knowledge of the topic.

Although Nabi's two manuscripts on the CFM (1999; 2002) have each been cited more than one hundred times by other scholars, to date the literature has yet to thoroughly test the propositions in the model or replicate Nabi's (2002) initial empirical findings. Clearly, more work is needed to see if the CFM can reliably predict the effects of fear appeals on audiences across various message contexts. However, the integration of message processing principles with the action tendencies of discrete emotions has helped advance theory on fear appeal research.

The Stage Model

Another addition to the body of fear appeal theories is the stage model (Das, de Wit, and Stroebe 2003; de Hoog, Stroebe, and de Wit 2007). The stage model combines concepts from information processing theories (e.g., the Elaboration Likelihood Model and the Heuristic Systematic Model, Chaiken 1980; Petty and Cacioppo 1986) with the concepts from the aforementioned literature on fear appeals. Specifically, the model argues that appraisals occur in stages, with threat appraisals typically occurring first and thereby eliciting negative affect, followed by coping appraisals in response to the suggestion of behavior change in the message. When either threat appraisal—perceived susceptibility or severity—is high, the stage model predicts that the audience will process the information in the fear appeal systematically (i.e., they will pay attention to the details of the arguments). However, when susceptibility and severity are low, the stage model predicts heuristic, cue-based processing will ensue.

As with the EPPM, the stage model focuses on the situation where both threat and efficacy perceptions are strong. In this situation, the stage model argues that message consumers will likely feel like their self-definitional belief in being healthy is being attacked. Therefore, the message sparks a defensive motivation in the audience. Audience members then systematically process the information in hopes of finding a flaw in the logic in order to alleviate the threat to their identity as a healthy individual. Finding none, as the health threat discussed in the appeal likely does exist, processing of the efficacy component in the message will be positively biased such that individuals are more likely to accept it as a plausible way to alleviate the threat, regardless of the quality of the message arguments. A final prediction of the stage model is that attitudes toward the target behavior are influenced heavily by perceived severity, whereas actual behavior does not depend on perceptions of severity as much as it does on how vulnerable the individual feels.

Although the stage model advances fear appeal theory by including predictions related to information processing (as did the CFM before it), Mongeau (2013) notes that scholars should be cautious before relying on the stage model when trying to predict fear appeal effects. He argues that the predictions in the model are "slippery . . . it is not clear whether main effects or interaction effects should influence responses" (193). Additionally, a meta-analysis, of studies that employed components of the stage model found some inconsistencies with the model. That is, in the meta-analysis severity did influence attitudes and self-efficacy did predict attitudes and behaviors, and not just attitudes as predicted by the stage model (de Hoog et al. 2007). The role of the emotion of fear, other than its impact on shaping perceptions of threat, is also not entirely clear in the stage model.

Moderators of Fear Appeal Effects

While theories about fear appeals largely examine mechanisms, or causal drivers, of effects, researchers have also been interested in additional variables that may alter audience reactions to fear appeals. Multiple individual differences are ripe for inclusion as moderators of fear appeal effects. For example, when faced with a threat, some individuals, known as monitors, want to seek out more information and find out as much as possible about the potential danger, whereas their counterparts—blunters—seek distraction and want to avoid information about the threat (Miller 1987). Monitors will more readily approach such information, experience less negative affect from consuming it, attend to it more deeply, and are more likely to exhibit message-consistent attitudes than are blunters (Miller, Shoda, and Hurley 1996). Which coping style (monitoring versus blunting) audiences employ will make a difference in how deeply they attend to information discussing a potential threat.

Dillard and Nabi (2006) note that this particular individual difference variable can impact which type of cancer prevention messages will be most effective with particular target audiences: "We might speculate that those with monitoring tendencies will be more emotionally reactive to cancer information generally. Thus, more subtle emotional appeals may be needed to prevent excessive, and perhaps counterproductive, emotional reactivity. Conversely, those with more blunting tendencies may be more likely to experience counterproductive emotional reactions, like reactance" (S127).

Another individual difference variable often looked at as a potential moderator of fear appeal effects is trait anxiety (Spielberger, Gorsuch, and Lushene 1970b). However, there is mixed evidence as to trait anxiety's impact on fear appeal effects. For instance, Witte and Allen (2000) did not find a significant relationship between trait anxiety and attitudes, intentions, or behaviors. Yet there are instances in the literature where trait anxiety did interact with components of fear appeals to alter the pattern of effects. Witte and Morrison (2000) found that trait anxiety did not relate significantly to threat perceptions, efficacy perceptions, or behavior related to fear appeals about condoms and AIDS prevention. However, the researchers did find that those participants low in trait anxiety exhibited significantly more defensive avoidance than did those high in trait anxiety. This finding indicates that there could possibly be a matching effect (Petty, Fabrigar, and Wegener 2003; Petty and Wegener 1998) such that those who are already in a semi-anxious state when presented with a fear appeal may be more accepting of the message. Need for cognition, or a general tendency to think in depth about a situation or stimulus (Cacioppo, Petty, and Kao 1984), has also been proposed as a moderator of fear appeal effects, with some empirical support. Ruiter, Verplanken, De Cremer, and Kok (2004) found in an experiment that participants high in need for cognition were significantly more likely to respond adaptively to a fear appeal than were those participants low in need for cognition.

The nature of the health threat discussed in a message can also moderate reactions to fear appeals. Nabi, Roskos-Ewoldsen, and Carpentier (2008) found that participants who expressed higher levels of subjective knowledge about cancer detection behaviors experienced less fear after exposure to a message about self-exams. The connection between the threat at the heart of the message and the likelihood of death may evoke terror management processes in audiences, as predicted by terror management theory (TMT), making message acceptance moderated by the worldviews (Hunt and Shehryar 2011) or the perceived ability of the target behavior to alleviate the threat and distract from death-related thoughts (Cooper, Goldenberg, and Arndt 2014). In support of the merging of EPPM and TMT concepts, Cooper et al. found that beachgoers primed to think about death were more likely to pursue sun-protective behaviors when they were then read efficacy messages highlighting the effectiveness of those behaviors, whereas beachgoers who were *not* primed to think of death exhibited similar behaviors regardless of whether the efficacy message was read to them or not.

An additional moderator to consider when assessing the effectiveness of fear appeals is time since message exposure. Emotions are strong but short-lived phenomena that can dissipate quickly (Izard 1977), and the passage of time after a fear appeal may change the way audiences react to it. Research on fear appeals meant to curb drunk driving provides evidence for this supposition. Lewis, Watson, and White (2008) found that interactions of threat and efficacy after viewing a fear appeal were significantly associated with persuasion variables, as measured immediately after exposure, whereas a positively framed message that avoided evoking fear was not as persuasive. However, two to four weeks later, the positive message was more persuasive than the fear appeal. It is possible that the adaptive purposes of positive versus negative emotions may explain these results. While negative emotions alert us to an immediate threat and focus attention, positive emotions promote building relationships and broadening one's horizons for longer-term prosperity (Fredrickson 1998; 2001). Especially for behaviors with strong social implications (e.g., drunk driving, where others can be killed or seriously injured and where the individual involved could face shame from other members of society), fear appeals may not provoke the long-term motivation or social orientation to alter behaviors long after message viewing in the ways that positive emotional appeals may.

Beyond the aforementioned variables, there are many others that researchers could and should test as potential moderators of fear appeal effects. As research reveals additional moderators, it will become easier to predict the specific contexts under which fear appeals (or fear-evoking messages in

general, be they strategic or not) shape audience reactions to health messages.

FEAR APPEALS: EFFECTIVE OR NOT, AND WHY?

What the aforementioned theories of fear appeal effects and discussion of
moderators reveal is a body of literature rife with inconsistencies and calls
for additional research. In such a situation, taking a broader view on the
literature can help researchers make sense of the conflicting results from one
study to the next. Meta-analyses and reviews of the literature point to a
general conclusion that fear appeals share a positive and linear association
with message acceptance (see Mongeau 2013). Boster and Mongeau (1984)
and later Mongeau (1998) found in both of their meta-analyses that fear
appeals resulted in moderate but significant associations between perceived
fear and the strength of the fear appeal. The authors also found that there was
a smaller but still significant relationship between the amount of fear evoked
and attitudes toward the target behavior as well as behavior change. Witte
and Allen (2000) likewise found in their meta-analysis a significant relationship between fear appeals and persuasion, but they also updated the literature
to test for threat and efficacy interactions and fear control outcomes across
studies. They found that there was a positive linear relationship between fear
manipulations and behavior ($r = .15$). However, they did not find the threat
by efficacy interactions predicted by the EPPM, and neither did de Hoog et
al. (2007) in a subsequent meta-analysis. The literature seems to coalesce
around a small but significant relationship between fear and persuasion, but
the mechanisms are not entirely clear.

It is also possible that methodological issues are clouding insights into
fear appeal effects (Mongeau 2013; O'Keefe 2003). While the EPPM has
been criticized for the lack of empirical support for many of its twelve
propositions (Popova 2012), other researchers have argued that methodological issues may be responsible and not necessarily the model itself. For instance, Peters, Ruiter, and Kok (2012) used stricter inclusion criteria in their
meta-analysis of fear appeal effects. The authors only analyzed studies that
employed full factorial orthogonal manipulations of threat and efficacy (i.e.,
manipulations of each construct were independently manipulated), and included a measurement of behavioral outcomes. The authors, while only testing the effects of six studies with these stringent inclusion criteria, found that
the interaction effects predicted by the EPPM were significant in their sample. That is, the threat component only had an effect on behavior when the
efficacy component was also strong, while the efficacy component only impacted behavior when the threat component was strong. Previously, Weinstein (2000) had also found support for the multiplicative relationship be-

tween threat and efficacy when using a within-subjects design. He suggested that larger samples would be necessary for between-subjects experiments to have adequate power to find the multiplicative relationship between the two variables predicted by the EPPM (Witte 1994).

However, the Peters et al. (2012) meta-analysis did not measure the impact of the emotion of fear, pointing to a broader problem in current fear appeal theorizing: a lack of measurement of emotional responses in addition to measures of cognitive appraisals of threat and efficacy. O'Keefe (2003) argues that fear reactions are too often left unmeasured in fear appeal research. When they are measured, he points out that researchers typically employ measures of fear arousal merely as a manipulation check and not as a mediator of message effects, as proposed by the EPPM and E-EPPM. To truly test the effects of fear-based appeals, researchers will need to measure actual fear reactions and apply rigorous statistical tests of mediation and moderation related to the emotion itself.

Other scholars have noted that fear appeals that include both threat and efficacy components can evoke emotions *other than* fear, with these additional emotions also influencing persuasive outcomes (Dillard, Plotnick, Godblod, Freimuth, and Edgar 1996; Nabi 2015; Popova 2012). Moreover, the efficacy component of a traditional fear appeal may cause audiences to feel relief or hope, thereby diminishing post-message fear and motivating different behaviors in audiences (Nabi). That is because feelings of relief and hope have different associated action tendencies than does fear (Lazarus 1991). Considering and measuring a multitude of emotional reactions to fear appeals could help improve knowledge related to why and when fear appeals do or do not lead to message acceptance.

It is also not entirely clear when or why message-relevant fear leads to more or less elaboration of the message, a variable that contributes to both persuasion and the longevity of message acceptance. Social psychologists have found that feelings of fear typically motivate individuals to pay greater attention to and systematically process relevant information (Forgas 2000; Raghunathan and Corfman 2004). In order to protect an individual from a perceived threat, the experience of fear promotes "tunnel vision" such that one's focus is placed squarely on threat-relevant details (Izard 1993). However, evidence in the communication literature found that individuals who saw low-fear messages processed the information systematically while those who saw high-fear messages processed information heuristically (Hale, Lemieux, and Mongeau 1995).

The stage model (de Hoog et al. 2008) argues a different perspective— that fear motivates deeper message processing because those exposed to the fear appeal are trying to think of ways to discredit the message that points out a self-relevant threat. Nabi (1999; 2002) offers some nuance to our understanding of how fear relates to message processing. In the CFM, the avoidance tendencies associated with fear are thought to lead audiences to avoid thinking deeply about the message. However, if the message offers cues of later reassurance, then even the fearful audience member will be motivated to pay attention to it and process the information. Given the contrasting hypotheses, much additional work is needed to clarify the conditions under which message-relevant fear promotes or prohibits message elaboration.

A study of attitude accessibility also offers insights as to when fear appeals may be processed systematically or heuristically. Roskos-Ewoldsen, Yu, and Rhodes (2004) demonstrated that while efficacy messages make attitudes toward a target behavior more accessible, high fear-arousing messages result in less accessible attitudes toward the threat. Because more accessible attitudes can cue an individual to believe there is something important in the environment, accessible attitudes are more likely to spur message deliberation than are less accessible attitudes (Roskos-Ewoldsen, Bichsel, and Hoffman 2002). If a fear appeal results in the efficacy information being more accessible, then perhaps that portion of the message will be more deeply processed than the initial threat component that aroused fear and decreased accessibility of threat attitudes.

In sum, there is evidence that fear appeals can be somewhat persuasive when they include an efficacy/coping component, but this is not always the case. Much work remains to understand why and under what circumstances persuasion can be enhanced. The evidence indicates that cognitive appraisals of threat and efficacy are important predictors of persuasion, as is the emotional reaction of fear. The specifics of the interrelations between these variables and potential moderator variables require more theorizing and empirical testing. For example, the efficacy components of a fear appeal could evoke hope in audiences, and the approach motivation associated with that discrete emotion may help explain some of the variance in fear appeal effects. Additional research is necessary to increase the explanatory powers of fear appeal theories and continue explaining more of the unexplained variance in fear appeal effects.

FEAR AND PREVENTION MESSAGES

Gaps in our understanding of why fear appeals work in some circumstances has not stopped researchers and practitioners from applying fear appeals to health contexts. Indeed, the study of message-relevant fear has been inextricably linked with health communication since the earliest social science investigation of fear appeals tested the impact of dental hygiene messages (Janis and Feshbach 1953). Since that time, studies of fear appeals and fear evoked by other forms of mass media permeate the health communication literature. In fact, a search of Google Scholar for the phrase "fear and health communication" returns more than 1.25 million results. Message-relevant fear is a particularly important emotion to consider in a preventative context because feelings of fear can make a seemingly far away health threat seem more realistic and more likely. In many situations, that addition of uncertainty about a healthy outcome can help motivate a health individual to take action to stay that way.

The EPPM, in particular, is often applied to fear appeals in preventative health contexts (Witte et al. 2000), from and teen pregnancy and sexually transmitted disease prevention (Roberto, Zimmerman, Carlyle, and Abner 2007) and HIV/AIDS prevention (Witte 1998) to cardiovascular disease prevention (McKay, Berkowitz, Blumberg, and Goldberg 2004) and skin cancer prevention (Stephenson and Witte 1998). Additional work in a prevention context as focused on what combination of threat and efficacy components in a prevention message are most effective. Following a message about HPV prevention, Carcioppolo et al. (2013) found that a one-to-one ration of threat-to-efficacy message components was the most persuasive approach. The authors found that this ratio was more effective because it resulted in higher reported levels of fear and risk susceptibility by participants than did other ratios. They also found that how the threat outcome was framed influenced the persuasiveness of the message. When the fear appeal focused on genital warts as the outcome of HPV, participants reported higher levels of response efficacy, which in turn fostered stronger prevention intentions. However, when the fear appeal focused on cervical cancer as the outcome of HPV, participants felt lower response efficacy and reported weaker intentions.

Campaign designers often employ fear in messages aimed at reducing or eliminating tobacco use (for more on campaigns about tobacco cessation, see chapter 11, this volume), a behavior change with huge prevention implications. For instance, the Centers for Disease Control and Prevention launched a national media campaign in 2012 called "Tips from Former Smokers," which used narratives from real former smokers and portrayed negative consequences of their past actions (e.g., a stoma in their throats, missing teeth, a premature child, immobility, etc.) and used graphic images alongside these testimonials (McAfee, Davis, Alexander Jr, Pechacek, and Bunnell 2013). Preliminary evaluations found that smokers who reacted to the ads with fear, disgust, or both emotions perceived the ads as highly effective (Jónsdóttir, Holm, Poltavski, and Vogeltanz-Holm 2014). Additionally, studies of social media responses to these fear appeals found strong evidence of message acceptance based on an analysis of EPPM constructs in the social media messages about "Tips" (Emery, Szczypka, Abril, Kim, and Vera 2014).

In a disease prevention context, it is important to note that the stage of change of the audience member viewing a fear appeal, including ones aimed at smoking cessation, may impact subsequent health behaviors. Cho and Salmon (2006) tested how different stages of readiness to change (Prochaska and DiClemente 1992) moderated the effectiveness of fear appeals about skin cancer prevention. They found that participants who were in the pre-contemplation stage were more likely to think defensively, to be fatalistic about skin cancer, to hold less favorable attitudes toward the prevention behaviors, and to report lower intentions to engage in preventative behaviors after viewing the fear appeal than those who were in later stages of change (i.e., had already intended to engage in or had previously engaged in the cancer prevention behaviors). Wong and Cappella (2009) applied a similar design to test the effectiveness of fear-evoking anti-smoking television PSAs. They found that threat and efficacy were both important predictors of message acceptance for smokers with low readiness to quit, whereas efficacy was the most important predictor among smokers with high readiness to quit. The authors point out the implications of this work for designing effective fear-evoking cancer prevention messages: "Tailoring messages to focus either on increasing motivation and/or confidence to quit smoking in line with the smoker's level of readiness to quit would be an important strategy for improving the effectiveness of fear appeals" (12).

However, there are concerns about the overuse of fear in anti-smoking and other health campaigns. Research in New Zealand found that anti-smoking fear campaigns were more effective with high self-efficacy audiences and that fear appeals contributed to a stigmatization of smokers that made it even more difficult for low-efficacy smokers to quit (Thompson, Barnett, and Pearce 2009). This finding is part of a larger argument, outlined in detail below, about the potential pitfalls of using fear appeals in an attempt to persuade audiences to take preventive health actions.

While fear appeal messages purposefully seek to arouse the negative emotion, health and medical news can inadvertently spur feelings of fear and anxiety by presenting information about real threats to well-being (see chapter 12 about health journalism, this volume). Fear is an increasingly common theme in news reports on all topics, from drugs and crimes to disease (Altheide and Michalowski 1999). News coverage of deadly communicable diseases, such as HIV/AIDS (Lupton 1994) and Creutzfeld-Jacob Disease (mad cow disease) (Washer 2006), tend to be particularly adept at arousing fear in the public.

Additionally, how the news media frame potential health threats can influence the emotions aroused in readers and viewers (e.g., Balzarotti and Ciceri 2014; Hoffner and Ye 2009; Lawrence 2004). For instance, Major (2009) found that in news stories about lung cancer and obesity thematic news frames featuring a broader context elicited higher levels of negative emotions and lower levels of positive emotions than did episodic news frames featuring the plights of individuals dealing with those health conditions. Additionally, she found that participants in her experiment experienced higher levels of negative and lower levels of positive emotions when they read loss-framed (i.e., emphasizing costs) news stories on these two health topics than when they read gain-framed (i.e., emphasizing benefits) stories. While this study did not differentiate fear from the other negative emotions used in the negative emotion index, the results indicate the importance of analyzing multiple formats of health news coverage in order to understand how audiences will respond to health news stories.

Fear is an especially important emotion in a preventative health context because these feelings can motivate health information seeking (see chapter 13 about health information seeking, this volume). The Theory of Motivated Information Management (TMIM, Afifi and Weiner 2004) posits that too much or too little uncertainty will result in feelings of anxiety. Anxiety levels impact outcome expectations and efficacy for finding information from other individuals, and these variables then shape the nature of information seeking. However, just because anxiety can lead individuals to seek out health information, these emotions do not necessarily foster beneficial outcomes after the search is finished. Baumgartner and Hartmann (2011) found that health anxiety is related to an increase in online health information seeking, but that health-anxious individuals experience more negative consequences from online health information searches than do those who were not as anxious. Additional research is needed to track how levels of fear and anxiety ebb and flow throughout a search for health information. Future work could also examine the differential impacts of pre- and post-search fear and anxiety on health information seekers.

While fear is commonly employed in health messages, theory-based approaches to constructing such messages are not always utilized in practice. Soames Job (1988) argues that many fear-based health campaigns are ineffective because they are not careful with where in the message the fear component is placed, and they often overemphasize punishment for noncompliance. To that point, he suggests that fear-based health campaign messages are most effective when they allow for the target behavior (e.g., smoking cessation) to be reinforced by a reduction in fear, which can be achieved by following five guidelines: (1) The fear-inducing portion of the message should occur before the portion suggesting the target behavior; (2) The fear-inducing portion of the message should be realistic and not overly extreme; (3) A very specific target behavior should be offered in the message; (4) The level of fear elicited in the message should match the intensity that performing the target behavior would be able to alleviate; and (5) This fear offset could occur as reinforcement for the target behavior, thereby confirming its effectiveness. Following these guidelines may be an effective way to help prevent the reactance that often accompanies fear appeals promoting health behaviors (Dillard and Shen 2005).

FEAR AND ENGAGEMENT WITH PUBLIC HEALTH POLICIES

Since the 1960s, fear has been omnipresent in American political advertisements (Brader 2006). Persuasive messages advocating for or against public policy have also contained their share of fear-evoking content. Political advertisements that evoke fear in voters have been shown to stimulate vigilance, increase reliance on contemporary evaluations of candidates, and promote persuasion (Brader 2005). Given its ability to mobilize audiences to act with regard to politics and/or policy, it is not surprising that fear appeals are also adopted in campaigns to sway public opinion about health and healthcare policy. Health care reform provides a modern example of the use of fear in this context. In March 2010, President Barack Obama signed into law the Patient Protection and Affordable Care Act, colloquially known as "Obamacare." Opponents, largely conservatives and Republicans, challenged the legislation in the courts (Dolgin and Dietrich 2011). In 2012, the Supreme Court upheld the majority of the act as constitutional (Kaiser Family Foundation 2012).

During the build up to passing the legislation into law, through legal challenges in the courts, and even after the Supreme Court's rulings, proponents and opponents of health care reform used various messages in an attempt to sway public opinion. Conservatives battling against the initiative employed fear-based reframing of features of the reform, like calling regulatory panels "death panels," and fear-evoking images, such as an Uncle Sam mascot with a creepy grin attempting to conduct a gynecological exam in one television advertisement and a prostate exam in another (Rozsa 2013).

Regardless of one's ideological leanings, it is clear that fear was an essential component of the campaign against the health care law, and future work is needed to see exactly how fear about this policy influenced public opinion and engagement with the reform. Overall, little work has directly addressed the implications of fear appeals on policy issues separate from campaigns for office. Of the work that has been done, there are conflicting results as to the link between negative political messages, their effectiveness, and distrust in government (c.f., Martinez and Delegal 1990). A meta-analysis of negative political campaigns revealed that negative campaigning is not an effective means of winning votes (Lau, Sigelman, and Rovner 2007). However, this meta-analysis did find that negative campaigns are more memorable and stimulate greater knowledge. Additionally, this body of literature indicates that negative campaigning does *not* depresses voter turnout. However, it is connected with lower levels of political efficacy, trust in government, and overall public mood. Most of this work addresses the context of individual candidates' campaigns for office, and much work remains to be done to test if these findings would hold true for influencing the effects of campaigns focused on increasing or decreasing public support for health-related policies.

THE ETHICS OF HEALTH MESSAGES THAT SCARE AUDIENCES

Many researchers have expressed concerns over the heavy reliance on fear-inducing messages as vehicles for disseminating health information and motivating health behavior changes. Hastings, Stead, and Webb (2004) outline reasons for concern about the commonplace use of fear appeals. In addition to concerns about the methodology used in many studies, many of which take place in controlled settings and not in the field, the researchers argue that fear appeals can also result in complacency among those who are not directly targeted (as fear requires a perception of self-relevance to be activated, and those who cannot find relevance in a fear appeal may falsely believe they are not at risk). Moreover, they posit that fear appeals may be contributing to increased social inequity between those who respond to fear campaigns, which are often the "worried well" (973) who are higher in socioeconomic status than those who do not respond to the appeals and tend to be less educated and poorer (Hastings et al. 2004). Hastings et al. argue that the frequent use of fear appeals can result in a chronic sense of heightened anxiety among those individuals lower in socioeconomic status who are also at greater risk for health issues.

Be it a campaign for individual behavior change or an advertisement advocating for changes in society-wide health policies, the use of fear in health messages is not a practice without its critics. These arguments point to the need to examine studies of individual and societal effects from a long-term perspective in order to get a broader view of the outcomes associated with fear appeals. If the use of fear appeals causes more harm than good in a society over time, it will be increasingly difficult for health message designers and researchers to justify their use. Furthermore, although meta-analyses do show some support for a positive relationship between fear arousal and persuasion, many other studies related to health communication have found that fear impeded persuasion and/or behavior change (e.g., Myrick and Oliver 2014; Yoo, Kreuter, Lai, and Fu 2014). As many scholars note (e.g., Ruiter et al. 2004), those wanting to evoke fear in audiences in order to persuade them should proceed with caution.

CONCLUSION

This chapter offers an overview of theoretical and empirical research related to fear and communication while also suggesting potential areas for future research and additional methodological rigor. In sum, fear is a negatively valenced emotion that results from appraisals of uncertainty in the face of a potential threat. A frightened individual is motivated to avoid danger and revise his or her plans to escape from a threat. Fear has been of great interest to communication scholars studying everything from persuasion and enter-tainment to journalism and policy messages. However, persuasive fear ap-peals, in particular, still suffer from a lack of conceptual clarity.

While meta-analysis indicates that there is a positive linear relationship between fear levels and outcomes that may aid in preventative health efforts, fear can also lead to maladaptive outcomes if individuals do not have the necessary coping skills to deal with the aversive implications of a threatening message, if individuals are not motivated to overcome reactance to messages that threaten their freedom, or if individuals are so frightened the avoidance tendencies of fear prevent audiences from even attending to the message in the first place. Mongeau (2013) sums up the state of fear appeal research as follows: "Fear appeals work, at least for most audiences and most contexts. Disagreements abound, however, concerning why fear appeals work (and why they don't)" (184).

There are also ethical concerns about using fear to scare people into taking action when the use of fear appeals is connected to deleterious effects on those lower in socioeconomic status, who also happen to be the people who would most benefit from improved health behaviors. Moreover, can fear-inducing messages promote sustained, long-term health behavior change? Additional research is needed to adequately address this question, but preliminary work indicates that positively toned health messages may be more beneficial in sustaining behavior change, at least in certain health con-texts, than are fear-inducing appeals.

Another consideration is the terminology associated with theories of fear appeal effects. The idea that fear control, or regulation of the emotion of fear, should be considered maladaptive runs contrary to functional theories of emotion that argue that each feeling evolved in order to serve an adaptive purpose for individuals. Fear's adaptive purpose is to help an organism avoid a threat. Behaviors related to message acceptance (i.e., calling a quit line after seeing an anti-smoking PSA) may very well fall under the guise of fear control as that behavior could provide a way to escape the threat. While the processes labeled as fear control in the EPPM—defensive avoidance, denial, message rejection, etc.—are clearly counterproductive to persuasion (and, in the case of the preventative health messages, positive health behavior changes), the semantics may give researchers the mistaken impression that the motivations associated with feelings of fear are entirely counter to behav-ior change. It is perhaps the action tendencies associated with fear that help explain the positive relationship between fear and persuasion in many meta-analyses, this despite a definitive answer on the role of more cognitive fac-tors (appraisals of threat and efficacy) in fear appeal effects.

From fear appeals to fear-evoking news stories, the emotion of fear is integrally tied to the study of emotions and health-related media effects. Continued work on theory development as well as rigorous field and longitudinal tests of the effects of fear-evoking messages are necessary to understand the relationships between message-induced fear and preventative health behaviors. As this body of literature continues to develop, researchers and message designers can put these new insights to use in helping to prevent illness and disease in ways that also take into account the ethics of trying to scare audiences into better health.

REFERENCES

Afifi, W. A., and J. L. Weiner. 2004. Toward a theory of motivated information management. *Communication Theory* 14(2):167–90. doi: 10.1111/j.1468-2885.2004.tb00310.x.

Altheide, D. L., and R. S. Michalowski. 1999. Fear in the news. *Sociological Quarterly* 40(3):475–503. doi: 10.1111/j.1533-8525.1999.tb01730.x.

Balzarotti, S., and M. R. Ciceri. 2014. News reports of catastrophes and viewers' fear: Threat appraisal of positively versus negatively framed events. *Media Psychology*, 1–21. doi: 10.1080/15213269.2013.826588.

Bandura, A. 1993. Perceived self-efficacy in cognitive development and functioning. *Educational Psychologist* 28(2):117–48. doi: 10.1207/s15326985ep2802_3.

Baumgartner, S. E., and T. Hartmann. 2011. The role of health anxiety in online health information search. *Cyberpsychology, Behavior, and Social Networking* 14(10):613–18. doi: 10.1089/cyber.2010.0425.

Boster, F. J., and P. A. Mongeau. 1984. Fear-arousing persuasive messages. In R. N. Bostrom and B. H. Westley (Eds.), *Communication Yearbook* (Vol. 8, pp. 330–75). Beverly Hills, CA: Sage.

Brader, T. 2005. Striking a responsive chord: How political ads motivate and persuade voters by appealing to emotions. *American Journal of Political Science* 49(2):388–405. doi: 10.1111/j.0092-5853.2005.00130.x.

———. 2006. *Campaigning for hearts and minds: How emotional appeals in political ads work*. Chicago, IL: University of Chicago Press.

Cacioppo, J. T., R. E. Petty, and C. F. Kao. 1984. The efficient assessment of need for cognition. *Journal of Personality Assessment* 48(3):306–7. doi: 10.1207/s15327752jpa4803_13.

Carcioppolo, N., J. D. Jensen, S. R. Wilson, W. B. Collins, M. Carrion, and G. Linnemeier. 2013. Examining HPV threat-to-efficacy ratios in the Extended Parallel Process Model. *Health Communication* 28(1):20–28. doi: 10.1080/10410236.2012.719478.

Chaiken, S. 1980. Heuristic versus systematic information processing and the use of source versus message cues in persuasion. *Journal of Personality and Social Psychology* 39(5):752–66.

Cho, H., and C. T. Salmon. 2006. Fear appeals for individuals in different stages of change: Intended and unintended effects and implications on public health campaigns. *Health Communication* 20(1):91–99. doi: 10.1207/s15327027hc2001_9.

Cooper, D. P., J. L. Goldenberg, and J. Arndt. 2014. Perceived efficacy, conscious fear of death and intentions to tan: Not all fear appeals are created equal. *British Journal of Health Psychology* 19(1):1–15. doi: 10.1111/bjhp.12019.

Das, E. H. H. J., J. B. F. de Wit, and W. Stroebe. 2003. Fear appeals motivate acceptance of action recommendations: Evidence for a positive bias in the processing of persuasive messages. *Personality and Social Psychology Bulletin* 29(5):650–64. doi: 10.1177/0146167203029005009.

de Hoog, N., W. Stroebe, and J. B. F. de Wit. 2007. The impact of vulnerability to and severity of a health risk on processing and acceptance of fear-arousing communications: A meta-analysis. *Review of General Psychology* 11(3):258–85. doi: 10.1037/1089-2680.11.3.258.

———. 2008. The processing of fear-arousing communications: How biased processing leads to persuasion. *Social Influence* 3(2):84–113. doi: 10.1080/15534510802185836.

Dillard, J. P. 1994. Rethinking the study of fear appeals: An emotional perspective. *Communication Theory* 4(4):295–323. doi: 10.1111/j.1468-2885.1994.tb00094.x.

Dillard, J. P., and R. L. Nabi. 2006. The persuasive influence of emotion in cancer prevention and detection messages. *Journal of Communication* 56:S123–S139. doi: 10.1111/j.1460-2466.2006.00286.x.

Dillard, J. P., C. A. Plotnick, L. C. Godblod, V. S. Freimuth, and T. Edgar. 1996. The multiple affective outcomes of AIDS PSAs: Fear appeals do more than scare people. *Communication Research* 23(1):44–72. doi: 10.1177/009365096023001002.

Dillard, J. P., and L. Shen. 2005. On the nature of reactance and its role in persuasive health communication. *Communication Monographs* 72(2):144–68. doi: 10.1080/03637750500111815.

Dolgin, J. L., and K. R. Dietrich. 2011. Social and legal debate about the Affordable Care Act. *University of Missouri Kansas City Law Review* 80(1):45–90.

Emery, S. L., G. Szczypka, E. P. Abril, Y. Kim, and L. Vera. 2014. Are you scared yet? Evaluating fear appeal messages in tweets about the tips campaign. *Journal of Communication* 64(2):278–95. doi: 10.1111/jcom.12083.

Esteves, F., C. Parra, U. L. F. Dimberg, and A. Öhman. 1994. Nonconscious associative learning: Pavlovian conditioning of skin conductance responses to masked fear-relevant facial stimuli. *Psychophysiology* 31(4):375–85. doi: 10.1111/j.1469-8986.1994.tb02446.x.

Forgas, J. P. 2000. Affect and information processing strategies: An interactive relationship. In J. P. Forgas (Ed.), *Feeling and thinking: The role of affect in social cognition*. Cambridge, UK: Cambridge University Press.

Fredrickson, B. L. 1998. What good are positive emotions? *Review of General Psychology* 2(3):300–319. doi: 10.1037/1089-2680.2.3.300.

———. 2001. The role of positive emotions in positive psychology: The broaden-and-build theory of positive emotions. *American Psychologist* 56(3):218–26. doi: 10.1037/0003-066X.56.3.218.

Goodall, C. E., and P. Reed. 2013. Threat and efficacy uncertainty in news coverage about bed bugs as unique predictors of information seeking and avoidance: An extension of the EPPM. *Health Communication* 28(1):63–71. doi: 10.1080/10410236.2012.689096.

Hale, J. L., R. Lemieux, and P. A. Mongeau. 1995. Cognitive processing of fear-arousing message content. *Communication Research* 22(4):459–74. doi: 10.1177/009365095022004004.

Hastings, G., M. Stead, and J. Webb. 2004. Fear appeals in social marketing: Strategic and ethical reasons for concern. *Psychology and Marketing* 21(11):961–86. doi: 10.1002/mar.20043.

Hoffner, C., and J. Ye. 2009. Young adults' responses to news about sunscreen and skin cancer: The role of framing and social comparison. *Health Communication* 24(3):189–98. doi: 10.1080/10410230902804067.

Hovland, C., I. L. Janis, and H. Kelly. 1953. *Communication and persuasion*. New Haven, CT: Yale University Press.

Hunt, D. M., and O. Shehryar. 2011. Integrating terror management theory into fear appeal research. *Social and Personality Psychology Compass* 5(6):372–82. doi: 10.1111/j.1751-9004.2011.00354.x.

Izard, C. E. 1977. *Human emotions*. New York: Plenum.

———. 1993. Four systems for emotion activation: Cognitive and noncognitive processes. *Psychological Review* 100(1):68–90. doi: 10.1037/0033-295X.100.1.68.

Janis, I. L., and S. Feshbach. 1953. Effects of fear-arousing communications. *Journal of Abnormal and Social Psychology* 48(1):78–92. doi: 10.1037/h0060732.

Jónsdóttir, H. L., J. E. Holm, D. Poltavski, and N. Vogeltanz-Holm. 2014. The role of fear and disgust in predicting the effectiveness of television advertisements that graphically depict the health harms of smoking. *Preventing Chronic Disease* 11:E218. doi: 10.5888/pcd11.140326.

Kaiser Family Foundation. 2012. A guide to the Supreme Court's Affordable Care Act decision *Focus on Health Reform* (pp. 1–10). Kaiser Family Foundation.

Lang, P. J., M. Davis, and A. Öhman. 2000. Fear and anxiety: Animal models and human cognitive psychophysiology. *Journal of Affective Disorders* 61(3):137–59. doi: http://dx.doi.org/10.1016/S0165-0327(00)00343-8.

Lau, R. R., L. Sigelman, and I. B. Rovner. 2007. The effects of negative political campaigns: A meta-analytic reassessment. *Journal of Politics* 69(4):1176–209. doi: 10.1111/j.1468-2508.2007.00618.x.

Lawrence, R. G. 2004. Framing obesity: The evolution of news discourse on a public health issue. *The Harvard International Journal of Press/Politics* 9(3):56–75. doi: 10.1177/1081180x04266581.

Lazarus, R. S. 1991. *Emotion and adaptation*. New York: Oxford University Press.

Leshner, G., F. Vultee, P. D. Bolls, and J. Moore. 2010. When a fear appeal isn't just a fear appeal: The effects of graphic anti-tobacco messages. *Journal of Broadcasting and Electronic Media* 54(3):485–507. doi: 10.1080/08838151.2010.498850.

Leventhal, H. 1970. Findings and theory in the study of fear communications. In L. Berkowitz (Ed.), *Advances in Experimental Social Psychology* (Vol. 5, pp. 119–86). New York: Academic Press.

Lewis, I. M., B. Watson, and K. M. White. 2008. An examination of message-relevant affect in road safety messages: Should road safety advertisements aim to make us feel good or bad? *Transportation Research Part F: Traffic Psychology and Behaviour* 11(6):403–17. doi: http://dx.doi.org/10.1016/j.trf.2008.03.003.

———. 2013. Extending the explanatory utility of the EPPM beyond fear-based persuasion. *Health Communication* 28(1):84–98. doi: 10.1080/10410236.2013.743430.

Lupton, D. 1994. *Moral threats and dangerous desires: AIDS in the news media*. New York: Routledge.

MacLeod, C. 1999. Anxiety and anxiety disorders. In T. Dalgleish and M. J. Power (Eds.), *Handbook of cognition and emotion* (pp. 447–77). West Sussex, England: John Wiley and Sons.

Major, L. H. 2009. Break it to me harshly: The effects of intersecting news frames in lung cancer and obesity coverage. *Journal of Health Communication* 14(2):174–88. doi: 10.1080/10810730802659939.

Martinez, M. D., and T. Delegal. 1990. The irrelevance of negative campaigns to political trust: Experimental and survey results. *Political Communication* 7(1):25–40. doi: 10.1080/10584609.1990.9962885.

McAfee, T., K. C. Davis, R. L. Alexander Jr., T. F. Pechacek, and R. Bunnell. 2013. Effect of the first federally funded US antismoking national media campaign. *The Lancet* 382(9909):2003–11. doi: 10.1016/S0140-6736(13)61686-4.

McKay, D. L., J. M. Berkowitz, J. B. Blumberg, and J. P. Goldberg. 2004. Communicating cardiovascular disease risk due to elevated homocysteine levels: Using the EPPM to develop print materials. *Health Education and Behavior* 31(3):355–71. doi: 10.1177/1090198104263353.

Miller, S. M. 1987. Monitoring and blunting: Validation of a questionnaire to assess styles of information seeking under threat. *Journal of Personality and Social Psychology* 52(2):345–53. doi: 10.1037/0022-3514.52.2.345.

Miller, S. M., Y. Shoda, and K. Hurley. 1996. Applying cognitive-social theory to health-protective behavior: Breast self-examination in cancer screening. *Psychological Bulletin* 119(1):70–94.

Mongeau, P. A. 1998. Another look at fear arousing messages. In M. Allen and R. Preiss (Eds.), *Persuasion: Advances through meta-analysis* (pp. 330–75). Cresskill, NJ: Hampton Press.

Mongeau, P. A. 2013. Fear appeals. In J. P. Dillard and L. Shen (Eds.), *The SAGE handbook of persuasion: Developments in theory and practice* (pp. 184–99). Thousand Oaks, CA: Sage.

Morales, A. C., E. C. Wu, and G. J. Fitzsimons. 2012. How disgust enhances the effectiveness of fear appeals. *Journal of Marketing Research* 49(3):383–93. doi: 10.1509/jmr.07.0364.

Myrick, J. G., and M. B. Oliver. 2014. Laughing and crying: Mixed emotions, compassion, and the effectiveness of a YouTube PSA about skin cancer. *Health Communication*, 1–10. doi: 10.1080/10410236.2013.845729.

Nabi, R. L. 1999. A cognitive-functional model for the effects of discrete negative emotions on information processing, attitude change, and recall. *Communication Theory* 9(3):292–320. doi: 10.1111/j.1468-2885.1999.tb00172.x.

———. 2002. Anger, fear, uncertainty, and attitudes: A test of the cognitive-functional model. *Communication Monographs* 69(3):204–16.

———. 2015. Emotional flow in persuasive health messages. *Health Communication* 30(2):114–24. doi: 10.1080/10410236.2014.974129.

Nabi, R. L., D. Roskos-Ewoldsen, and F. D. Carpentier. 2008. Subjective knowledge and fear appeal effectiveness: Implications for message design. *Health Communication* 23(2):191–201. doi: 10.1080/10410230701808327.

O'Keefe, D. J. 2003. Message properties, mediating states, and manipulation checks: Claims, evidence, and data analysis in experimental persuasive message effects research. *Communication Theory* 13(3):251–74. doi: 10.1111/j.1468-2885.2003.tb00292.x.

Öhman, A. 2009. Of snakes and faces: An evolutionary perspective on the psychology of fear. *Scandinavian Journal of Psychology* 50:543–52.

Peters, G.-J. Y., R. A. C. Ruiter, and G. Kok. 2012. Threatening communication: A critical re-analysis and a revised meta-analytic test of fear appeal theory. *Health Psychology Review* 7(sup1):S8–S31. doi: 10.1080/17437199.2012.703527.

Petty, R. E., and J. T. Cacioppo. 1986. The elaboration likelihood model of persuasion. *Advances in Experimental Social Psychology* 19:123–205.

Petty, R. E., L. R. Fabrigar, and D. T. Wegener. 2003. Emotional factors in attitudes and persuasion. In R. J. Davidson, K. R. Scherer, and H. H. Goldsmith (Eds.), *Handbook of affective sciences* (pp. 752–72). Oxford: Oxford University Press.

Petty, R. E., and D. T. Wegener. 1998. Matching versus mismatching attitude functions: Implications for scrutiny of persuasive messages. *Personality and Social Psychology Bulletin* 24(3):227–40.

Popova, L. 2012. The Extended Parallel Process model: Illuminating the gaps in research. *Health Education and Behavior* 39(4):455–73. doi: 10.1177/1090198111418108.

Prochaska, J. O., and C. C. DiClemente. 1992. Stages of change in the modification of problem behaviors. *Progress in behavior modification* 28:183–218.

Raghunathan, R., and K. Corfman. 2004. Sadness as pleasure-seeking prime and anxiety as attentiveness prime: The "different affect–different effect" (DADE) model. *Motivation and Emotion* 28(1):23–41. doi: 10.1023/B:MOEM.0000027276.32709.30.

Rintamaki, L. S., and Z. J. Yang. 2014. Advancing the Extended Parallel Process model through the inclusion of response cost measures. *Journal of Health Communication*, 1–16. doi: 10.1080/10810730.2013.864722.

Roberto, A. J., R. S. Zimmerman, K. E. Carlyle, and E. L. Abner. 2007. A computer-based approach to preventing pregnancy, STD, and HIV in rural adolescents. *Journal of Health Communication* 12(1):53–76. doi: 10.1080/10810730601096622.

Rogers, R. W. 1975. A protection motivation theory of fear appeals and attitude change. *The Journal of Psychology* 91(1):93–114. doi: 10.1080/00223980.1975.9915803.

Roseman, I. J. 2011. Emotional behaviors, emotivational goals, emotion strategies: Multiple levels of organization integrate variable and consistent responses. *Emotion Review* 3(4):434–43. doi: 10.1177/1754073911410744.

Roseman, I. J., C. Wiest, and T. S. Swartz. 1994. Phenomenology, behaviors, and goals differentiate discrete emotions. *Journal of Personality and Social Psychology* 67(2):206–21. doi: 10.1037/0022-3514.67.2.206.

Roskos-Ewoldsen, D. R., J. Bichsel, and K. Hoffman. 2002. The influence of accessibility of source likability on persuasion. *Journal of Experimental Social Psychology* 38(2):137–43. doi: http://dx.doi.org/10.1006/jesp.2001.1492.

Roskos-Ewoldsen, D. R., J. H. Yu, and N. Rhodes. 2004. Fear appeal messages affect accessibility of attitudes toward the threat and adaptive behaviors. *Communication Monographs* 71(1):49–69. doi: 10.1080/0363452042000228559.

Rozsa, M. 2013. The anti-Obamacare ads have been nothing but fear-mongering drivel. *Policy Mic.* http://mic.com/articles/75369/the-anti-obamacare-ads-have-been-nothing-but-fear-mongering-drivel.

Ruiter, R. A. C., B. Verplanken, D. De Cremer, and G. Kok. 2004. Danger and fear control in response to fear appeals: The role of need for cognition. *Basic and Applied Social Psychology* 26(1):13–24. doi: 10.1207/s15324834basp2601_2.

So, J. 2013. A further extension of the Extended Parallel Process Model (E-EPPM): Implications of cognitive appraisal theory of emotion and dispositional coping style. *Health Communication* 28(1):72–83. doi: 10.1080/10410236.2012.708633.

Soames Job, R. F. 1988. Effective and ineffective use of fear in health promotion campaigns. *American Journal of Public Health* 78(2):163–67. doi: 10.2105/AJPH.78.2.163.

Spielberger, C. D., R. L. Gorsuch, and R. E. Lushene. 1970a. *STAI manual for the state-trait anxiety inventory.* Palo Alto, CA: Consulting Psychologists Press.

———. 1970b. State-Trait Anxiety Inventory.

Stephenson, M. T., and K. Witte. 1998. Fear, threat, and perceptions of efficacy from frightening skin cancer messages. *Public Health Review* 26(2):147–74.

Thompson, L. E., J. R. Barnett, and J. R. Pearce. 2009. Scared straight? Fear-appeal anti-smoking campaigns, risk, self-efficacy and addiction. *Health, Risk and Society* 11(2):181–96. doi: 10.1080/13698570902784281.

Turner, M. M., R. N. Rimal, D. Morrison, and H. Kim. 2006. The role of anxiety in seeking and retaining risk information: Testing the risk perception attitude framework in two studies. *Human Communication Research* 32(2):130–56. doi: 10.1111/j.1468-2958.2006.00006.x.

Washer, P. 2006. Representations of mad cow disease. *Social Science and Medicine* 62(2):457–66. doi: http://dx.doi.org/10.1016/j.socscimed.2005.06.001.

Weinstein, N. D. 2000. Perceived probability, perceived severity, and health-protective behavior. *Health Psychology* 19(1):65–74. doi: 10.1037/0278-6133.19.1.65.

Witte, K. 1992. Putting the fear back into fear appeals: The extended parallel process model. *Communication Monographs* 12(4):329–49. doi: 10.1080/03637759209376276.

———. 1994. Fear control and danger control: A test of the Extended Parallel Process Model (EPPM). *Communication Monographs* 61(2):113. doi: 10.1080/03637759409376328.

———. 1998. A theoretically based evaluation of HIV/AIDS prevention campaigns along the trans-Africa highway in Kenya. *Journal of Health Communication* 3(4):345–63. doi: 10.1080/108107398127157.

Witte, K., and M. Allen. 2000. A meta-analysis of fear appeals: Implications for effective public health campaigns. *Health Education and Behavior* 27(5):591–615.

Witte, K., G. Meyer, and D. Martell. 2000. *Effective health risk messages: A step-by-step guide.* Thousand Oaks, CA: Sage.

Witte, K., and K. Morrison. 2000. Examining the influence of trait anxiety/repression-sensitization on individuals' reactions to fear appeals. *Western Journal of Communication* 64(1):1–27. doi: 10.1080/10570310009374661.

Wong, N. C. H., and J. N. Cappella. 2009. Antismoking threat and efficacy appeals: Effects on smoking cessation intentions for smokers with low and high readiness to quit. *Journal of Applied Communication Research* 37(1):1–20. doi: 10.1080/00909880802593928.

Yoo, J. H., M. W. Kreuter, C. Lai, and Q Fu. 2014. Understanding narrative effects: The role of discrete negative emotions on message processing and attitudes among low-income African American women. *Health Communication* 29(5):494–504. doi: 10.1080/10410236.2013.776001.

Yzer, M. C., B. G. Southwell, and M. T. Stephenson. 2013. Inducing fear as a public communication campaign strategy. In R. E. Rice and C. K. Atkin (Eds.), *Public communication campaigns* (Fourth ed., pp. 163–76). Los Angeles: Sage.

Chapter Three

Guilt

Imagine the following scenario: You skipped your yoga class after work and, instead, went home and sat out on the couch. You watched television for hours, not getting any exercise at all that day. You know your doctor said you needed to exercise for both stress relief and heart health, but you just could not muster up the gumption to get it done that particular day. At least you decide to make dinner at home instead of ordering a high-calorie pizza. However, you have a craving for something sweet and end up eating a half-pint of chocolate ice cream that night.

Now, imagine another possible scenario: You again skipped your yoga class, but instead of going home to the couch, this time you head to the local bar to meet up with some friends. After a fun evening of drinks and revelry, you drive home and are a little more "buzzed" than you should have been behind the wheel of a car. The next day, while browsing the Internet, you read a story about a young girl killed by a different drunk driver. The story includes heart-wrenching quotes from her grieving parents.

If either of these scenarios had actually occurred, how would you feel? Especially consider how you would feel a bit later, after the sugar high from the cheesecake or the buzz of your drink has worn off. "Guilty" is the likely response most individuals would give. As these hypothetical situations illustrate, the emotion of guilt is frequently tied to behaviors that promote illness—behaviors like eating ice cream or drinking with friends—that are often more pleasurable and/or easier to enact than are tedious health behaviors.

For some individuals, guilt from performing unhealthy actions can motivate positive health behavior changes. For others, health-related messages, such as the news article about the drunk driving crash or a public service announcement from Mothers Against Drunk Driving (MADD), evoke feelings of guilt for past behaviors. Feelings of guilt about drinking and driving in past situations can then encourage individual behavior change (e.g., I will never drive while drunk again) and also advocacy for policy changes (e.g., signing a petition asking lawmakers to lower the minimum blood alcohol content allowed for operating a vehicle). Anticipating future feelings of guilt when contemplating an action (e.g., if I eat this ice cream, I feel really bad about myself afterward) can also alter an individual's present behavior. This chapter explores the psychological qualities and functions of guilt, research on the effects of guilt in communication processes, and how the emotion may influence reactions to prevention and health policy messages.

PSYCHOLOGICAL QUALITIES OF GUILT

Guilt is a negatively valenced emotion (Izard 1977; Lazarus 1991). Gaylin (1979) states that guilt "signals us when we have transgressed from codes of behavior which we personally want to sustain. . . . Feeling guilty informs us we have failed our own ideals" (52). Guilt is one of the self-conscious emotions, along with embarrassment, pride, and shame (Lewis 2008). Emotions in the self-conscious family typically take time to develop in humans as they require certain cognitive abilities before they can be fully experienced. Until a child can understand and remember its culture's codes of behavior, then it will be difficult for that child to understand that she has violated the code. Unlike other types of emotions, particularly those whose initial experiences occur much earlier in life (e.g., joy, sadness, or fear), the events that evoke self-conscious emotions can differ largely from person to person or culture to culture.

Violation of an individual's set of standards, rules, or goals (SRGs) are what determine when an individual will feel guilty (Stipek, Recchia, McClintic, and Lewis 1992). As Lazarus (1991) wrote, the core relational theme of guilt is feeling as though one has acted in a morally deficient way. The SRGs that define the boundaries of what is or is not morally reprehensible are largely shaped by the culture and society in which an individual lives. SRGs are incorporated into individual self-concepts at a very early age through social learning (Stipek et al. 1992). Each individual has a unique set of SRGs; however, members of similar groups (e.g., members of the same religion, those who live in the same geographic area, those who share a professions or cultural heritage, etc.) are likely to have overlapping SRGs. The ability to self-evaluate one's behavior as either meeting or not meeting these standards, rules, or goals is crucial for experiencing any of the self-conscious emotions.

Individuals are most likely to experience guilt when they judge their behavior as failing to live up to one of their own SRGs. Guilt is the emotion experienced when one believes *a specific behavior* does not live up to one's SRGs (Lewis 1992). Unlike guilt, shame occurs when individuals perceive themselves as being *generally* bad people. Because guilt, unlike shame, is the result of evaluating a specific action, it motivates those experiencing it to try to correct or mitigate the behavior that caused the guilt. Accordingly, the action tendency of guilt is to take corrective action to repair the failure or prevent it from happening again (Barrett, Zahn-Waxler, and Cole 1993; Lazarus 1991; Lewis 2008). Since guilt motivates people to take corrective action, which helps alleviate negative feelings, it is a less intense emotion than shame. Shame is, instead, associated with a lack of action and/or maladaptive behavior. While all of the self-conscious emotions may impact how audiences respond to prevention-focused health messages, it is the active and restorative nature of guilt that makes it of particular interest to health communication scholars.

As discussed above, feelings of guilt manifest after someone evaluates his or her actions as having violated a valued SRG. However, an individual does not have to *actually* violate an SRG to experience guilt. Existential guilt occurs when an individual compares her own well-being to the well-being of others (Izard 1977). This type of guilt can encourage those experiencing it to take action in order to close the gap between others' well-being and her own.

A second type of guilt is reactive guilt, which occurs when individuals feel regret over past transactions (Lewis 2008). This is the type of guilt likely experienced in the scenario where a person eats a high-calorie dessert and later has to confront the bathroom scale. Particularly for typical or minor transgressions (e.g., overeating, skipping an exercise session), this type of guilt is likely a shared experience common to many members in a society that shares SRGs.

In addition to existential and reactive guilt, there is anticipated guilt (Lewis 2008; Lindsey 2005). Merely foreseeing a possible violation of one's standards can spur feelings of guilt. This is the guilt that could be evoked by the story about drunk driving; the reader feels anticipatory guilt thinking about the possibility of causing an accident. The anticipation of possible feelings of guilt in the future is enough to motivate the reader to call a taxi next time he is out on the town in order to avoid the aversive emotional state of guilt. Interestingly, though, people are often inaccurate when they predict the impact of health-related behaviors on their emotional state (Connolly and Reb 2005). Therefore, anticipated guilt might be more or less than the actual guilt someone would experience if he or she violated an SRG.

Guilt can also be differentiated on the basis of who is harmed by the violation of an SRG. As demonstrated in the hypothetical examples, guilt can occur when an individual participates in an activity that harms himself (e.g., overeating). However, guilt can also be elicited by behaviors that harm others, such as drunk driving (Tangney and Dearing 2002). If one's SRGs overlap at all with other individuals' SRGs, which they often do since SRGs are mostly learned from others, then current guilt or anticipation of guilt can motivate people to comply with social norms (Hoffman 1982).

Many researchers argue that humans evolved to experience guilt because the emotion has socially adaptive properties. Neuroimaging studies have confirmed that feelings of guilt accompanied by social consequences lead to greater activation in certain guilt-associated brain regions than do feelings of guilt that are experienced without social consequences (Morey et al. 2012). This body of work has demonstrated that there is an overlap in the patterns of brain activation for feelings of guilt and feelings of empathy, strengthening the argument that feelings of guilt (current or anticipated), while unpleasant, do serve an important social function in motivating altruistic behavior (Batson 2011; Morey et al. 2012).

As the literature on guilt reveals, the emotion is highly dependent on specific individuals, specific situations, and the context of that situation. Feelings of guilt depend on the individual's SRGs, on whether the violation of an SRG is current or anticipatory, and whether the self or others are/will be harmed by the violation. However, individuals also have general tendencies toward feeling guilty or not, which is known as dispositional guilt (Tangney, Stuewig, and Mashek 2007). Individuals who have particularly high levels of dispositional guilt over a long period of time may develop a chronic state of guilt and even other difficulties, such as depression (Tangney, Stuewig, and Mashek 2007).

Given that guilt occurs when one perceives a violation, or possible future violation, of a standard, rule or goal, the role of good health and well-being as important values in modern society makes health behavior an apt arena for studying guilt effects. Because good health signifies virtue, those who are unhealthy may be made to feel guilty or unworthy by others or by the society as a whole (Fitzgerald 1994; Wikler 1987). Despite the clear link between guilt and health behavior, guilt has not been as thoroughly studied for its impact on health or the processing of health messages as have other emotions.

However, the psychology of guilt has many ramifications for individual health behaviors (Consedine and Moskowitz 2007). For instance, given the social function of guilt, if social norms are health-promoting (e.g., the norm is to exercise regularly and eat fresh vegetables), then one might expect feelings of guilt to motivate individuals to undertake healthy behaviors. Indeed, the health behavior literature confirms this view. Studies show that adolescents and young adults who feel guilty are less likely to smoke cigarettes, drink, or use marijuana (Dearing, Stuewig, and Tangney 2005; Quiles, Kinnunen, and Bybee 2002), while those who experience guilt related to sex are more likely to use condoms (Wayment and Aronson 2002). Researchers have also linked guilt to increased motivation to exercise and improve one's diet (Eyler and Vest 2002; Sukhdial and Boush 2004).

Anticipated guilt also has a strong relationship with lower levels of a number of risky health behaviors (Consedine and Moskowitz 2007). Despite the fact that individuals are not terribly accurate in predicting how guilty they might feel in the future, anticipated guilt is still an important consideration in understanding why individuals make the health-related choices they do. An underestimation of future guilt might result in poor short-term decisions (e.g., I won't feel all that guilty if I eat this huge slice of cheesecake tonight). However, an overestimation of future guilt could also be unhealthy. For example, constantly overestimating how guilty one might feel after overeating could eventually lead to disordered eating or an eating disorder.

GUILT AND COMMUNICATION

Given its many potential impacts on behavior, guilt is an important emotion to study in a communication context. O'Keefe (2000) defines a guilt appeal as a message that attempts to evoke some amount of guilt in the receiver and also offers a recommended action to reduce or alleviate the guilt. These appeals typically have two parts: The first aims to evoke guilt by drawing the audiences' attention to a moral inconsistency while the second describes the target behavior the audience should take to remedy this indiscretion and reduce their feelings of guilt (O'Keefe 2002).

Research indicates that guilt appeals message designers commonly use them in attempts to persuade audiences. A content analysis of advertisements in popular magazines found that guilt appeals are frequently employed by advertisers, at about the same rate as other persuasive strategies (e.g., the use of humor, sexual imagery, or comparisons with other products) (Huhmann and Brotherton 1997). Huhmann and Brotherton also found that charities and health-related products were the sectors that most frequently employed guilt appeals in magazines. A more recent analysis of food advertisements in parenting magazines found that food products with objectively poor nutritional quality (based on total fat, saturated fat, sodium, protein, sugar and fiber) were significantly more likely than advertisements for healthier products to suggest the less-than-healthy foods were "no guilt" products (Manganello, Clegg Smith, Sudakow, and Summers 2013).

Guilt appeals can be explicit or more subtle and implicit, and meta-analysis indicates that the subtle approach is more effective in persuading audiences (O'Keefe 2000). O'Keefe posits that explicit, intense guilt appeals may backfire because they elicit additional emotions of anger, annoyance, or resentment toward the message source. According to O'Keefe, the mechanism through which effective guilt appeals operate is by creating an inconsistency between the message target's own standards and her actions.

Research on advertising provides evidence of guilt's ability to influence communication processes and outcomes. In a test of consumer responses to fear-inducing charity appeals modeled on the tenets of the Extended Parallel Process Model (Witte 1992), Basil, Ridgway, and Basil (2008) found that participants experiencing empathy *and* efficacy in response to charity messages also felt guilty. But those same participants additionally reported reduced maladaptive responses to the fear appeal. Without appraisals of efficacy, though, participants in the study were more likely to report maladaptive responses to the fear appeal. Furthermore, participants' feelings of guilt were positively and significantly related to intentions to donate to the charity featured in the fear appeal. This study demonstrates that (1) intended emotional tone of a message (e.g., a fear appeal) can spur feelings of guilt in audiences; and (2) guilt can encourage persuasion, given the right circumstances, such as when they feel efficacious.

The amount of guilt generated by a message can moderate the effectiveness of this emotion in fostering persuasion. Coulter and Pinto (1995) found via an experiment that moderate guilt appeal advertisements targeting working mothers were more persuasive than either low- or high-guilt appeals. The researchers discovered that high-intensity guilt appeals actually resulted in feelings of anger and perceptions that the company was manipulating them, which corresponded with decreased persuasion. Statistical analyses revealed that anger mediated the relationship between the level of guilt and consumer attitudes and purchase intentions. Trying to find which message features elicit the "sweet spot" between those extremes—the optimal amount of message-relevant guilt for various persuasive contexts—is an important goal of future research in this area, as would be testing which content and structural features of messages can induce guilt in audiences.

GUILT AND PREVENTION MESSAGES

Guilt appeals can be found in messages targeting many types of behaviors related to health. A few prevention contexts, in particular, have been addressed by many researchers. For example, guilt appeals are especially common in messages advocating against drinking and drug use (Agrawal and Duhachek 2010). A review of mass media campaigns for reducing drinking and driving found them to be, in general, effective at reducing drunk driving behaviors (Elder et al. 2004). Why, exactly, do guilt-based appeals work to promote anti-drinking and anti-drug messages? For health messages, some research indicates that anticipated guilt, versus present guilt, is a key variable for motivating message compliance. Messages that increase the audiences' perceptions of risk related to anti-drug messages were more likely to increase anticipated feelings of guilt and also compliance with the messages (Becker-Olsen and Briones 2009).

Anticipated guilt also has a direct relationship to motivation to behave in a way to protect others, especially when a message includes components that detail a threat to others, effective ways to avoid that threat (i.e., response-efficacy) and encouragement that the audience is capable of avoiding the threat (i.e., self-efficacy). Massi (2005) found that when those three message components are present—threat, response-efficacy, and self-efficacy—audiences experience anticipated guilt but little or no negative reactions to the message. This anticipated guilt then prompts intentions to change behavior as well as actual behavior change. In the world of health communication, anticipated guilt is one key mechanism to provide audiences with the motivation to change their behaviors.

Individual differences may also influence the effectiveness of guilt appeals aimed at encouraging prevention behaviors. Becker-Olsen and Briones (2009) found that individuals with higher levels of dispositional guilt were more persuaded by drug prevention messages than were those with lower levels of dispositional guilt. This finding indicates that guilt-based anti-drinking and/or anti-drug campaigns may seem effective because a large segment of the population is prone to feeling guilty, and therefore are easily moved by such appeals.

Given the connection between guilt appeals and persuasion, it is helpful to also understand what message features and/or frames may elicit the emotion. As mentioned earlier, guilt can occur when a violation occurs (or might occur in the future), one that would harm either the self or others. Research demonstrates that messages discussing threats to others are often better at eliciting guilt and motivating behavior change than are self-directed messages. For instance, in a study of messages advocating testing for sexually transmitted diseases, Hullett (2004) found that other-directed messages were more likely to prime values (and therefore, goals to live up to one's values). By making values, akin to SRGs, salient, these other-focused messages also appeared more relevant to audiences. Perceived relevance then increased feelings of guilt and positive attitudes toward the message, which then increased participants' intentions to actually get tested.

In the appraisal theory view of emotions, perceived relevance is necessary for the initial evocation of an emotion (Lazarus 1991). Therefore, Hullett's (2004) findings on message relevance as a precursor to feelings of guilt fit well within the theoretical confines of emotion theory and provide future areas of research for guilt appeals. Guilt appeals tailored to individuals via computer technology would likely be even more effective at motiving healthy and/or prosocial behaviors (see chapter 14 on eHealth, this volume) given the relationship between health message tailoring and relevance (Rimal and Adkins 2003).

While some guilt appeals may persuade audiences to change their health behaviors, those audience members who recognize and dislike the attempt to persuade via guilt are unlikely to be persuaded due to psychological reactance. According to psychological reactance theory, if people believe that a message is trying to limit their freedom by forcing a response, they will feel threatened and be motivated to restore their freedom (Brehm 1966; Quick and Considine 2008; Quick and Stephenson 2008). This will lead to negative reactions to the message, including feelings of anger at those trying to limit their freedom.

Given that many prevention messages focus on stopping a bad behavior (e.g., smoking, drinking, drug abuse), appeals that aim to make those who perform the behaviors feel guilty, even ashamed, are especially prone to backfire. For instance, in a field experiment testing emergency preparedness messages, Turner and Underhill (2012) found that high-intensity guilt appeals resulted in the highest levels of anger toward the source of the message. In an example from the health communication literature, Agrawal and Duhachek (2010) found that when participants already felt guilt prior to viewing anti-drinking advertisements, a guilt-framed appeal lead to defensive processing of the message, which then resulted in an *increase* in drinking behaviors. It is possible that the pre-existing guilt of the participants prior to message exposure could have carried over and amplified post-message guilt such that the total amount of guilt became too explicit and then created hostility toward the message (O'Keefe 2002).

However, research also shows that individuals who view guilt-evoking advertisements do not necessarily develop negative attitudes toward those messages unless they perceive the ads as manipulative (Cotte, Coulter, and Moore 2005). In an experiment testing the differences between guilt and shame toward STD testing, Boudewyns, Turner, and Paquin (2013) demonstrated that messages evoking shame were associated with anger and manipulative intent, whereas guilt-evoking messages were not. It is possible that some studies finding guilt appeals or high levels of post-message guilt to be ineffective may have actually confounded high levels of guilt with feelings of shame, which are more likely to result in reactance and anger. Future work is needed to tease out the differences between the two in a media effects context as well as to understand which components can evoke guilt without shame.

While the focus of this chapter so far has been on persuasive guilt appeals, health and medical reporting, social media messages about health and patient-provider communication can also serve as instigators of guilt. Copious news coverage of a particular health issue may make news consumers who are either prone to guilt or who are currently violating the health standard discussed in the news more prone to consider changing the behavior. In a social media context, if members of one's social network are reinforcing a health value that a user is violating, that too could spark feelings of guilt and possibly motivate behavior change if the guilt is not too little or too much. For instance, if many of one's friends are posting Facebook messages about working out, that might be enough to induce guilt and motivate the user to do a few jumping jacks between computer sessions. The tone that health care providers use with their patients can also induce guilt, while some patients may not even bring up sensitive topics (e.g., their tobacco- or alcohol-related habits) because they anticipate feeling guilty (Simmons et al. 2009). Additional research is needed to better understand the impact of guilt and anticipatory guilt in these non-persuasive domains.

GUILT AND ENGAGEMENT WITH PUBLIC HEALTH POLICIES

Because guilt can be elicited based on a perception that one's behavior toward others does not comply with moral guidelines, guilt is also a pertinent emotion to examine in the context of messages advocating for health-related policies that may help other individuals. Although little research currently examines this specific context, work in political communication provides insight into the ways in which notions of guilt can be used to sway public opinion. Feldman and Steenbergen (2001) argue that humanitarianism, a moral obligation to help others, is part of the American sociopolitical ethos. Their research found that a sense of humanitarianism could explain public support for specific welfare programs, this despite the public's general suspicion of expanding government and a strong beliefs in self-independence. If helping others is a moral obligation, then not helping others can result in guilt. If individuals do not advocate for health policies that would help prevent disease, especially among vulnerable populations, messages encouraging support for such policies may find guilt appeals effective.

The framing of public issues can also be tied to guilt in ways that influence public opinion and policy reactions. Entman (2004) examined media framing and official spin in two real situations in which a passenger plane was shot down by a military force and all the passengers were accidentally killed. The first incident was in 1983 when a Soviet Air Force fighter jet destroyed a Korean Air Lines flight and the second was in 1988 when a U.S. Navy ship shot down an Iran Air flight. Entman found that U.S. news sources framed the Soviet incident in terms of guilt and moral bankruptcy, while they framed the very similar U.S. incident in terms of the complexity of operating military technology, deemphasizing moral judgments.

Extrapolating the implications of Entman's (2004) findings to messages about public health policy might suggest that news about health policies that would correct an injustice perpetrated by a non-government entity (e.g., to-bacco companies) may be more impactful if audiences feel guilty after con-suming them. On the other hand, news about policy issues that implicate the government (e.g., a mishandling of a viral epidemic) may result in greater public support if technical information is emphasized. Knowing these circumstances for probable guilt elicitation and likely public reactions may help policy advocates to plan more effective counter appeals or other forms of strategic messaging that work to emphasize the guilt of not helping indi-viduals in need.

GUILT AND ETHICS

A final consideration for including guilt in preventative health and health policy messages is the ethics of making audiences feel guilty (Guttman and Salmon 2004). Depending on the context, preventative health messages try-ing to evoke guilt in order to prevent disease (e.g., messages promoting condom use to prevent sexually transmitted infections) may inadvertently create stigma (e.g., a stigma of STIs that prevents people from using con-doms or seeking testing). Simmons et al. (2009) argue that stigma and guilt experienced by relapsed smokers who tried to quit create barriers for efforts to prevent future relapses. Additionally, if messages do not include a promi-nent efficacy component then the audience will not have a good behavioral outlet for feelings of guilt evoked by the message.

Issues of stigma and efficacy from preventative health messages may not be a pressing concern for highly educated or affluent audiences who can find the efficacy information they need on their own and can rather easily arrange to see a health care provider to ask any further questions. However, for low-income audiences and those with little education or health knowledge, using preventative health messages to evoke guilt without providing feasible and efficacious behavioral paths to alleviate the guilt would be irresponsible (Guttman and Salmon 2004). A study of attitudes toward breastfeeding in a low-income population found that while the mothers were aware of the bene-fits of breastfeeding, they experienced feelings of guilt and shame from not being able to do so given various medical and economic constraints (Gutt-man and Zimmerman 2000). Health message designers should be aware of health disparities and pre-message levels of efficacy in their target population prior to employing a guilt appeal.

CONCLUSION

Guilt is a negatively valenced discrete emotion evoked by a violation of one's standards, rules, or goals. The action tendency associated with guilt is to make reprimands and behave in a way to prevent future guilt. There are many different kinds of guilt, starting with dispositional versus situational guilt. Present guilt is also different from anticipatory guilt, with anticipatory guilt being a mechanism behind the effectiveness of many guilt appeals.

The extant research points to both the persuasive abilities of low-to-moderat-level guilt appeals as well as the necessity of using caution when trying to use guilt-evoking message content to persuade. Health communication researchers and message creators who decide to use guilt appeals should be sure to extensively pre-test the messages with the target audiences in order to ensure the message does not induce too little or too much guilt. Nor should the guilt-evoking message evoke shame if the goal is to motivate positive behavior changes given shame's tendency to demotivate individuals.

It is also important that message designers be cognizant of possible reactance and anger toward those who use guilt appeals. The appearance of being overly manipulative can negate any good information contained in a health message. Additionally, high levels of dispositional guilt or high levels of situational guilt carrying over from temporally proximate events can both influence how an audience member will respond to a guilt appeal. While it may be impossible for a health message sent via a mass medium, like traditional broadcast television, to differ based on individual audiences, advances in computer tailoring provide promising avenues for developing more effective health-focused guilt appeals.

Many avenues for additional research on guilt in the context of preventative health message effects exist. Future research could examine how the aggregate levels of guilt from health-related guilt appeals and guilt-evoking news content in one's media diet as well as interpersonal health-related communication might jointly influence health behaviors. Additionally, more research is needed to understand exactly which features of a message are most likely to induce guilt in audiences (O'Keefe 2002).

Few, if any, individuals are immune to the moments described in the hypothetical situations at the beginning of this chapter. Humans are imperfect creatures, and all have failed to meet their own or others' standards at some point. On a day of weakness, an individual may give in, eat a large slice of decadent cheesecake, and later that day experience guilt after stepping on the bathroom scale. However, on other days, the anticipation of the guilt that would be caused by stepping on the scale post-cheesecake could lead the individual to choose fruit for dessert instead. Those who want to understand the effects of health messages on audiences would be wise to include measures of message-relevant and trait levels of guilt in their calculus.

REFERENCES

Agrawal, N., and A. Duhachek. 2010. Emotional compatibility and the effectiveness of anti-drinking messages: A defensive processing perspective on shame and guilt. *Journal of Marketing Research* 47(2):263–73. doi: 10.1509/jmkr.47.2.263.

Barrett, K. C., C. Zahn-Waxler, and P. M. Cole. 1993. Avoiders vs. amenders: Implications for the investigation of guilt and shame during toddlerhood? *Cognition and Emotion* 7(6):481–505. doi: 10.1080/02699939308409201.

Basil, D. Z., N. M. Ridgway, and M. D. Basil. 2008. Guilt and giving: A process model of empathy and efficacy. *Psychology and Marketing* 25(1):1–23. doi: 10.1002/mar.20200.

Batson, C. D. 2011. *Altruism in humans.* New York: Oxford University Press.

Becker-Olsen, K., and R. L. Briones. 2009. Towards a drug free America: Guilt processing and drug prevention. *Journal of Research for Consumers* (16):1–17. doi: jrconsumers.com.libproxy.lib.unc.edu/Academic_Articles/issue_16/Drug_Free_America_academic.pdf.

Boudewyns, V., M. M. Turner, and R. S. Paquin. 2013. Shame-free guilt appeals: Testing the emotional and cognitive effects of shame and guilt appeals. *Psychology and Marketing* 30(9):811–25. doi: 10.1002/mar.20647.

Brehm, J. W. 1966. *A theory of psychological reactance.* New York: Academic Press.

Connolly, T., and J. Reb. 2005. Regret in cancer-related decisions. *Health Psychology* 24(4, Suppl):S29–S34. doi: 10.1037/0278-6133.24.4.S29.

Consedine, N. S., and J. T. Moskowitz. 2007. The role of discrete emotions in health outcomes: A critical review. *Applied and Preventive Psychology* 12(2):59–75. doi: 10.1016/j.appsy.2007.09.001.

Cotte, J., R. A. Coulter, and M. Moore. 2005. Enhancing or disrupting guilt: The role of ad credibility and perceived manipulative intent. *Journal of Business Research* 58(3):361–68. doi: 10.1016/S0148-2963(03)00102-4.

Coulter, R. H., and M. B. Pinto. 1995. Guilt appeals in advertising: What are their effects? *Journal of Applied Psychology* 80(6):697–705. doi: 10.1037/0021-9010.80.6.697.

Dearing, R. L., J. Stuewig, and J. P. Tangney. 2005. On the importance of distinguishing shame from guilt: Relations to problematic alcohol and drug use. *Addictive Behaviors* 30(7):1392–404. doi: 10.1016/j.addbeh.2005.02.002.

Elder, R. W., R. A. Shults, D. A. Sleet, J. L. Nichols, R. S. Thompson, and W. Rajab. 2004. Effectiveness of mass media campaigns for reducing drinking and driving and alcohol-involved crashes: A systematic review. *American Journal of Preventive Medicine* 27(1):57–65. doi: 10.1016/j.amepre.2004.03.002.

Entman, R. M. 2004. *Projections of power: Framing news, public opinion, and U.S. foreign policy.* Chicago, IL: The University of Chicago Press.

Eyler, A. A., and J. R. Vest. 2002. Environmental and policy factors related to physical activity in rural white women. *Women and Health* 36(2):109–19. doi: 10.1300/J013v36n02_08.

Feldman, S., and M. R. Steenbergen. 2001. The humanitarian foundation of public support for social welfare. *American Journal of Political Science* 45(3):658–77.

Fitzgerald, F. T. 1994. The tyranny of health. *New England Journal of Medicine* 331(3):196–98. doi: doi:10.1056/NEJM199407213310312.

Gaylin, W. 1979. *Feelings: Our vital signs.* New York: Harper and Row.

Guttman, N., and D. R. Zimmerman. 2000. Low-income mothers' views on breastfeeding. *Social Science & Medicine* 50(10):1457–73. doi: 10.1016/S0277-9536(99)00387-1.

Guttman, N., and C. T. Salmon. 2004. Guilt, fear, stigma and knowledge gaps: Ethical issues in public health communication interventions. *Bioethics* 18(6):531–52. doi: 10.1111/j.1467-8519.2004.00415.x.

Hoffman, M. 1982. Development of prosocial motivation: Empathy and guilt. In N. Eisenberg (Ed.), *The development of prosocial behavior* (pp. 281–313). New York: Academic Press.

Huhmann, B. A., and T. P. Brotherton. 1997. A content analysis of guilt appeals in popular magazine advertisements. *Journal of Advertising* 26(2):35–45. doi: 10.1080/00913367.1997.10673521.

Hullett, C. R. 2004. Using functional theory to promote sexually transmitted disease (STD) testing: The impact of value-expressive messages and guilt. *Communication Research* 31(4):363–96. doi: 10.1177/0093650204266103.

Izard, C. E. 1977. *Human emotions*. New York: Plenum.

Lazarus, R. S. 1991. *Emotion and adaptation*. New York: Oxford University Press.

Lewis, M. 1992. *Shame: The exposed self.* New York: The Free Press.

———. 2008. Self-conscious emotions: Embarrassment, pride, shame, and guilt. In M. Lewis, J. M. Haviland-Jones, and L. F. Barrett (Eds.), *Handbook of emotions* (Third ed.). New York: Guilford Press.

Lindsey, L. L. M. 2005. Anticipated guilt as behavioral motivation: An examination of appeals to help unknown others through bone marrow donation. *Human Communication Research* 31(4):453–81. doi: 10.1111/j.1468-2958.2005.tb00879.x.

Manganello, J. A., K. Clegg Smith, K. Sudakow, and A. C. Summers. 2013. A content analysis of food advertisements appearing in parenting magazines. *Public Health Nutrition* 16(12):2188–96. doi:10.1017/S1368980012005216.

Massi, L. L. 2005. Anticipated guilt as behavioral motivation. *Human Communication Research* 31(4):453–81. doi: 10.1111/j.1468-2958.2005.tb00879.x.

Morey, R. A., G. McCarthy, E. S. Selgrade, S. Seth, J. D. Nasser, and K. S. LaBar. 2012. Neural systems for guilt from actions affecting self versus others. *NeuroImage* 60(1):683–92. doi: 10.1016/j.neuroimage.2011.12.069.

O'Keefe, D. J. 2000. Guilt and social influence. *Communication Yearbook*, 23:67–101.

———. 2002. Guilt as a mechanism of persuasion. In J. P. Dillard and M. W. Pfau (Eds.), *The persuasion handbook: Developments in theory and practice* (pp. 329–44). Thousand Oaks, CA: Sage.

Quick, B. L., and J. R. Considine. 2008. Examining the use of forceful language when designing exercise persuasive messages for adults: A test of conceptualizing reactance arousal as a two-step process. *Health Communication* 23(5):483–91. doi: 10.1080/10410230802342150.

Quick, B. L., and M. T. Stephenson. 2008. Examining the role of trait reactance and sensation seeking on perceived threat, state reactance, and reactance restoration. *Human Communication Research* 34(3):448–76. doi: 10.1111/j.1468-2958.2008.00328.x.

Quiles, Z. N., T. Kinnunen, and J. Bybee. 2002. Aspects of guilt and self-reported substance use in adolescence. *Journal of Drug Education* 32(4):343–62. doi: 10.2190/VN3D-5M0A-47BN-3Y3T.

Rimal, R. N., and A. D. Adkins. 2003. Using computers to narrowcast health messages: The role of audience segmentation, targeting, and tailoring in health promotion. In T. L. Thompson, A. M. Dorsey, K. I. Miller, and R. Parrott (Eds.), *Handbook of health communication* (pp. 497–513). Mahwah, NJ, US: Lawrence Erlbaum Associates Publishers.

Simmons, V. N., E. B. Litvin, R. D. Patel, P. B. Jacobsen, J. C. McCaffrey, G. Bepler, . . . T. H. Brandon. 2009. Patient–provider communication and perspectives on smoking cessation and relapse in the oncology setting. *Patient Education and Counseling* 77(3):398–403. doi: 10.1016/j.pec.2009.09.024.

Stipek, D., S. Recchia, S. McClintic, and M. Lewis. 1992. Self-evaluation in young children. *Monographs of the Society for Research in Child Development* 57(1):i–95. doi: 10.2307/1166190.

Sukhdial, A., and D. M. Boush. 2004. Eating guilt: Measurement and relevance to consumer behavior. *Advances in Consumer Research* 31:575–76. doi: http://www.acrwebsite.org.libproxy.lib.unc.edu/volumes/v31/acr_vol31_166.pdf.

Tangney, J. P., and R. L. Dearing. 2002. *Shame and guilt*. New York: The Guilford Press.

Tangney, J. P., J. Stuewig, and D. J. Mashek. 2007. Moral emotions and moral behavior. *Annual Review of Psychology* 58:345–72. doi: 10.1146/annurev.psych.56.091103.070145.

Turner, M. M., and J. C. Underhill. 2012. Motivating emergency preparedness behaviors: The differential effects of guilt appeals and actually anticipating guilty feelings. *Communication Quarterly*, 60(4):545–59. doi: 10.1080/01463373.2012.705780.

Wayment, H. A., and B. Aronson. 2002. Risky sexual behavior in American white college women: The role of sex guilt and sexual abuse. *Journal of Health Psychology* 7(6):723–33. doi: 10.1177/1359105302007006876.

Wikler, D. 1987. Who should be blamed for being sick? *Health Education and Behavior* 14(1):11–25. doi: 10.1177/109019818701400104.

Witte, K. 1992. Putting the fear back into fear appeals: The extended parallel process model. *Communication Monographs* 12(4):329–49.

Chapter Four

Anger

Fists clenched, teeth grinding, red color infusing the cheeks, difficulty standing still, perhaps a trickle of sweat running down the temple—the physical manifestations of anger are easy to spot (Tavris 1989). Even cartoon characters have ways to express anger as animators draw them with steam coming out of their ears. Anger is an intense emotion, one deeply tied to the social nature of human beings. Studies show that feelings of anger can capture our attention better than most other emotions (Hansen and Hansen 1988; Tavris 1989). Even from a very young age, individuals can recognize anger in others (Haviland and Lelwica 1987).

Given its prominent positioning as an inevitable part of the human experience, communication researchers can benefit from understanding the role of anger in determining the effects of preventative health messages on audiences. A health message may evoke anger toward a disease, toward a company producing harmful products, toward a public policy, or toward the groups that propose limits on the audience members' freedom to do as he or she pleases. The links between post-message anger and subsequent behavior make it an especially crucial emotion to understand in the public health context.

PSYCHOLOGICAL QUALITIES OF ANGER

Anger occurs when one believes there has been an injury or injustice committed against oneself or a close associate (Lazarus 1991). In essence, people feel angry when they are blocked from achieving their goals. Lazarus states that the action tendency of anger is to seek retribution for the offense incurred or to remove whatever is blocking goal progress. Frijda, Kuipers, and ter Schure (1989) found that anger was associated with the desire to change one's current situation. Unlike other negative emotions that come with avoidance motivations, anger is associated with approach motivations; feeling angry encourages individuals to move toward whatever is causing the injury or injustice in order to remove or harm it (Carver and Harmon-Jones 2009; Harmon-Jones and Sigelman 2001; Roseman, Wiest, and Swartz 1994).

Given that anger is associated with appraisals of individual control (Lazarus 1991), it is understandable that the action tendencies associated with this emotion are related to taking control of the situation by any means necessary. The actions prompted by feelings of anger can be constructive or destructive, depending on the intensity of the emotion (Turner 2007). For example, some individuals become overly aggressive or violent when angry, while others are better able to repress violent urges (Guerrero 1994; Tavris 1989).

Anger is also rooted in appraisals of certainty such that the person experiencing anger is fairly confident she knows the cause of the anger and is, therefore, more likely to blame another person than to blame situational factors or oneself (Keltner, Ellsworth, and Edwards 1993; Ortony, Clore, and Collins 1988; Roseman 1984). These co-occurring appraisals of certainty and control cause angry individuals to be rather optimistic in assessing possible risks (Lerner and Keltner 2000; 2001). Additionally, feelings of anger have been shown to lead individuals to predict a greater likelihood that anger-evoking events will occur in the future (DeSteno, Petty, Rucker, Wegener, and Braverman 2004).

In addition to fostering optimistic risk perceptions and distorted likelihood estimates, anger has been associated with heuristic processing of information (Lerner and Tiedens 2006). That is, those experiencing anger are less likely to elaborate on messages presented to them and are, instead, more likely to rely on heuristic cues or stereotypes for making decisions (Bodenhausen, Sheppard, and Kramer 1994; Tiedens and Linton 2001). However, some research has found message-relevant anger *increases* processing depth as compared to other negative emotions, like fear, sadness, and revulsion (Nabi 2002). More work is necessary to determine the exact conditions and individual difference factors that determine whether feelings of anger either increase or decrease the depth of message processing.

The experience of anger itself, more so than most emotions, has been directly linked to negative health effects, such as increased pain, more frequent physician visits, coronary heart disease, immune functioning, and even premature death (Consedine and Moskowitz 2007). However, Consedine and Moskowitz point out that anger may also have some health benefits. Because the action tendency of anger is to remove whatever obstacle is blocking a goal, the angry individual may be motivated to work to remove barriers to individual and/or public health (Consedine, Magai, and Horton 2005; McKeen, Chipperfield, and Campbell 2004).

ANGER AND COMMUNICATION

There are multiple ways in which a message leads audience members to feel angry. First, the message itself could portray an event that an individual appraises as goal relevant, goal incongruent, certain, and blameworthy of another, resulting in anger directed at the entity or individual the message says is to blame. Second, audiences could respond with similar appraisals directed at the *source* of a message for discussing an activity or regulation that would limit the audience members' freedom (Dillard and Shen 2005). For instance, if someone who believes that childhood vaccines are linked with autism sees a government-sponsored PSA promoting vaccination, that viewer may become angry at the message source (i.e., the government) for what he believes is a risky action that parents should make and not the government (see the discussion of reactance, below).

Communication researchers have investigated some of the ways in which feelings of anger might enhance or inhibit persuasion. One way is via anger's influence on information processing. Whereas previous psychological research indicated that negative emotions fostered more systematic message processing and positive emotions fostered more heuristic message processing, Mitchell, Brown, Morris-Villagran, and Villagran (2001) found that feelings of anger, sadness, and happiness (manipulated via different videos prior to exposure to the target video message) did not moderate message processing. That is, no matter their emotional states, participants who saw strong arguments about bone marrow donation were more persuaded than those who saw weak arguments, in line with the tenets of dual-process theories of persuasion (Chaiken 1980; Petty and Cacioppo 1986). However, both angry and sad participants recalled more about the weak messages than the strong messages and had fewer negative thoughts about strong messages, whereas happy participants recalled more about the strong messages but had more negative thoughts about strong messages. Furthermore, happy participants reported more negative thoughts about the weak message than did sad participants, but fewer negative thoughts than did angry participants.

These results supported the view that discrete emotions come with different action tendencies, with anger (in particular) associated with more negative thoughts, even cynicism (Mitchell et al. 2001). Although the anger manipulation did not stem from the target message in this study, it was still message relevant (just relevant to the immediately prior media message) and also may provide insight as to how placing anger-inducing content at the beginning of a message may shape processing of subsequent parts of a message.

Nabi (2003) later confirmed that the experience of different negative emotions, including anger, promotes differences in information accessibility, processing, behavioral intentions, and policy preferences. In her study, she found that participants who were primed to feel angry about a familiar social problem found information related to blame and retribution (information that matches the appraisal tendencies of anger) than were fearful participants. In this study, Nabi argued that emotions act as frames because they privilege certain types of subsequent information, that is, they make aspects of reality more salient (Entman 1993). The increased salience of emotion-relevant information, in turn, shapes attitudes and decisions. When the content of a message angers its audience, then the emotions-as-frames perspective predicts that information related to appraisals and action tendencies of anger will be more accessible and subsequent messages related to those action tendencies will be favored and/or more persuasive.

Differences in message content have also been shown to interact with feelings of anger to impact persuasiveness. In a study of the effects of gain and loss frames (i.e., messages that present information in terms of benefits or costs, respectively), Yan, Dillard, and Shen (2012) investigated when and why feelings of anger may promote message acceptance. They found that a gain frame message about a hepatitis C detection test was more persuasive when audience members were made to feel either happy or angry prior to encountering the message than when they were afraid. Using meditational analyses, the researchers revealed that this effect occurred because feelings of either anger or happiness both activated the behavioral activation system (BAS), which makes the emphasis on benefits within the gain frame a better match for the participants' approach-focused motivational state, thereby improving attitudes and intentions toward the detection test.

As with the study by Mitchell et al. (2001), this study did not directly test the effects of anger resulting from the target message, but it does illuminate the role of pre-existing anger in shaping message-related outcomes. Additional research is needed to test how pre-existing and message-relevant anger might jointly impact message processing, memory, attitudes, and behavioral outcomes related to message consumption. It is possible that excitation transfer could lead to the experience of message-relevant anger becoming more intense after exposure to a previously angering message or situation (Zillmann 1971). However, data is needed to verify this hypothesis in a discrete emotion context.

While each of the aforementioned empirical studies provides important insights as to the role of anger in communication processes, there are also theories that can help media effects researchers predict anger's impact on audiences. Below is a discussion of three specific conceptual guides that are relevant when researching the impact of message-relevant anger.

Psychological Reactance Theory

Perhaps the most studied anger-related concept in the realm of communication is psychological reactance (reactance, for short). Reactance is an adverse response that occurs when someone perceives a threat to her freedom (J. W. Brehm 1966). Psychological reactance theory (PRT) states that the greater the perceived threat to an individual's freedom, and the more importance that individual places on freedom, the stronger the individual's reactance will be (Brehm). Reactance, in turn, motivates individuals to take action to restore their freedom (Quick and Stephenson 2008).

In a communication context, reactance is often directed at the *source* of the message that threatens freedom. Messages that are dogmatic and vivid and/or controlling in nature are particularly likely to spark reactance in audiences (Miller, Lane, Deatrick, Young, and Potts 2007; Quick and Stephenson 2008). In addition to situational reactance (i.e., the type of reactance evoked by a particular context, including a media message), some individuals have higher levels of trait reactance and are, therefore, predisposed to respond with greater state reactance to a perceived threat to their freedom than are those low in levels of this trait (S. S. Brehm and Brehm 1981; Hong 1992).

Dillard and Shen (2005) conceptualize reactance to messages as a combination of the emotion of anger and negative cognitions. In a test of this framework, they found that messages that included a threat to freedom fostered reactance in message consumers, which in turn shaped both attitudes toward alcohol consumption and flossing. Rains and Turner (2007) confirmed the viability of this model (reactance as a combination of anger and negative cognitions) and also found that the higher the magnitude of the request in a persuasive message, the greater the reactance reported by their participants. A meta-analysis of 20 studies on psychological reactance again confirmed that the concept is well represented as a combination of anger and negative cognitions (Rains 2013).

Researchers have also tested how restoring the sense of freedom threatened by messages can ameliorate the negative effects of reactance on message acceptance and behavior change. J. W. Brehm (1966) argued that restoring a sense of autonomy and self-determination in the threatened individual should dampen, even eliminate, psychological reactance. Such restoration may take the form of actually performing the behavior threatened in the message (e.g., smoking after a message advocates for tobacco cessation), or it may involve watching someone else perform the threatened behavior (e.g., watching a movie where the characters smoke).

The Anger Activism Model

Another conceptual framework that deals directly with the impact of anger on message acceptance and behavior is the Anger Activism Model (AAM). The AAM proposes that messages that evoke anger can lead to attitude and behavior change when the audience is friendly toward the position advocated in a message and also has strong perceptions that their actions can make a difference (Turner 2007). Turner argues that anger appeals (i.e., persuasive messages that purposefully try to evoke anger in audiences to convince them to accept an argument or take action) are only persuasive if they also provide audiences with information that improves their perceptions of efficacy. That is, an effective anger appeal should persuade audiences that complying with the message's target recommendation will effectively fulfill their anger-induced desire to seek retribution.

Turner (2007) further segments four groups of individuals based on their levels of anger and efficacy. She labels those who feel very angry and highly efficacious as activists. Activists are highly committed to undertake the behaviors promoted by the anger appeal. Those who are less angry but still feel highly efficacious are empowered. The empowered hold supportive attitudes but are less likely to take action because they do not perceive the issue to be as important. The third group in the AAM, angry audiences, is comprised of individuals who have strong feelings of anger but do not feel efficacious. Angry audiences hold positive attitudes toward the advocated position but are less likely to engage in related behaviors due to their lack of efficacy. Finally, disinterested individuals are those who are both less angry and less efficacious than their counterparts, and neither their attitudes nor behavioral intentions are strong.

Cognitive Functional Model

In addition to PRT and the AAM, another theoretical framework for understanding how anger might influence the way audiences process and respond to media messages is the Cognitive Functional Model (CFM) (Nabi 1999; 2002). Nabi argues that messages with certain core relational themes evoke corresponding emotions. Which type of discrete negative emotion a message evokes then determines how motivated audiences will be to attend to the message. Motivation to attend to a message as well as audience expectations about the amount of reassuring information that will be found in a message jointly determine how likely audiences are to accept or reject that message's central argument. In the case of message-induced anger, Nabi posits that audiences will be motivated to pay attention to a message because anger is an approach emotion. It is then the expectation that the message will have information consistent with anger's action tendency (need for retribution) that determines if an angry person will subsequently attend to this message.

The example Nabi (2002) offers in her manuscript deals with messages about drunk driving. She provides an example for applying the CFM within this context:

> [I]f receivers view a PSA that emphasizes how convicted drunk drivers continue to carry valid driver's licenses, the perceived injustice will evoke anger and the desire for retribution. Receivers then consider whether the remainder of the message will offer retributive information. Provided some expectation that it will, even if uncertain, receivers will maintain motivation to attend to the message carefully. Only if they believe the message will not contain valid or useful suggestions for retribution will motivation for message processing diminish. (206–7)

While existing tests of the CFM have not been entirely supported (Nabi 2002), additional work in a variety of communication contexts is needed to fully flesh out the viability of each of its predictions. Nonetheless, the CFM is grounded in well-established work on discrete emotions (Lazarus 1991) and cognitive information processing (Petty and Cacioppo 1986), and it provides a wealth of avenues for future research on the role of negative emotions, including anger, in media effects.

Research on reactance, the AAM, and the CFM all provide conceptual guidance to those hoping to understand the role of anger in media effects. These models, as well as additional empirical evidence about anger's effects on audiences' responses to messages, have been found across multiple communication contexts. Below, the focus is on the role of anger in shaping reactions to prevention-focused health messages, specifically.

ANGER AND PREVENTION MESSAGES

There are multiple ways in which anger can influence audience reactions to prevention-focused health messages. As such, health message designers frequently create content aimed at evoking the emotion. For example, multiple anti-smoking PSAs have attempted to make audiences feel anger toward tobacco companies (Dillard and Nabi 2006; Hicks 2001). Messages that purposefully try to spur feelings of anger in audiences often do so with the hopes of motivating individuals to take action. An anger appeal is a message designed to communicate that a negative event has been or will be caused intentionally by another person and that attention is needed to combat this action (Nabi 1999; Turner 2012). Turner contends that anger appeals are the least studied of emotional message appeals; however, existing research points to the utility of trying to evoke anger if the majority of the target audience already believes that rights have been violated (e.g., when tobacco companies mislead uneducated consumers about the risks of their products).

Anger can also influence audience perceptions of prevention messages because of the aforementioned biases in risk perceptions associated with the feeling. That is, angry individuals typically are optimistic in the face of risk. Lerner and Keltner (2001) found that feelings of anger (more so than feelings of fear) were closely associated with expectations that good things would happen to participants later in life and that bad things would not happen. This finding comports with subsequent research demonstrating that feelings of anger are, in fact, associated with greater sense of personal efficacy than are feelings of other negative emotions (Griffin et al. 2008). The implications of these findings for perceptions of health risks are evident: those individuals experiencing feelings of anger may be less likely than those who are not angry to acknowledge their true level of risk for various illnesses, especially if they have yet to encounter (or acknowledge) any symptoms.

In many health communication situations, anger is not purposefully used as a persuasive tool but is rather an unintended effect of a health message that threatens the audience's freedom to do whatever they please. In this situation, anger can inhibit the persuasiveness of a health message by causing reactance. As Dillard and Nabi (2006) note, viewers of a tobacco PSA might also become angry at the message producers for bringing up an uncomfortable issue, which in turn could prevent message acceptance. In fact, some research on responses to health PSAs has found viewers who felt angry after seeing a PSA perceived it to be less effective (Dillard and Peck 2001). Dillard and Peck posit that because the action tendency of anger is to remove an obstacle, if audiences perceive the message itself to be an obstacle, then by rejecting the message the audience is simply acting upon their emotion-induced motivation. This is a particularly important consideration in the context of prevention messages where the target audience may feel fine and healthy despite performing the behavior that the message claims is dangerous and unhealthy. Without personal experience with the harmful effects of the behavior discussed in a message, audiences may be much quicker to become angry at any attempt to stop them from doing something they find pleasurable.

Because reactance fosters a resistance to persuasion (S. S. Brehm and Brehm 1981), it is a critical consideration for those designing prevention messages, particularly in communities or cultures that place a high value on freedom. Many health messages ask individuals to trade some type of freedom, be it smoking in public, siting on the couch, or buying any size soda without paying an extra tax, in return for public health benefits. This implicit request to relinquish at least one freedom means there is high probably that some, if not many, audience members will respond with reactance toward health messages and their creators.

Multiple studies have found that health messages, particularly those that are forceful or insistent on behavior change, result in audience reactance toward the message. For example, Quick and Considine (2008) found that the use of forceful language to persuade gym-goers to lift weights or participate in group exercise classes was met initially with reactance and then with a motivation to restore freedom, as predicted by psychological reactance theory. In this situation, the members of a fitness center who were told they had to participate in a specific type of exercise (either weightlifting or group exercise, depending on the condition) and that the benefits were undeniable, felt their freedom was threatened more so than those who saw a message asking them to consider one of the types of exercise because there was good evidence to support it as an effective way to improve physical and mental health. Given the importance of exercise to preventing a wide range of maladies and illnesses, this study indicates that providing audiences with a variety of ways to engage in physical activity should be a more successful messaging strategy for avoiding reactance, and thereby promoting exercise.

Using non-forceful language is one way to avoid reactance. However, as J. W. Brehm (1966) proposed, there are multiple ways to restore reactance and improve message acceptance. Most of Brehm's suggestions, though, deal with ways the individual herself can counteract reactance. Other media-related research indicates that restoration of freedom can also include derogating the source of the freedom-threatening message (e.g., questioning the credibility of the messages source) (Miller et al. 2007). Miller and colleagues argued that a simple form of message-based restoration is to remind audiences that they have a choice in their behavior. In their study, which also examined the effects of a message advocating for regular exercise, they found that language such as "you should" and "you ought to" resulted in greater reactance than did non-controlling language. The authors also found concrete, specific information about exercise resulted in more positive attitudes toward the behavior than did abstract language. This finding indicates that, perhaps, knowing the specifics prevents audiences from ruminating and fixating on over-exaggerated threats to their freedom that do not exist in reality.

Similarly, using non-threatening language in a health message can also prevent audiences from feeling as though their freedom is threatened. Veldhuis, Konijn, and Seidell (2014) found that simply providing adolescent female magazine readers with information about the weight status of models on the cover (i.e., telling readers the models were thinner than a normal woman) was more effective at preventing negative body perceptions than was warning the magazine readers about the dangers of seeing images of underweight models for one's self-image. The informative label ("These models are underweight") was also more effective at preventing negative body perceptions than was no label on the images of underweight magazine models. The authors note that the informational label gave adolescent magazine readers the knowledge of possible negative consequences without denigrating their own self-image the way a warning message did. While this study did not directly study or measure reactance, the fact that a warning was *not* the most effective way to promote preventative health outcomes implies that using freedom-threatening language may fall short as a health education strategy. This finding begs future research on the language used in warning labels on products like tobacco aimed at preventing cancer and cardiovascular conditions (e.g., Zhao, Nan, Yang, and Iles 2014), as well as proposed labels on products such as sugar-sweetened beverages that aim to prevent obesity, diabetes, and tooth decay (Capewell 2014).

Another option for mitigating the negative effects of reactance is using messages to induce empathy in audiences. Broadly defined, empathy is the process of understanding others, and it has both affective and cognitive components (see the appendix for a more detailed discussion of empathy) (Lazarus 1991; Zillmann 1991). Affective and cognitive components of empathy are closely related (Batson 2011; Batson, Chang, Orr, and Rowland 2002). These components involve the vicarious experience of another's emotions as well as cognitive perspective taking, respectively (Shamay-Tsoory, Aharon-Peretz, and Perry 2009). Media messages, particularly those featuring relatable individuals, are able to evoke empathy in audiences because humans have special neurons, called mirror neurons, that can mimic the experiences of an observed other (Rizzolatti 2008). Researchers have found that when people observe actions or emotional experiences in others, mirror neurons fire in their brains in similar patterns as if they were actually experiencing the emotions themselves (Jabbi, Swart, and Keysers 2007).

Shen (2010) found that when participants viewed PSAs about drunk driving and smoking, the experience of empathy for the individuals depicted in the PSAs resulted in lower reported reactance. Those participants who experienced empathy also found the PSAs more persuasive, thanks to the lowering of reactance. Other research provides guidance to message designers as to how to evoke empathy, in cases where preventative message designers are concerned their messages may spark reactance. For example, reader empathy for the victim in a news story about crime increased when the stories included personal information about the victim (Anastasio and Costa 2004). Additionally, Oliver, Dillard, Bae, and Tamul (2012) found that narrative news stories, as opposed to non-narrative fact-driven news stories, induced feelings of compassion in participants, which in turn increased empathic attitudes towards the stigmatized groups discussed in the stories. Together, these studies indicate that including personal information about a relevant individual's experience and/or using a narrative format for health messages may evoke empathic attitudes that in turn reduce reactance and foster preventative behavior changes.

In addition to inducing empathy in audiences, the process of emotion regulation (Gross 1998; 2002) can also help inform messaging strategies for reactance reduction. Emotion regulation occurs when an individual's appraisal of the person-environment relationship changes. A message that results in appraisals contrary to the pattern of appraisals found in anger may help regulate those initial feelings of anger. Changes in audiences' feelings of anger throughout the course of a message (i.e., emotion regulation) may be behind the effects of the aforementioned strategies' ability to mitigate reactance. That is, if the initial portion of a message evokes anger, subsequent message components that foster different appraisals may help regulate that anger.

However, research to date rarely tests changes in an audience member's discrete emotional reactions across the course of a message, making it difficult to test or support this proposition with current data (Nabi 2015). Additionally, researchers should consider that a reduction in message-relevant anger and/or reactance may result in audience complacency. This is because anger, while not always persuasive, is an approach-oriented emotion with a strong motivation to take action. Further research on the nuances of emotion regulation as they relate to anger, reactance, and preventative health messages effects is sorely needed to more fully understand which strategies for reducing reactance are most effective for particular types of audiences and why.

Beyond thinking about reactance, anger-evoking content can be used purposefully to design health messages that best match audiences' likely reactions to such messages. Turner's (2007) categorization of audience reactions to anger appeals would be very useful for tailoring such messages to various audiences that, via pre-testing or other formative work, are known to be either high or low in efficacy (see chapter 14 about eHealth, this volume, for a discussion of message tailoring). It is also important to reiterate in a health message context that, according to the AAM, when audience members disagree with the message's main argument, then increased message-relevant anger is associated with a linear decrease in attitudes toward the message's position. This means that persuasive health messages that aim to purposefully evoke feelings of anger should be sure to target the messages toward those who already agree, at least somewhat, with the advocated position.

The tailoring of anger-based health appeals to pro-attitudinal audiences could be done by tracking the content online information searches and websites use, much in the same way commercial websites display targeted advertisements for consumer products to Internet users. Because anger is a short-lived emotion, advanced technology that can target these types of health messages to receptive Internet users prior to the emotion dissipating (perhaps as a pop-up window on a browser, for example) should be the most effective in taking advantage of anger's potentially persuasive powers.

The CFM also provides researchers with valuable insight as to how negative emotions, such as anger, influence the processing of prevention-focused health messages. A big part of the battle is getting healthy (or seemingly healthy) individuals to take action to prevent future health problems and to pay attention to and carefully consider prevention-oriented messages. The CFM predicts that feelings of anger may encourage increased attention to such a message, as it is an approach emotion. However, in order for a prevention-focused health message to keep the attention of angry audience members, it would likely benefit from the inclusion of reassurance or efficacy statements, too. As with the AAM, the CFM underscores the important connection between efficacious anger appeals and efficacy. The CFM may also be particularly useful for understanding how anger impacts the effects of audiovisual and longer, more narrative prevention-oriented messages because these types of messages provide more space for cues of subsequent message reassurance. However, additional work is needed to verify this supposition.

ANGER AND ENGAGEMENT WITH PUBLIC HEALTH POLICIES

While a health-related message may induce anger about one's own situation, it can also induce anger toward public health policies and large organizations (such as government entities or corporations) that can also directly impact public health. Turner (2012) notes that anger appeals may be particularly fruitful in advocating for changes in public health policies that might protect disadvantaged populations. Evidence also indicates that anger may be a particularly powerful emotional force for motivating political participation (e.g., Marcus 2000), implying that the emotion could also be used to motivate audiences to engage with health policy messages. Using both experimental and survey data, researchers have found that anger, more so than anxiety or enthusiasm, is the best emotional predictor of political mobilization (Valentino, Brader, Groenendyk, Gregorowicz, and Hutchings 2011).

The ability of anger to motivate individuals to approach a situation makes it a valuable emotion for policy message designers to consider if they want to engage audiences in health-related policy issues. The "truth" campaign is one example of health-related messaging that aimed to evoke anger toward tobacco companies for duplicitous marketing practices in order to motivate young people to both avoid tobacco products but also support anti-tobacco policies (Hicks 2001) (see chapter 11 about health campaigns, this volume).

Feelings of anger also influence how people attribute responsibility for social problems, including those related to public health. The act of attributing responsibility for a social problem shapes how individuals assign blame for these problems and, in turn, what policy solutions they believe will be most effective for alleviating the problem (e.g., Coleman, Thorson, and Wilkins 2011; Iyengar 1991; Niederdeppe, Shapiro, and Porticella 2011). When individuals are angry, they are more likely to blame individuals than to blame situational factors for a problem (Keltner et al. 1993). If a health message about lung cancer makes the reader angry, then he may be less likely to support policy measures that address societal causes of lung cancer, like clean air regulations, smoking bans, or high taxes on cigarette products. Instead, research indicates that the angry audience member would be more likely to blame the individuals who smoke for their problems.

Existing research supports these suppositions. In the aforementioned study about emotional responses to social issues, Nabi (2003) found that participants who were angry were more likely to suggest individuals (and not societal factors) were at fault for drunk driving, and to suggest stronger punishments for offenders and greater education about the individual consequences of drunk driving (and not protection solutions, like breathalyzers in cars or more shuttles) than were participants who felt fearful. Nabi's study also that found these differences between participants who felt anger or fear only occurred when participants had already developed schema, or mental models, for the social problem. Basically, prior experience or familiarity with the topic moderated the effect of anger on the attribution of responsibility. This finding implies that for health policy issues that are well known to audiences (e.g., links between smoking and cancer), the emotions these policy messages evoke can have important consequences for which types of policies the public will support. However, for health topics that are novel or less familiar to the audience, the emotional framing of the message may have less impact on policy support, and therefore they give policy message designers more leeway in constructing those messages.

The topic of a health policy message itself should also be considered as a potential source of anger in audiences. Given the links between policies and politics, ideological leanings can interact with message content to produce reactance and dampen message acceptance. Because conservatism is associated with placing a higher value on self-reliance (Graham, Haidt, and Nosek 2009), messages that pin the cause of health issues on societal—and not individual—level factors may be incongruent with the moral foundations of conservatism. This can be especially true for issues of health disparities, or differences in health based on race, ethnicity, or economics. In fact, conservatives are less likely to recognize health differences based on these factors than are liberals (Booske, Robert, and Rohan 2011).

Gollust and Cappella (2014) examined different reactions to messages about the societal causes of health disparities based on political orientation and message characteristics. They found that Republicans (who are typically conservative), across different types of messages emphasizing social causes or personal causes of health disparities, were less angered by these messages than were Democrats (who are typically liberal). Additionally, one of the messages in the experiment attributed the cause of health disparities entirely to individual failings of those with poor health. This message evoked the most anger from Democrats and the least anger from Republicans. In conclusion, the authors note that the message that discussed social determinants of health disparities but also acknowledged individual factors produced the least amount of counterarguing for both Republicans and Democrats, and relatively low levels of anger for both parties as well (as compared to anger elicited by the other conditions). Therefore, this combination approach to messages about policy solutions related to health disparities may be the most fruitful for gaining bipartisan public support.

Beyond persuasive health messages, emotional reactions, including anger, to news accounts about public health policies can shape audience reactions to these policies. In a study of audience reactions to a representative sample of actual news stories about alcohol-related crimes, accidents, and injuries, Goodall and Reed (2013) found that the mere mention of alcohol as a cause increased anger reactions. Anger in response to these news stories was associated with increased blame for individuals (versus placing blame on societal factors) and support for policies that controlled individual behavior (versus policies that change social contexts). This study demonstrates that both persuasive and news media can result in message-relevant anger in audiences and help determine how they will respond to health-related policies.

CONCLUSION

Anger is a negatively valenced discrete emotion that occurs when one is blocked from reaching one's goal. Anger can also occur when one perceives an injustice or injury to oneself or to a close associate. Feelings of anger motivate individuals to try to remove the obstacle facing them and possibly take revenge against the offender. This emotion is characterized by appraisals of certainty—an angry person is certain of the cause of his or her negative emotional state—and appraisals of situational control that indicate that someone else is to blame.

In a preventative health communication context, gaining insight into the role of anger is particularly important because psychological reactance leads many audience members to feel angry toward those who advocate for health behavior changes. Preventative health messages that tell audiences how to act—and therefore take away the individuals' perception that they are free to act how they please—result in resistance to persuasion and even derogation of the source of the health message. This is a common risk in preventative health communication—health messages frequently direct people *not to do* something they previously felt free to do and enjoyed doing. Research indicates that evoking empathy as well as making it clear that audiences have a choice in their actions can help mitigate the negative effects of psychological reactance on health message acceptance. Future work could also investigate the role of emotion regulation strategies in lessening anger in order to lessen reactance and increase persuasion.

Additionally, work testing the role of anger in preventative health communication should examine if and how anger-induced optimistic risk bias may lead audiences to dismiss important health risks. Additional research could test if the sense of optimism associated with feelings of anger could be transferred from perceptions of individual risk to perceptions of the likelihood that individuals could overcome significant barriers to improving their health. For instance, if a smoker sees a news report of tobacco companies' hiding evidence of the severely addictive nature of nicotine and becomes angry, could subsequent smoking cessation messages be crafted such that the anger is harnessed to increase the smoker's optimism that she will be successful in her efforts to quit smoking instead of the anger being directed toward those who advocate against tobacco use? Further research is necessary to test if and how optimistic expectations can be targeted toward positive health behaviors and which message and structural features could be utilized toward these ends.

In sum, there is great potential for feelings of anger to be harnessed for persuasive prevention-focused health messages. Moreover, anger can result from consuming news about preventative health issues and policies. The emotion can motivate individuals to approach a situation and can also lead to a more optimistic post-message outlook. However, anger is also associated with psychological reactance and might contribute to backlash against messages that instruct audiences to avoid particular health-related actions. More research is needed to test the best contexts and message features for employing anger, and understanding its effects, for preventative health and policy support.

REFERENCES

Anastasio, P. A., and D. M. Costa. 2004. Twice hurt: How newspaper coverage may reduce empathy and engender blame for female victims of crime. *Sex Roles* 51(9–10):535–42. doi: 10.1007/s11199-004-5463-7.

Batson, C. D. 2011. *Altruism in humans.* New York: Oxford University Press.

Batson, C. D., J. Chang, R. Orr, and J. Rowland. 2002. Empathy, attitudes, and action: Can feeling for a member of a stigmatized group motivate one to help the group? *Personality and Social Psychology Bulletin* 28(12):1656–66. doi: 10.1177/014616702237647.

Bodenhausen, G. V., L. A. Sheppard, and G. P. Kramer. 1994. Negative affect and social judgment: The differential impact of anger and sadness. *European Journal of Social Psychology* 24(1):45–62. doi: 10.1002/ejsp.2420240104.

Booske, B. C., S. A. Robert, and A. M. K. Rohan. 2011. Awareness of racial and socioeconomic health disparities in the United States: The National Opinion Survey on Health and Health Disparities, 2008–2009. *Preventing Chronic Disease* 8(4):A73.

Brehm, J. W. 1966. *A theory of psychological reactance.* New York: Academic Press.

Brehm, S. S., and J. W. Brehm. 1981. *Psychological reactance: A theory of freedom and control.* New York: Academic Press.

Capewell, S. 2014. Sugar sweetened drinks should carry obesity warnings. *BMJ* 348:g3428. doi: 10.1136/bmj.g3428.

Carver, C. S., and E. Harmon-Jones. 2009. Anger is an approach-related affect: Evidence and implications. *Psychological Bulletin* 135(2):183–204. doi: 10.1037/a0013965.

Chaiken, S. 1980. Heuristic versus systematic information processing and the use of source versus message cues in persuasion. *Journal of Personality and Social Psychology* 39(5):752–66.

Coleman, R., E. Thorson, and L. Wilkins. 2011. Testing the effect of framing and sourcing in health news stories. *Journal of Health Communication* 16(9):941–54. doi: 10.1080/10810730.2011.561918.

Considine, N. S., C. Magai, and D. Horton. 2005. Ethnic variation in the impact of emotion and emotion regulation on health: A replication and extension. *The Journals of Gerontology Series B: Psychological Sciences and Social Sciences* 60(4):P165–P173. doi: 10.1093/geronb/60.4.P165.

Considine, N. S., and J. T. Moskowitz. 2007. The role of discrete emotions in health outcomes: A critical review. *Applied and Preventive Psychology* 12(2):59–75. doi: 10.1016/j.appsy.2007.09.001.

DeSteno, D., R. E. Petty, D. D. Rucker, D. T. Wegener, and J. Braverman. 2004. Discrete emotions and persuasion: The role of emotion-induced expectancies. *Journal of Personality and Social Psychology* 86(1):43–56. doi: 10.1037/0022-3514.86.1.43.

Dillard, J. P., and R. L. Nabi. 2006. The persuasive influence of emotion in cancer prevention and detection messages. *Journal of Communication* 56:S123–S139. doi: 10.1111/j.1460-2466.2006.00286.x.

Dillard, J. P., and E. Peck. 2001. Persuasion and the structure of affect: Dual systems and discrete emotions as complementary models. *Human Communication Research* 27(1):38–68. doi: 10.1111/j.1468-2958.2001.tb00775.x.

Dillard, J. P., and L. Shen. 2005. On the nature of reactance and its role in persuasive health communication. *Communication Monographs* 72(2):144–68. doi: 10.1080/03637750500111815.

Entman, R. M. 1993. Framing: Toward clarification of a fractured paradigm. *Journal of Communication* 43(4):51–58. doi: 10.1111/j.1460-2466.1993.tb01304.x.

Frijda, N. H., P. Kuipers, and E. ter Schure. 1989. Relations among emotion, appraisal, and emotional action readiness. *Journal of Personality and Social Psychology* 57(2):212–28. doi: 10.1037/0022-3514.57.2.212.

Gollust, S. E., and J. N. Cappella. 2014. Understanding public resistance to messages about health disparities. *Journal of Health Communication* 19(4):493–510. doi: 10.1080/10810730.2013.821561.

Goodall, C. E., and P. Reed. 2013. Threat and efficacy uncertainty in news coverage about bed bugs as unique predictors of information seeking and avoidance: An extension of the EPPM. *Health Communication* 28(1):63–71. doi: 10.1080/10410236.2012.689096.

Goodall, C. E., M. D. Slater, and T. A. Myers. 2013. Fear and anger responses to local news coverage of alcohol-related crimes, accidents, and injuries: Explaining news effects on policy support using a representative sample of messages and people. *Journal of Communication* 63(2):373–92. doi: 10.1111/jcom.12020.

Graham, J., J. Haidt, and B. A. Nosek. 2009. Liberals and conservatives rely on different sets of moral foundations. *Journal of Personality and Social Psychology* 96(5):1029–46. doi: 10.1037/a0015141.

Griffin, R. J., Z. Yang, E. ter Huurne, F. Boerner, S. Ortiz, and S. Dunwoody. 2008. After the flood: Anger, attribution, and the seeking of information. *Science Communication* 29(3):285–315. doi: 10.1177/1075547007312309.

Gross, J. J. 1998. The emerging field of emotion regulation: An integrative review. *Review of General Psychology* 2(3):271–99.

Gross, J. J. 2002. Emotion regulation: Affective, cognitive, and social consequences. *Psychophysiology* 39:281–91.

Guerrero, L. K. 1994. "I'm so mad I could scream": The effects of anger expression on relational satisfaction and communication competence. *Southern Communication Journal* 59(2):125–41. doi: 10.1080/10417949409372931.

Hansen, C. H., and R. D. Hansen. 1988. Finding the face in the crowd: An anger superiority effect. *Journal of Personality and Social Psychology* 54(6):917–24. doi: 10.1037/0022-3514.54.6.917.

Harmon-Jones, E., and J. Sigelman. 2001. State anger and prefrontal brain activity: Evidence that insult-related relative left-prefrontal activation is associated with experienced anger and aggression. 5. 80, from http://psycnet.apa.org/journals/psp/80/5/797/.

Haviland, J. M., and M. Lelwica. 1987. The induced affect response: 10-week-old infants' responses to three emotion expressions. *Developmental Psychology* 23(1):97–104. doi: 10.1037/0012-1649.23.1.97.

Hicks, J. J. 2001. The strategy behind Florida's "truth" campaign. *Tobacco Control* 10(1):3–5. doi: 10.1136/tc.10.1.3.

Hong, S.-M. 1992. Hong's psychological reactance scale: A further factor analytic validation. *Psychological Reports* 70(2):512–14. doi: 10.2466/pr0.1992.70.2.512.

Iyengar, S. 1991. *Is anyone responsible? How television frames political issues.* Chicago: University of Chicago Press.

Jabbi, M., M. Swart, and C. Keysers. 2007. Empathy for positive and negative emotions in the gustatory cortex. *NeuroImage* 34(4):1744–53. doi: http://dx.doi.org/10.1016/j.neuroimage.2006.10.032.

Keltner, D., P. C. Ellsworth, and K. Edwards. 1993. Beyond simple pessimism: Effects of sadness and anger on social perception. *Journal of Personality and Social Psychology* 64(5):740–52. doi: 10.1037/0022-3514.64.5.740.

Lazarus, R. S. 1991. *Emotion and adaptation.* New York: Oxford University Press.

Lerner, J. S., and D. Keltner. 2000. Beyond valence: Toward a model of emotion-specific influences on judgment and choice. *Cognition and Emotion* 14(4):473–93. doi: 10.1080/026999300402763.

———. 2001. Fear, anger, and risk. *Journal of Personality and Social Psychology* 81(1):146–59. doi: 10.1037/0022-3514.81.1.146.

Lerner, J. S., and L. Z. Tiedens. 2006. Portrait of the angry decision maker: How appraisal tendencies shape anger's influence on cognition. *Journal of Behavioral Decision Making* 19:115–37.

Marcus, G. E. 2000. Emotions in politics. *Annual Review of Political Science* 3(1):221–50. doi: 10.1146/annurev.polisci.3.1.221.

McKeen, N. A., J. G. Chipperfield, and D. W. Campbell. 2004. A longitudinal analysis of discrete negative emotions and health-services use in elderly individuals. *Journal of Aging and Health* 16(2):204–27. doi: 10.1177/0898264303262648.

Miller, C. H., L. T. Lane, L. M. Deatrick, A. M. Young, and K. A. Potts. 2007. Psychological reactance and promotional health messages: The effects of controlling language, lexical concreteness, and the restoration of freedom. *Human Communication Research* 33(2):219–40. doi: 10.1111/j.1468-2958.2007.00297.x.

Mitchell, M., K. Brown, M. Morris-Villagran, and P. Villagran. 2001. The effects of anger, sadness and happiness on persuasive message processing: A test of the negative state relief Model. *Communication Monographs* 68(4):347–59. doi: 10.1080/03637750128070.

Nabi, R. L. 1999. A cognitive-functional model for the effects of discrete negative emotions on information processing, attitude change, and recall. *Communication Theory* 9(3):292–320. doi: 10.1111/j.1468-2885.1999.tb00172.x.

———. 2002. Anger, fear, uncertainty, and attitudes: A test of the cognitive-functional model. *Communication Monographs* 69(3):204–16.

———. 2003. Exploring the framing effects of emotion. *Communication Research* 30(2):224–47. doi: 10.1177/0093650202250881.

———. 2015. Emotional flow in persuasive health messages. *Health Communication* 30(2):114–24. doi: 10.1080/10410236.2014.974129.

Niederdeppe, J., M. A. Shapiro, and N. Porticella. 2011. Attributions of responsibility for obesity: Narrative communication reduces reactive counterarguing among liberals. *Human Communication Research* 37(3):295–323. doi: 10.1111/j.1468-2958.2011.01409.x.

Oliver, M. B., J. P. Dillard, K. Bae., and D. J. Tamul. 2012. The effect of narrative news format on empathy for stigmatized groups. *Journalism and Mass Communication Quarterly* 89(2):205–24. doi: 10.1177/1077699012439020.

Ortony, A., G. L. Clore, and A. Collins. 1988. *The cognitive structure of emotions.* New York: Cambridge University Press.

Petty, R. E., and J. T. Cacioppo. 1986. The elaboration likelihood model of persuasion. *Advances in Experimental Social Psychology* 19:123–205.

Quick, B. L., and J. R. Considine. 2008. Examining the use of forceful language when designing exercise persuasive messages for adults: A test of conceptualizing reactance arousal as a two-step process. *Health Communication* 23(5):483–91. doi: 10.1080/10410230802342150.

Quick, B. L., and M. T. Stephenson. 2008. Examining the role of trait reactance and sensation seeking on perceived threat, state reactance, and reactance restoration. *Human Communication Research* 34(3):448–76. doi: 10.1111/j.1468-2958.2008.00328.x.

Rains, S. A. 2013. The nature of psychological reactance revisited: A meta-analytic review. *Human Communication Research* 39(1):47–73. doi: 10.1111/j.1468-2958.2012.01443.x.

Rains, S. A., and M. M. Turner. 2007. Psychological reactance and persuasive health communication: A test and extension of the intertwined model. *Human Communication Research* 33(2):241–69. doi: 10.1111/j.1468-2958.2007.00298.x.

Rizzolatti, G. 2008. *Mirrors in the brain: How our minds share actions, emotions.* Oxford; New York: Oxford University Press.

Roseman, I. J. 1984. Cognitive determinants of emotion: A structural theory. *Review of Personality and Social Psychology* 5:11–36.

Roseman, I. J., C. Wiest, and T. S. Swartz. 1994. Phenomenology, behaviors, and goals differentiate discrete emotions. *Journal of Personality and Social Psychology* 67(2):206–21. doi: 10.1037/0022-3514.67.2.206.

Shamay-Tsoory, S. G., J. Aharon-Peretz, and D. Perry. 2009. Two systems for empathy: A double dissociation between emotional and cognitive empathy in inferior frontal gyrus versus ventromedial prefrontal lesions. *Brain* 132(3):617–27. doi: 10.1093/brain/awn279.

Shen, L. 2010. Mitigating psychological reactance: The role of message-induced empathy in persuasion. *Human Communication Research* 36(3):397–422. doi: 10.1111/j.1468-2958.2010.01381.x.

Tavris, L. 1989. *Anger: The misunderstood emotion.* New York: Touchstone.

Tiedens, L. Z., and S. Linton. 2001. Judgment under emotional certainty and uncertainty: The effects of specific emotions on information processing. *Journal of Personality and Social Psychology* 81(6):973–88.

Turner, M. M. 2007. Using emotion in risk communication: The Anger Activism Model. *Public Relations Review* 33(2):114–19. doi: 10.1016/j.pubrev.2006.11.013.

———. 2012. Using emotional appeals in health messages. In H. Cho (Ed.), *Health communication message design: Theory and practice* (pp. 59–72). Thousand Oaks, CA: SAGE.

Valentino, N. A., T. Brader, E. W. Groenendyk, K. Gregorowicz, and V. L. Hutchings. 2011. Election night's alright for fighting: The role of emotions in political participation. *The Journal of Politics* 73(1):156–70. doi: 10.1017/S0022381610000939.

Veldhuis, J., E. A. Konijn, and J. C. Seidell. 2014. Counteracting media's thin-body ideal for adolescent girls: Informing is more effective than warning. *Media Psychology* 17(2):154–84. doi: 10.1080/15213269.2013.788327.

Yan, C., J. P. Dillard, and F. Shen. 2012. Emotion, motivation, and the persuasive effects of message framing. *Journal of Communication* 62(4):682–700. doi: 10.1111/j.1460-2466.2012.01655.x.

Zhao, X., X. Nan, B. Yang, and I. A. Iles. 2014. Cigarette warning labels: Graphics, framing, and identity. *Health Education* 114(2):101–17. doi:10.1108/HE-06-2013-0024.

Zillmann, D. 1971. Excitation transfer in communication-mediated aggressive behavior. *Journal of Experimental Social Psychology* 7(4):419–34. doi: 10.1016/0022-1031(71)90075-8.

———. 1991. Empathy: Affect from bearing witness to the emotions of others. In J. B. D. Zillmann (Ed.), *Responding to the screen: Reception and reaction processes* (pp. 135–67). Hillsdale, NJ; England: Lawrence Erlbaum Associates, Inc.

Chapter Five

Sadness

Feeling blue, down in the dumps, or in the doldrums—the ways of describing sadness are many, likely because it is an experience with which everyone can relate. Sadness has been examined in literature about tragic lovers and in the front pages of newspapers after the death of a public figure. It is a negatively valenced emotional state that no human can escape at one point or another. In a health context, thinking of others with an illness or becoming sick oneself can evoke the feeling. The purpose of this chapter is to explore the psychological qualities of and research related to feelings of message-relevant sadness. This chapter discusses the role of sadness in the context of preventative health communication and policy and includes a discussion of possibilities for future directions for research.

PSYCHOLOGICAL QUALITIES OF SADNESS

Sadness occurs when one experiences the loss, or absence, of a desired reward (Lazarus 1991). The core relational theme of sadness is an irrevocable loss and a sense of helplessness about harm or loss (Smith and Lazarus 1993). When individuals feel sad, they are likely to believe that something—be it a person, a relationship, a meaningful possession, or even a personal achievement—is missing in their lives (Raghunathan and Pham 1999).

Smith and Lazarus (1993) maintain that the important appraisal components of sadness are that the situation is motivationally relevant, incongruent with goals, low problem-focused coping potential exists, and the individual has little expectation that his or her lot will change anytime soon. Furthermore, sadness is strongly associated with appraisals of situational control, as opposed to individual agency (Smith and Ellsworth 1985). This means a sad individual tends to believe there is little she can do to change the current

71

situation. This sad person also expects the situation to remain gloomy for the foreseeable future.

Frequent intense feelings of sadness can be a symptom of depression or other mental illness; however, feeling sad is *not* the equivalent of being clinically depressed (Consedine and Moskowitz 2007). Nonetheless, sadness may not be the healthiest of emotions. For older adults, feelings of sadness predict nursing home admissions (Harris and Cooper 2006) and death (Cooper, Harris, and Mcgready 2002). In Cooper et al.'s study, sadness was a stronger predictor of death in the elderly than was clinical depression. For patients who are already ill, feeling sad (as opposed to feeling happy) has been linked to having more aches and pains (Salovey and Bimbaum 1989).

In addition to its influence on physical health, sadness also has implications for behavioral outcomes. The adaptive function of sadness is to help individuals adjust to a loss (Dillard, Plotnick, Godblod, Freimuth, and Edgar 1996). The action tendency of sadness is a noticeable lack of action; sad individuals expend less energy than the less melancholy (Brehm, Brummett, and Harvey 1999). Instead, sad individuals withdraw and become self-focused, searching within themselves for ways to cope with the less-than-ideal situation (Dillard et al. 1996). As Lazarus (1991) notes, sadness is more about resignation than struggle. This tendency toward inaction differentiates sadness from many other negative emotions, like anger or fear, which predispose a sense of urgency. In fact, sadness has been associated with a reduction in appetite and a decreased need for calories, which makes sense given that the sad individual is not terribly active and does not need as many calories as an active individual would (Macht 1999).

Despite the lack of motivation to take action, feelings of sadness can influence people to eventually take action. For instance, Raghunathan and Pham (1999) found that feeling sad primed participants in their experiment to develop an implicit goal to replace the reward that was lost. This prime resulted in sad participants opting for more rewarding, but also more risky, options when placed in trade-off situations than did participants in the experiment who felt anxious.

Sadness can also serve a learning function. Feeling sad signals to an individual that her plan has failed and perhaps a new plan is needed (Dillard and Peck 2000). A sad individual is, therefore, motivated to change or rearrange goals and priorities in order to avoid future failure. Feeling sad prompts individuals to focus their attention inward, which can then lead to an awareness of health symptoms, perceiving these symptoms as severe, and subsequently seeking early treatment or prevention of an even more severe illness (Consedine and Moskowitz 2007). This could be one outcome of the rearranging of priorities prompted by feelings of sadness (Johnson-Laird and Oatley 1992). Therefore, while sadness might not directly motivate immediate health behavior change, the emotion's impact on goal rearrangement can indirectly prompt changes in health-related thoughts and/or actions that subsequently shape behaviors.

An additional way that sadness may indirectly impact health is through social networks and social ties. When people observe sadness in another individual, they are likely to respond to the sad person by offering social support (Averill 1968). Research demonstrates that people who witness sadness in another's facial expression are more likely to exhibit helping behaviors (Eisenberg et al. 1989). Indeed, emotions serve a number of important social functions, including aiding individuals in their quests to strengthen relationships or solve problems with those relationships. (Keltner and Haidt 1999).

Another feature of sadness is that it can foster deeper elaboration, or systematic processing, of information. Bodenhausen, Sheppard, and Kramer (1994) found that, compared to angry participants, sad participants were less likely to make stereotypical judgments in a social judgment task and were less likely to rely on heuristic cues in a persuasion context than were angry participants. Additionally, the study indicated that sad individuals may be less likely to judge stigmatized groups for which public policies are often crucial for improving health, well-being, such as people with a mental illness, with a sexually transmitted disease, who smoke, or who are obese.

Furthermore, social psychologists have found that feeling sad increases one's expectation that sad events will also happen in the future (DeSteno, Petty, Wegener, and Rucker 2000). This finding is consistent with health-related work by Salovey and Bimbaum (1989), which found that sad participants were less likely than happy participants to see themselves as invulnerable to future health issues. DeSteno, Petty, Rucker, Wegener, and Braverman (2004) also found that messages with emotional overtones that match a participant's current emotional state are more persuasive than those that mismatch one's current state. The relationship between emotional state and the emotional tone of the message was mediated by emotion-specific expectancies. That is, sad audiences were more persuaded by sad messages than they were by messages with angry emotional overtones because they expected more sad events to occur in the future.

SADNESS AND COMMUNICATION

While there is not a voluminous body of literature focused on the effects of sadness in a health communication context, an extensive collection of theory and research on the impact of emotions, including sadness, exists in the larger corpus of communication research. One such theoretical framework is that of mood management, which argues that viewers choose to consume different types of media in order to either improve aversive emotional states or maintain positive states (Zillmann 1988; Zillmann and Bryant 1985). Mood management goals can motivate audiences to choose certain genres of media over others in the hope that they will be able to regulate their emotions (for a review, see Oliver 2003).

Advances in theory have revealed that media audiences are motivated not only by hedonistic, pleasure-seeking goals, but also by a desire to find meaningfulness and connect with the human experience (Oliver 2008; Oliver and Bartsch 2010; 2011; Oliver and Raney 2011). Understanding that individuals will consume non-hedonic media because they appreciate the lessons embedded in the content helps explain why, despite the fact that they know the media contains upsetting content, many people are want to tearjerkers, tragic stories, and other sadness-evoking media (Oliver 1993). For instance, Oliver (1993) found that many individuals, but particularly women, enjoy watching sad films and will voluntarily watch them despite the negative emotional state they can induce. Her data suggest that people who are more likely to enjoy sad films have higher levels of trait empathy and femininity than those who do not enjoy sad films as much. And while audiences may not say that they truly enjoy watching a tearjerker movie, they do say that they appreciate sad media and often continue to think about the content of this meaningful media experience long after viewing it (Bartsch and Oliver 2011).

Beyond mood management predictions about whether or not someone will consume sadness-evoking media content, Nabi's (1999; 2002) cognitive functional model provides guidance as to how feelings of sadness can influence the way audiences interact with messages. According to the CFM, sadness, because of its appraisal components, encourages effortful thought and deliberation of the situation. This tendency to think about the situation translates into more thorough processing of a persuasive message. Because sadness is viewed as an approach-oriented emotion in the CFM (due to the tendency of sad people to dwell on what is making them sad), Nabi argues that the message does not need cues of reassurance to ensure that sad audiences will be motivated to continue viewing it. In short, sadness can increase message elaboration, and therefore if the message contains strong arguments, the CFM predicts it will be persuasive in this situation.

SADNESS AND PREVENTION MESSAGES

There is limited existing research on the role of sadness in health-related media processes and effects; however, some does exist. Dillard and Peck (2000) found that feelings of sadness increased audiences' perceived effectiveness of a PSA about drug use. Also in the context of PSA effects, Dillard et al. (1996) demonstrated that fear appeals in PSAs about AIDS that were meant to mainly frighten audiences instead evoked a wide range of emotions in addition to fear, one of which was sadness. Alongside feelings of fear, feelings of sadness in response to the AIDS PSAs in their study were associated with message acceptance in the first experiment but not in the second. Dillard et al. propose that the PSAs used as stimuli in the second study may not have evoked enough sadness in participants, therefore limiting the persuasive potential of sadness in this situation.

Raghunathan and Pham's (1999) aforementioned study of the positive relationship between sadness and preferences for risk-taking also has implications for health communication research. The authors discovered that sad participants in their study were more likely to seek rewarding yet risky options when placed in trade-off situations. This combination of risk and reward could be applied to health messages such that prevention or early detection behaviors that prevent advanced disease but are viewed as "risky" (e.g., wearing a condom or getting a mammogram) because of the social ramifications or pain involved may become more attractive if a health message first uses a storyline or particular music that causes feelings of sadness in the audience. The initial sadness evoked by the first part of the message may motivate those sad individuals to reappraise the risks of the target health behaviors and to find them more rewarding than they would have if they saw the message in a neutral state.

For example, an individual who likes to tan outdoors might feel sad after reading a news story about a woman who frequented tanning salons, developed melanoma, and died. This resultant sadness at the death of this very relatable person could motivate the reader to search online for information about preventing skin cancer. Whereas she previously found the idea of visiting a dermatologist cumbersome, in light of the story in the news and her current emotional state, the individual may now call and schedule an appointment. The appointment would seem more rewarding in this state, whereas before it seemed like a nuisance. Future research could investigate the potential of messages or combination of messages that start by evoking sadness and end with suggesting prevention behaviors. Further work is also needed to discover which features of a message are best at eliciting sadness and to understand how much sadness is best to evoke in audiences given that too much or too little sadness may result in inaction.

Mood management research may also have implications for understanding how sadness can promote behavior change through prevention-focused health messages. Although the majority of mood management research has taken place in the realm of entertainment studies, there are potential implications for applying these principles in order to motivate people to view preventative health messages. For instance, if individuals will watch a sad movie in order to connect with others and partake in the human experience, it also implies that they would be willing to consume messages that discuss tragic health outcomes, which could contain information on prevention ac-

tions. And because consuming media in order to appreciate the human experiences helps foster deeper cognitive reflection of the content (Bartsch and
Oliver 2011), health information embedded in sad narratives may be better
remembered and make a more significant impact on audiences than would
health information presented in a less poignant context.

Given the important connection between message exposure and the effectiveness of health messages, such as health campaigns, fixing audience attention on prevention messages is the first and crucial step to using messages to
change behavior (Randolph and Viswanath 2004). As Randolph and Viswanath argue, health messages compete in a very crowded media market for
audiences' attention. Therefore, theoretical perspectives that help researchers
understand how to motivate selective exposure to health messages, such as
mood management principles that explain why individuals watch sad movies, may help get the public to notice prevention messages. Future research
is needed to test these assumptions and to see if there are any moderators that
might make sadness-evoking preventative health messages either more or
less likely to be viewed by audiences.

Based on principles of mood management, Carpentier et al. (2008) studied how healthy adolescents, as compared to adolescents with mood depressive disorder, use media to help regulate their moods. The researchers found
that adolescents with mood depressive disorder were significantly more likely to use media than were healthy adolescents. Additionally, the data indicated that adolescents who were experiencing a negative mood (similar to sadness) were more likely to consume more media one week later than were
those adolescents who were not in a negative mood. However, the adolescents' situational mood as well as having a previous diagnosis of a mood
disorder did *not* predict the use of specifically sad media by teenagers in the
study.

These findings indicate that principles of mood management could help
inform the best timing and channel section for the placement of prevention-
focused health messages directed at adolescents, and other segments of the
population. For instance, if there is a tragic event in a community, such as a
school shooting or natural disaster, sadness resulting from these events may
motivate different types of media selection than in a less-sad atmosphere.
And they might consume additional media in order to cope with the feelings
of sadness (Nabi, So, and Prestin 2011). Therefore, prevention-focused messages urging adolescents to seek help if they experience early symptoms of
post-traumatic stress order, or to encourage others to get help if they observe
those symptoms, could be promoted in media channels commonly used by
adolescents during that time period. That is one of many possibilities for
utilizing mood management principles from entertainment research to improve the reach and relevance of preventative health communication.

Mood management research also suggests that women may be more responsive, and may even seek out, health messages embedded in sad story lines, whereas men may be less likely to come across sad health messages, or to appreciate them when they do. This situation could be particularly likely in the context of entertainment education where health messages are embedded into popular entertainment programs and sometimes result in sad endings, meant to show the audience the negative consequences of not taking prevention actions (Piotrow and de Fossard 2004; Singhal and Rogers 1999). Research is needed to test such a propositions and to describe the processes behind these effects and potential moderators like gender.

Another application of mood management to prevention-focused health messages is that research demonstrates that sad individuals are likely to consume media that evokes a similar emotional state so that they can observe others who are doing worse than they are (Bartsch, Mangold, Viehoff, and Vorderer 2006). For example, lonely elderly individuals have been shown to prefer viewing a story about another lonely elder instead of a story about a happy, socially integrated elder (Mares and Cantor 1992). Downward social comparison has also been observed with heartbroken youth who prefer to listen to melancholy songs about love instead of happy love songs (Knobloch and Zillmann 2003). Bartsch and her colleagues (2006) point out that this type of socially comparative media consumption can act as a form of emotional coping for media consumers. Viewing media about individuals worse off than the audience member does not change the individual's actual situation, but it does put that situation into a more meaningful context. As Bartsch et al. write, "The stigmatizing significance of the problem is changed if one realizes that the problem is quite common, or if one manages to transfer the stigma to someone who 'really' has this problem when compared to oneself" (267).

The ability of sad media to change audience perspectives, even reduce stigma, has direct implications for communicating preventative health messages to the public. For instance, if an individual is worried about asking a sexual partner to use a condom due to the awkwardness and stigma associated with it, perhaps watching a video narrative about someone in a worse situation who has an unwanted pregnancy and/or a sexually transmitted infection would help the individual cope with her anxiety and eventually decide on a good strategy for taking action next time. Similarly, merely discussing stigmatized conditions like sexually transmitted infections may be easier for those who have watched such media narratives about others who have already dealt with such conditions. The possibilities for applying mood management principles concerning sad emotional states, specifically, to preventative health messaging contexts are many and beg further exploration.

In addition to mood management, Nabi's (1999; 2002) CFM can also guide research on the role of sadness in preventive message effects. Based on the CFM, health researchers hoping to target sad audiences likely do *not* need to use flashy approaches or unnecessary fear in order to maintain the audiences' attention. For example, imagine family members who are sad because their aunt just had a severe heart attack, likely caused by an unhealthy diet and a sedentary lifestyle in addition to a possible genetic component. These family members are the individuals who most need to take preventive action to prevent heart disease, but the sadness may be preventing much action. However, if hospital personnel presented the family members with a pamphlet containing information on how to achieve better heart health, their sad states should foster deep, and not superficial, message processing of the information. The pamphlet would not need to be flashy or rely on heuristic strategies to get attention but could instead focus on ways to prevent future losses.

Moreover, according to the CFM's predictions about the role of sadness in persuasive messages, a persuasive health appeal that aims to make the audience feel some degree of sadness should be well suited for health organizations that cannot afford expensive or ostentatious production practices. The organization would likely not need to spend money hiring a celebrity spokesperson, for instance. That is because the audience, once induced by the beginning of the message to feel sad, would be better persuaded by strong arguments than by famous faces or professional-grade animated graphics. So far, more tests of the CFM's main hypotheses are needed in order to see whether or not its predictions hold up in various health contexts, including these hypothetical scenarios. Yet the model can act as a conceptual guidepost for message creators hoping to understand how sadness may influence acceptance (or rejection) of prevention-focused health messages.

Research on the frames used in health media can also assist health communication researchers in understanding how sadness influences audience reactions to prevention information. Prospect theory states that individuals will react differently to the same set of facts depending on how that information is framed (Kahneman and Tversky 1979). Specifically, when decisions are framed as something to be gained, a potential benefit, that individuals tend to respond in risk-averse ways. However, when a decision is framed as a potential loss or costly, then individuals are more risk-seeking in their actions, opting for decisions that tend to be risky. Specifically related to health and the emotion of sadness, Major (2011) found that loss-framed health news stories evoked greater feelings of sadness, along with feelings of fear and guilt, than did gain-framed stories on the same topics (one news story was about obesity and the other was about lung cancer). However, she did not find that feelings of sadness influenced whom newsreaders blamed for the health diseases (individuals or society). More research is needed to test if sadness on its own, without strong co-occurring feelings of fear or guilt, might have different interactions with message frames, and therefore different effects on the reactions to health messages.

Research has also shown that an individual's mood can influence framing effects (Hirt, McDonald, Levine, Melton, and Martin 1999). While sadness is a discrete emotion and not a mood, the mood manipulations in such studies likely evoked discrete feelings of sadness, too. For instance, Wegener, Petty, and Klein (1994) induced a negative mood in participants by having them watch a sad video about a child with cancer. Based on the propositions of appraisal theory (Lazarus 1991; Smith and Lazarus 1993) and emotion contagion (Hatfield, Cacioppo, and Rapson 1993; Neumann and Strack 2000), this type of induction would likely result in a stimuli-specific reaction of sadness. Furthermore, the researchers found that for participants high in need for cognition (i.e., people who enjoy a certain amount of mental exertion and tend to elaborate messages presented to them), watching the video about a child with cancer resulted in the loss-framed message being more persuasive than the gain-framed message.

A study by Keller, Lipkus, and Rimer (2003) demonstrated that messages about breast cancer and mammography were more persuasive for individuals in a sad mood if those messages were framed as a gain (i.e., benefits of having a mammogram) instead of as a loss (i.e., the possible costs of not having a mammogram). These contradictory findings indicate that more research is needed to truly understand the impact of pre-existing sadness on responses to differentially framed health messages. By testing and measuring the discrete emotion of sadness—versus a more diffuse negative mood—perhaps greater precision can be brought to testing the juxtaposition of sadness and health message framing. The presence of effects in extant research indicates that the emotion does, indeed, have an impact on framing effects. However, what exactly that impact is, or what moderators that could account for this opposite result, remains unclear and points to the need for additional research in this arena.

Another study examining young adults' reactions to news coverage of the death of Apple CEO Steve Jobs from pancreatic cancer revealed that those who felt sad in response to the news of his passing were more likely to seek information about Jobs's health or how he died than were those who did not feel sad in response to the news (Myrick, Willoughby, Noar, and Brown 2013). Additionally, those in the study who experienced sadness after hearing of Jobs's death from cancer were more likely to talk to others about health issues. Respondents who identified with Jobs were more likely to experience sadness in response to his death, suggesting that the role of sadness in reactions to health messages can be linked to engagement or involvement with media persona or characters. In this particular study, feelings of sadness were able to motivate two important health-related communication behaviors—information seeking and interpersonal communication—that are important precursors to making positive health behavior changes.

Another study of the public's reactions to a celebrity death provides additional insights as to the potential role of sadness in health message effects. Kim, Gilbert, Edwards, and Graeff (2009) analyzed public tweets about pop star Michael Jackson's death in June of 2009. News of Jackson's death resulted in what the authors' called "a large wave of digital mourning" (4). The authors found in tweets about Jackson collected within two weeks of his death, Twitter users employed far more words associated with negative emotions than they did in a random sample of tweets not about his death. While the focus of the study was largely on methodological approaches to coding social media messages for expressions of sadness, the findings demonstrate that people do turn to social media to express their emotions in relation to celebrity deaths. Because expressions of sadness can foster others to provide social support, this use of social media may indirectly help with grieving and coping with sad feelings in a healthy way. Additionally, because many people also use social media to search for health information (Fox 2011), these celebrity death situations could be an opportunity for health organizations to post messages on social media with information on how to potentially prevent or treat the ailments of these public figures.

SADNESS AND ENGAGEMENT WITH PUBLIC HEALTH POLICIES

Little research has examined the role of sadness in public support for public health policies. However, clues reside in the literature on fundraising, where non-profit organizations often use sadness-toned messages to persuade audiences to donate money. Few who watch television for an extended period of time can escape the commercials of a child suffering from malnourishment or a cleft pallet or the advertisements showing video of downtrodden kittens and sad-looking puppies needing rescue from a shelter. As these ads demonstrate, appeals meant to make the audience feel sad are commonplace in the area of charitable giving, and may be a useful avenue for health and medical organizations hoping to raise money to lobby for and/or research policy change.

Research in social psychology provides evidence for the potential effectiveness of such appeals. For example, work on emotional contagion has shown that seeing sadness reflected in the faces of others, even others on television, can cause audiences to also feel sad and sympathetic toward others (Small and Verrochi 2009). Neuroscience research has pointed to the existence of mirror neurons that foster this reflection of the emotions of others within ourselves (Rizzolatti 2008; Wolf, Gales, Shane, and Shane

2001). Small and Verrochi (2009) demonstrated that this emotional contagion effect is more likely to lead audiences to give to a charity when viewers see sad expressions on others' faces (and subsequently feel sad themselves) than when they see happy expressions on the faces of others. The researchers also emphasize that the contagion effects of viewing sadness on charitable behavior is automatic and not deliberately thoughtful.

There is also research to indicate that health organizations should be careful in trying to evoke sadness in their appeals, as some audiences may see it as manipulative or may want to avoid those negative emotional states. This is particularly so when audiences stop to think about their feelings of sadness, unlike the automatic processes discussed above. A study on the effects of deliberation on sad appeals found that when audiences stop and deliberate on their feelings of sadness, the effectiveness of the emotion in motivating charitable behavior dissipates (Wilson and Schooler 1991). For health and policy organizations hoping to raise funds via media campaigns, this research would suggest that short and readily understood sadness appeals may be more effective than long ones that draw attention to the persuasive strategy and give audiences too much time to contemplate just how sad the message is making them feel. As mentioned above, future research is needed to assess what the optimum level of message-relevant sadness is to promote persuasion, be it for fostering public support for health policy or for encouraging individual health behavior change.

CONCLUSION

While unpleasant, negative emotions such as sadness serve an important function for human beings. These emotions alert individuals to the fact that something in their environment or within themselves is causing distress. Sadness, with its pull toward introspection and contemplation, can alert individuals to possible health symptoms they may have otherwise overlooked. Sadness can also enhance the perceived benefits, or rewards, from undertaking behaviors that were previously thought to be risky, perhaps motivating individuals to undertake difficult, painful, or socially awkward preventative behaviors that could improve or maintain health. Furthermore, feelings of sadness may encourage others in one's environment to provide social support, be it in person or via media channels. Because social support is an important predictor of positive health outcomes, this indirect effect of sadness may be particularly important in an era of social media and interactive communication technologies.

Literature in social psychology and communication provide many potential paths for researchers to take in order to advance the literature on the connections between feelings of sadness and health message effects. For instance, research on mood management and meta-emotions has largely been applied to the study of entertainment media, but it may also provide insight as to how to get the public to pay attention to health messages that may contain unpleasant or even saddening information. Sadness evoked by health messages can also influence how we process health information and ultimately help shape our decisions to do something with that information, or not. Much more research is needed to test these potential routes for research given that sadness is a relatively understudied emotion in the realm of health communication. Although most people do not enjoy feeling blue, messages that put audiences in the doldrums may, if employed in the proper context, be able to improve our ability to communicate with audiences about prevention behaviors.

REFERENCES

Averill, J. R. 1968. Grief: Its nature and significance. *Psychological Bulletin* 70(6, Pt. 1):721–48. doi: 10.1037/h0026824.

Bartsch, A., R. Mangold, R. Viehoff, and P. Vorderer. 2006. Emotional gratifications during media use—An integrative approach. *Communications* 31(3):261. doi: 10.1515/COMMUN.2006.018.

Bartsch, A., and M. B. Oliver. 2011. Making sense of entertainment: On the interplay of emotion and cognition in entertainment experience. *Journal of Media Psychology: Theories, Methods, and Applications* 23(1):12–17. doi: 10.1027/1864-1105/a000026.

Bodenhausen, G. V., L. A. Sheppard, and G. P. Kramer. 1994. Negative affect and social judgment: The differential impact of anger and sadness. *European Journal of Social Psychology* 24(1):45–62. doi: 10.1002/ejsp.2420240104.

Brehm, J. W., B. H. Brummett, and L. Harvey. 1999. Paradoxical sadness. *Motivation and Emotion* 23(1):31–44. doi: 10.1023/A:1021379317763.

Carpentier, F. R. D., J. D. Brown, M. Bertocci, J. S. Silk, E. E. Forbes, and R. E. Dahl. 2008. Sad kids, sad media? Applying mood management theory to depressed adolescents' use of media. *Media Psychology* 11(1):143–66. doi: 10.1080/15213260701834484.

Consedine, N. S., and J. T. Moskowitz. 2007. The role of discrete emotions in health outcomes: A critical review. *Applied and Preventive Psychology* 12(2):59–75. doi: 10.1016/j.appsy.2007.09.001.

Cooper, J. K., Y. Harris, and J. Mcgready. 2002. Sadness predicts death in older people. *Journal of Aging and Health* 14(4):509–26. doi: 10.1177/089826402237181.

DeSteno, D., R. E. Petty, D. D. Rucker, D. T. Wegener, and J. Braverman. 2004. Discrete emotions and persuasion: The role of emotion-induced expectancies. *Journal of Personality and Social Psychology* 86(1):43–56. doi: 10.1037/0022-3514.86.1.43.

DeSteno, D., R. E. Petty, D. T. Wegener, and D. D. Rucker. 2000. Beyond valence in the perception of likelihood: The role of emotion specificity. *Journal of Personality and Social Psychology* 78(3):397–416. doi: 10.1037/0022-3514.78.3.397.

Dillard, J. P., and E. Peck. 2000. Affect and persuasion: Emotional responses to public service announcements. *Communication Research* 27(4):461–95. doi: 10.1177/009365000027004003.

Dillard, J. P., C. A. Plotnick, L. C. Godblod, V. S. Freimuth, and T. Edgar. 1996. The multiple affective outcomes of AIDS PSAs: Fear appeals do more than scare people. *Communication Research* 23(1):44–72. doi: 10.1177/009365096023001002.

Eisenberg, N., R. A. Fabes, P. A. Miller, J. Fultz, R. Shell, R. M. Mathy, and R. R. Reno. 1989. Relation of sympathy and personal distress to prosocial behavior: A multimethod study.

Journal of Personality and Social Psychology 57(1):55–66. doi: 10.1037/0022-3514.57.1.55.

Fox, S. 2011. *The Social Life of Health Information*. Washington, DC: Pew Research Center's Internet and American Life Project.

Harris, Y., and J. K. Cooper. 2006. Depressive symptoms in older people predict nursing home admission. *Journal of the American Geriatrics Society* 54(4):593–97. doi: 10.1111/j.1532-5415.2006.00687.x.

Hatfield, E., J. T. Cacioppo, and R. L. Rapson. 1993. Emotional contagion. *Current Directions in Psychological Science* 2(3):96–99. doi: 10.2307/20182211.

Hirt, E. R., H. E. McDonald, G. M. Levine, R. J. Melton, and L. L. Martin. 1999. One person's enjoyment is another person's boredom: Mood effects on responsiveness to framing. *Personality and Social Psychology Bulletin* 25(1):76–91. doi: 10.1177/0146167299025001007.

Johnson-Laird, P. N., and K. Oatley. 1992. Basic emotions, rationality, and folk theory. *Cognition and Emotion* 6(3–4):201–23. doi: 10.1080/02699939208411069.

Kahneman, D., and A. Tversky. 1979. Prospect theory: An analysis of decision under risk. *Econometrica* 47(2):263–91. doi: 10.2307/1914185.

Keller, P. A., I. M. Lipkus, and B. K. Rimer. 2003. Affect, framing, and persuasion. *Journal of Marketing Research* 40(1):54–64. doi: 10.2307/30038835.

Keltner, D., and J. Haidt. 1999. Social functions of emotions at four levels of analysis. *Cognition and Emotion* 13(5):505–21. doi: 10.1080/026999399379168.

Kim, E., S. Gilbert, M. J. Edwards, and E. Graeff. 2009. Detecting sadness in 140 characters: Sentiment analysis and mourning Michael Jackson on Twitter (pp. 1–15). Boston, MA: Web Ecology Project.

Knobloch, S., and D. Zillmann. 2003. Appeal of love themes in popular music. *Psychological Reports* 93(3):653–58. doi: 10.2466/pr0.2003.93.3.653.

Lazarus, R. S. 1991. *Emotion and adaptation*. New York: Oxford University Press.

Macht, M. 1999. Characteristics of eating in anger, fear, sadness and joy. *Appetite* 33(1):129–39. doi: http://dx.doi.org/10.1006/appe.1999.0236.

Major, L. H. 2011. The mediating role of emotions in the relationship between frames and attribution of responsibility for health problems. *Journalism and Mass Communication Quarterly* 88(3):502–22. doi: 10.1177/107769901108800303.

Mares, M.-L., and J. Cantor. 1992. Elderly viewers' responses to televised portrayals of old age: Empathy and mood management versus social comparison. *Communication Research* 19(4):459–78. doi: 10.1177/009365092019004004.

Myrick, J. G., J. F. Willoughby, S. M. Noar, and J. Brown. 2013. Reactions of young adults to the death of Apple CEO Steve Jobs: Implications for cancer communication. *Communication Research Reports* 30(2):115–26. doi: 10.1080/08824096.2012.762906.

Nabi, R. L. 1999. A cognitive-functional model for the effects of discrete negative emotions on information processing, attitude change, and recall. *Communication Theory* 9(3):292–320. doi: 10.1111/j.1468-2885.1999.tb00172.x.

———. 2002. Anger, fear, uncertainty, and attitudes: A test of the cognitive-functional model. *Communication Monographs* 69(3):204–16.

Nabi, R. L., J. So, and A. Prestin. 2011. Media-based emotional coping: Examining the emotional benefits and pitfalls of media consumption. In K. Döveling, C. von Scheve, and E. A. Konijn (Eds.), *The Routledge handbook of emotions and mass media* (pp. 116–33). New York: Routledge.

Neumann, R., and F. Strack. 2000. "Mood contagion": The automatic transfer of mood between persons. *Journal of Personality and Social Psychology* 79(2):211–23. doi: 10.1037/0022-3514.79.2.211.

Oliver, M. B. 1993. Exploring the paradox of the enjoyment of sad films. *Human Communication Research* 19(3):315–42. doi: 10.1111/j.1468-2958.1993.tb00304.x.

———. 2003. Mood management and selective exposure. In J. Bryant, D. Roskos-Ewoldsen, and J. Cantor (Eds.), *Communication and emotion* (pp. 85–106). Mahway, NJ: Lawrence Erlbaum Associates.

———. 2008. Tender affective states as predictors of entertainment preference. *Journal of Communication* 58(1):40–61. doi: 10.1111/j.1460-2466.2007.00373.x.

Oliver, M. B., and A. Bartsch. 2010. Appreciation as audience response: Exploring entertainment gratifications beyond hedonism. *Human Communication Research* 36(1):53–81. doi: 10.1111/j.1468-2958.2009.01368.x.

———. 2011. Appreciation of entertainment: The importance of meaningfulness via virtue and wisdom. *Journal of Media Psychology: Theories, Methods, and Applications* 23(1):29–33. doi: 10.1027/1864-1105/a000029.

Oliver, M. B., and A. A. Raney. 2011. Entertainment as pleasurable and meaningful: Identifying hedonic and eudaimonic motivations for entertainment consumption. *Journal of Communication* 61:984–1004.

Piotrow, P. T., and E. de Fossard. 2004. Entertainment-education as a public health intervention. In A. Singhal, M. J. Cody, E. M. Rogers, and M. Sabido (Eds.), *Entertainment-education and social change: History, research, and practice* (pp. 41–60). Mahwah, NJ: Lawrence Erlbaum Associates.

Raghunathan, R., and M. T. Pham. 1999. All negative moods are not equal: Motivational influences of anxiety and sadness on decision making. *Organuzational Behavior and Human Decision Processes* 79(1):56–77. doi: 10.1006/obhd.1999.2838.

Randolph, W., and K. Viswanath. 2004. Lessons learned from public health mass media campaigns: Marketing health in a crowded media world. *Annual Review of Public Health* 25:419–37. doi: 10.1146/annurev.publhealth.25.101802.123046.

Rizzolatti, G. 2008. *Mirrors in the brain: How our minds share actions, emotions.* Oxford; New York: Oxford University Press.

Salovey, P., and D. Bimbaum. 1989. Influence of mood on health-relevant cognitions. *Journal of Personality and Social Psychology* 57(3):539–51. doi: 10.1037/0022-3514.57.3.539.

Singhal, A., and E. M. Rogers. 1999. *Entertainment-education: A communication strategy for social change.* Mahwah, NJ: Lawrence Erlbaum Associates.

Small, D. A., and N. M. Verrochi. 2009. The face of need: Facial emotion expression on charity advertisements. *Journal of Marketing Research (JMR)* 46(6):777–87. doi: 10.1509/jmkr.46.6.777.

Smith, C. A., and P. C. Ellsworth. 1985. Patterns of cognitive appraisal in emotion. *Journal of Personality and Social Psychology* 48(4):813–38. doi: 10.1037/0022-3514.48.4.813.

Smith, C. A., and R. S. Lazarus. 1993. Appraisal components, core relational themes, and the emotions. *Cognition and Emotion* 7(3–4):233–69.

Wegener, D. T., R. E. Petty, and D. J. Klein. 1994. Effects of mood on high elaboration attitude change: The mediating role of likelihood judgements. *European Journal of Social Psychology* 24(1):25–43.

Wilson, T. D., and J. W. Schooler. 1991. Thinking too much: Introspection can reduce the quality of preferences and decisions. *Journal of Personality and Social Psychology* 60(2):181–92. doi: 10.1037/0022-3514.60.2.181.

Wolf, N. S., M. E. Gales, E. Shane, and M. Shane. 2001. The developmental trajectory from amodal perception to empathy and communication: The role of mirror neurons in this process. *Psychoanalytic Inquiry* 21(1):94.

Zillmann, D. 1988. Mood management through communication choices. *American Behavioral Scientist* 31(3):327–40. doi: 10.1177/000276488031003005.

Zillmann, D., and J. Bryant. 1985. *Selective exposure to communication.* Hillsdale, NJ: Erlbaum Associates.

Chapter Six

Humor

In a public service announcement for the American Heart Association, actress Elizabeth Banks portrays a flustered working mom trying to make her kids and husband breakfast when suddenly she clutches her chest, starts to sweat profusely, and eventually collapses to the floor (American Heart Association 2014). Banks realizes she is having a heart attack once her young son shows her the symptoms listed on a smartphone screen, but she waits to call 911 until she has finished making peanut butter and jelly sandwiches and the kids have left for school. When the 911 operator tells her the paramedics will be there in two minutes, she asks if they can take longer so she can have time to clean the house first.

In a press release about the PSA, Banks explained her motives for starring in the satirical video: "While the film is funny, having a heart attack is not something to be laughed at. However, I'm using humor to help uncover the truth about heart disease, to get people interested in learning more about their hearts—and our movement" (Huffington Post 2012). Her statement speaks more broadly as to why prevention advocates might employ humor in their health messages: It can grab attention and serve as a gateway to more serious conversations about potentially scary threats. Despite their popularity and prevalence in the media landscape, it is unclear just how effective humor-based messages are in actually changing audience behaviors. Research to date has yet to show clear mechanisms for humor's effects on message outcomes, and many show no change in subsequent behavior after seeing a humorous health message. However, the literature on positive discrete emotions, humor, and laughter provide researchers with some insights into the possible consequences of and processes behind humor effects as well as promising avenues for future work on humor and media effects.

While humor is not in and of itself an emotion, its evocation is undeniably tied to positive emotional states. Therefore, it is an important aspect of understanding the relationship between emotions and audience reactions to prevention-focused health messages. This chapter first outlines the psychological qualities and functions of humor before providing background on the discrete emotions of happiness and joy. Additionally, this chapter discusses laughter and its associations with humor and emotion. Then the chapter describes the literature on humor and communication before addressing the ties between humor and health communication, specifically. Finally, the chapter provides suggestions for message design and future research into the role of humor in prevention-oriented health messages.

PSYCHOLOGICAL QUALITIES OF HUMOR

Describing exactly what is and is not humorous has been a struggle for researchers (Wild, Rodden, Grodd, and Ruch 2003). Martin (2006) defines humor as "a broad term that refers to anything that people say or do that is perceived as funny and tends to make others laugh, as well as the mental processes that go into both creating and perceiving such an amusing stimulus, and also the affective response involved in the enjoyment of it" (5). This lengthy definition begets the notion that humor is a multifaceted experience including a social component, cognitive processes, emotional responses, and physiological reactions (Martin).

Researchers have generally come to agree that an unexpected or incongruent message or expression presented in a non-serious or playful setting are the ingredients for laughter-evoking humor (Gervais and Wilson 2005). Even infants will laugh and smile when they encounter unexpected stimuli, such as a peek-a-boo face or a tickle, when they also perceive their environment to be safe (McGhee 1979; Sroufe and Waters 1976). As such, the experience or perception of humor is often precipitated by a sense of surprise or an out-of-the-ordinary situation (Alden, Mukherjee, and Hoyer 2000). In short, appraisals of a situation as unexpected, non-serious, and playful can lead observers to find that situation humorous (Martin 2006).

Humor is fundamentally a social phenomenon, one that can be shaped by culture and context. People laugh more often when they are around others than when alone (Martin and Kuiper 1999). And although humor may share certain cognitive structures across international boundaries, specific content will be more humorous to audiences in certain countries if it resonates with cultural dimensions (e.g., collectivism versus individualism) (Alden, Hoyer, and Lee 1993). Across countries and generations, humor encourages people to play with each other, an evolutionarily adaptive outcome that fosters bonding, creativity, and even stress relief (Martin 2006).

HUMOR AND EMOTION

As discussed above, affect is a central component of the experience of humor. However, debates abound about the specific emotional state associated with humor. Some researchers argue that humor is a feeling akin to mirth (Martin 2006), while others have suggested amusement is the discrete emotional state associated with humor (Shiota, Campos, Keltner, and Hertenstein 2004). However, many of these definitions of humor overlap considerably with conceptualizations of other positive emotions, like happiness or joy. Therefore, it is worthwhile to explore the psychological properties of these emotions in order to develop a fuller sense of the emotional ramifications of media-based humor.

Happiness

The core relational theme of happiness is that one has gained, or is in the process of gaining, whatever one desires (Lazarus 1991). Feeling happy signals to an individual that a goal has been met or that good progress is being made toward achieving a goal. Therefore, happiness is most likely to be the result of humor that makes one feel good about oneself or that reinforces a particular belief or worldview. Lazarus suggests that the action tendency of happiness is a sense of pleasure or of security as well as a tendency to share positive outcomes or strategies with others.

Joy

Happiness is similar to but distinct from joy. Lazarus (1991) posits that joy, as compared to happiness, is "a more acutely intense reaction to a more specific event, but the two words overlap a great deal" (265). Frijda (1986) suggests that the action tendency associated with joy "is in part aimless, unasked-for readiness to engage in whatever interaction presents itself and in part readiness to engage in enjoyments" (89). Joy encourages play of all types: physical, social, intellectual, or artistic (Fredrickson 1998).

Fredrickson (1998) describes the benefit of the high-arousal emotion of joy: "Joy, then, not only broadens an individual's momentary thought-action repertoire through the urge to play, but also, over time and as a product of recurrent play, joy can have the incidental effect of building an individual's physical, intellectual, and social skills. Importantly, these new resources are durable and can be drawn on later, long after the instigating experience of joy has subsided" (305). Given the positive physical and psychological outcomes of joy and its motivation to take physical action, this happiness-related emotion may also be a beneficial response to humor-evoking preventative health messages.

Laughter

The most visible manifestation of humor is the laugh. Laughter, though seemingly frivolous in nature, serve important social functions and have strong evolutionary roots (Gervais and Wilson 2005). It is a universal human behavior, found the world over, and serves as a form of communication (Provine 2000). Laughter can even improve one's physical health (Rosner 2002). However, it is important to distinguish between two types of laughter in order to differentiate the functions of each type: Duchenne and non-Duchenne. Duchenne laughter is prompted by a specific stimulus and has an emotional valence, whereas non-Duchenne laughter is self-generated and devoid of emotion (Keltner and Bonanno 1997; Wild et al. 2003). Keltner and Bonanno found that Duchenne laughter was related to reduced feelings of anger, increased feelings of enjoyment, improved social relations, and even positive responses from strangers, while non-Duchenne laughter did not predict any of these outcomes. Gervais and Wilson (2005) point out that non-Duchenne laughter is a learned reproduction of Duchenne laughter. Individuals may use non-Duchenne laughter strategically in the hope of improving social ties while others produce it as an uncontrollable expression of nervousness. Some individuals even develop the habit of using non-Duchenne to punctuate statements.

Both types of laughter are behaviors connected to the social nature of human existence. According to Provine and Fischer (1989), individuals are 30 times more likely to laugh when they are in a social setting than when they are alone. Because of the importance of others in evoking laughter, cultural norms and learning are crucial factors in determining when laughter will be evoked and how it will be interpreted (Gervais and Wilson 2005; Goodson 2003). Therefore, messages designed to make the audience laugh must also follow appropriate cultural norms to elicit a good guffaw. Even then, if an individual has a past negative experience with content that is meant to be humorous, the learned response may not be laughter.

As previously mentioned, it is Duchenne laughter that coincides with an emotional reaction to a stimulus. Gervais and Wilson (2005) note that the exact nature of this emotional response has received many different titles, from mirth or amusement to joy or exhilaration. The common theme throughout these labels is that the emotional reaction associated with Duchenne laughter is a positively valenced one. Humor and laughter are both tied to increases in positive emotion and improvements in mood (Neuhoff and Schaefer 2002). Gervais and Wilson also argue that while laughing can have a positive effect on the psyche, it is Duchenne laughter's ability to induce positive affect in others that serves its central communicative purpose. This type of laughter is contagious and can also synchronize the emotions of group members (Provine 1992).

HUMOR AND COMMUNICATION

Humor has been studied in multiple communication contexts, including public speaking (Gruner 1985), persuasion (Markiewicz 1974), political communication, (Nabi, Moyer-Gusé, and Byrne 2007), workplace communication (Booth-Butterfield, Booth-Butterfield, and Wanzer 2007), advertising (Sternthal and Craig 1973), and educational communication (Bryant and Zillmann 1989; Kaplan and Pascoe 1977), to name a few.

Meyer (2000) refers to the use of humorous messages as a double-edged sword for group cohesion. While humor serves to bring together communicators via mutual identification and clarification of positions and values, he argues that it can also serve to divide people. That is because two other functions of humor in the communication process are to enforce norms and differentiate acceptable versus unacceptable behaviors or people. Meyer argues that these conflicting functions mean that humor can be used to delineate social boundaries or broaden them, depending on the context.

Research is mixed on the relationship between humorous messages and behavior change, but there is evidence that humor can facilitate intermediary communication processes, such as attention and attitude change, that can help facilitate persuasion and message-relevant behaviors. Advertising has long used humor as a tactic to communicate with consumers about products and brands. In a review of the literature on humor in advertising, Weinberger and Gulas (1992) arrived at four main conclusions. First, humorous advertisements tend to attract audience attention better than non-humorous ones. Second, humor does not help improve audience comprehension of advertisements. Third, the use of humor increases audiences liking of the source of the message, but it is not clear if humor also affects judgments of source credibility. Finally, humorous advertisements are more persuasive for products that are feeling-oriented, such as perfume, or for low involvement products that do not require much consideration before purchasing, such as nondurable goods. While these conclusions are helpful for health message designers, more research is needed to see how well they apply to health contexts (Turner 2012).

A more recent meta-analysis of the use of humor in advertising found that humor is associated with an increase in positive affect but also encourages audiences to denigrate the credibility of the source of the product or brand information (Eisend 2009). In another meta-analysis of the mechanisms behind humor effects in advertising, Eisend (2011) examined whether affect-oriented or cognition-oriented models, or a combination of the two, were better at explaining humor's effects on audiences. He found the combined affect-cognition model was the best predictor of humor's effects on audiences' advertising-related attitudes. Across the studies used in his analysis, humor enhanced positive affect and decreased negative affect, with positive affect predicting positive attitudes toward the advertisement and negative affect predicting negative attitudes. Humor was also associated with a decrease in negative cognitions about the advertisement and an increase in positive cognitions about the advertisement.

Beyond its use in advertisements, humor occurs frequently in public discourse. Another line of research on humor and communication resides in the realm of political communication. Since the time of Benjamin Franklin's political cartoons (Olson 1987), humor and satire have been used in attempts to sway citizens to support, or not support, a candidate or policy. In modern times, programs such as the *Daily Show* (Fox, Koloen, and Sahin 2007; Polk, Young, and Holbert 2009) and the *Colbert Report* (Hmielowski, Holbert, and Lee 2011; LaMarre, Landreville, and Beam 2009) have used humor to make political points and to attract viewers. Higher levels of exposure to political humor shows such as the *Daily Show* and the *Colbert Report* has been linked to higher levels of distrust in politicians, indicating that political comedians' arguments were at least partially adopted by the audience (Baumgartner 2007).

Nabi et al. (2007) studied the mechanisms behind audience reactions to political humor. The researchers found that humor led to greater liking of the source, closer information processing, and reduced counter-arguing against the comedian's message. However, they also found that humorous political messages led audiences to discount the message as merely a joke, not an argument to be taken seriously. Additionally, the use of humor in political messages resulted in a sleeper effect such that immediately after message exposure participants who saw the humorous message were no more persuaded than were the participants who saw a serious political message. However, the humorous message given by a famous comedian proved more persuasive than the serious message when participants were asked for their views on the political issue one week later. This experiment provides important insights as to the nuances of both why and when humor may be persuasive.

Turner (2012) notes that humor appeals are less easily defined than other types of emotional messages because humor can result in audiences experiencing a variety of positive emotions, such as joy or surprise, even hope under the right circumstances. However, she goes on to define humor appeals as "persuasive appeals that purposefully use positive affect, through the use of humor, to connect positive feelings with the issue being addressed in the message" (66). While non-persuasive health messages may seem humorous to some, the most likely context for a humorous preventative health message is that of a strategic message, such as a PSA or other health campaign.

Moreover, the presence of laughter in a message may impact audience's emotional reactions given laughter's communicative function (Gervais and Wilson 2005). Duchenne laughter presented within a message may amplify the positive emotional impact of that message because this type of laughter is contagious and spreads easily between those in a group. Additionally, this elicitation of positive affect via observations of laughter may encourage audiences to broaden their horizons and build their resources and relationships, as suggested by the broaden-and-build perspective on positive emotions (Fredrickson 1998; 2001). Future research into this behavioral outcome of positive emotion and humor will help elucidate the exact ways in which laughter may impact audience reactions to preventative health messages.

HUMOR AND PREVENTION MESSAGES

While there is a significant body of literature about the ways in which humor can be used to cope with or encourage recovery from illness (e.g., Christie and Moore 2005; Johnson 2002; Lunsford et al. 2006), less work has investigated how humorous messages influence prevention-focused health behaviors. There are many possible benefits of using positive emotional appeals, like humor appeals to promote preventative health behaviors. The use of positive emotions in health messages can help overcome defensive processing because positively toned messages tend to induce positive responses in audiences (Monahan 1995). Because positive emotions motivate people to approach stimuli that may help them achieve their goals, health messages infused with positive emotions may more easily convince audiences to move toward health-related goals.

Monahan (1995) argues that positive emotions in health messages, including humorous messages, will be most convincing when the audience meets three prerequisites: 1) The audience has little pre-existing knowledge of a health issue; 2) The audience is unlikely to be persuaded to comply with the target behavior based solely on the rational arguments for the behavior; and 3) The audience is highly involved with, or committed to, the health issue. Additional work is needed to test how these prerequisites operate in real-world contexts and for messages that evoke different positive emotions, but they do provide a nice concise framework for early-stage message design.

Some work has identified conditions under which humorous prevention-oriented health messages may be more or less persuasive. Turner (2012) notes "the contexts in which one might use humor instead of other kinds of emotional appeals is when the behavior being depicted is positive and created by a human being (vs. a natural phenomenon)" (67). She continues to state that message designers would be well served to recognize that the use of humor can make light of an issue and therefore they should shy away from using it for emotionally charged or very serious health contexts like HIV/AIDS or drunk driving.

Turner's (2012) example of an effective humor-based preventative health message is the *Healthy Penis* campaign. In response to a marked increase in cases of syphilis in the city, the San Francisco Department of Public Health started the campaign in hopes of encouraging syphilis testing and awareness among gay and bisexual men (Ahrens et al. 2006; Vega and Roland 2005). The campaign included cartoons and outreach workers dressed in humorous attire and was so effective that the campaign was later implemented in Seattle, WA, San Jose, CA, Cleveland, OH, and Winnipeg, Canada, with similar spin-off campaigns operating in Los Angeles, CA, Portland, OR, and Philadelphia, PA (Healthy Penis 2014). In this case, the disease in question was preventable and treatable if detected in time, and therefore not as serious as HIV/AIDS, and the general context made humor an efficacious health messaging strategy.

Another example of when humor can be persuasive in the right situation comes in the context of road safety. Qualitative research on road safety messages found that audiences perceived humorous messages emphasizing how one should drive as effective as long as the messages included an efficacy component and did not focus on overly serious negative outcomes (Lewis, Watson, White, and Tay 2007). Lewis, Watson, and White (2008) also found that time after message exposure, in addition to message context, can moderate the effectiveness of road safety appeals. Immediately after viewing a road safety message, fear-inducing messages appeared to be more effective than did humorous messages. However, over time the humorous message became more persuasive, consistent with Nabi et al.'s (2007) findings of a sleeper effect with humorous political messages.

Additionally, Blanc and Brigaud (2013) studied how humorous print advertisements aimed at preventing alcohol and tobacco use and obesity affected readers. Compared to health advertisements that were not judged as funny, advertisements employing humor were viewed for a longer amount of time and were judged as more persuasive by participants. Additionally, in a delayed recognition task that took place one week after message exposure, participants were more likely to recognize humorous than non-humorous prevention-oriented health advertisements. Although this study did not measure actual health behaviors, it provides a strong indication that in a sea of media, humor may be one effective way to gain audience attention and to encourage audiences to stop for a moment and ponder preventative health actions.

However, humor can also lead audiences to downgrade the severity of a medical condition, and therefore inadvertently lead them to downplay prevention behaviors in favor of risky behaviors. For instance, Moyer-Gusé, Mahood, and Brookes (2011) examined how the use of humor in a popular television comedy, *Scrubs*, affected audience members' perceived severity of an unintended pregnancy as well as their intentions to engage in unprotected sex. The researchers found that while pregnancy-related humor reduced counterarguing against the underlying entertainment education message (i.e., practice safe sex), the jokes on the show encouraged audiences to trivialize the condition of an unintended pregnancy.

Additionally, male participants in the study were more likely to demonstrate increased intentions to have unprotected sex after viewing the *Scrubs* episode than were women, indicating that the negative impact of humor on preventative health behaviors may depend on both the gender of the audience member and on the behavior in question. In this case, pregnancy might be a more important, and personally relevant, issue for women than for men, pointing to personal relevance as a possible moderator of humor effects. Future work could test this proposition in a variety of health contexts as well as with tailored health messages that emphasize personal relevance (see chapter 14 about eHealth, this volume).

Other research supports the existence of gender differences in humor effects on prevention-focused attitudes and behaviors. Conway and Dubé (2002) found that humorous messages promoting sunscreen and condom use (both prevention behaviors) were more persuasive than non-humorous messages for participants of either gender who reported high levels of masculinity. There was no difference in the effectiveness of the humorous and non-humorous messages for low-masculinity participants. Additional work is needed to understand why exactly men and women respond differently to humorous health messages.

Understanding why humorous health messages are persuasive and building theory in this area is an important endeavor for being able to better predict the contexts where humorous message content may be the best approach for promoting health behavior change. Although not directly focused on prevention, Nabi (in press) found that humorous messages about self-detection of breast and testicular cancer could motivate individuals to process a message, promote positive attitudes toward the target health behavior, and help mitigate anxiety about performing detection behaviors. This finding was similar to one in the consumer behavior literature where the combination of humor and fear-evoking material was more persuasive than a fear appeal alone (Mukherjee and Dubé 2012). While there was not a significant difference between humorous and non-humorous messages used in her study in fostering increased intentions to perform self-exams, she did find that, in a path model, the relationship between self-exam intentions and behaviors was stronger and statistically significant for participants who read the humorous message, whereas the relationship between intentions and behavior was not significant for those who saw the serious message. This study indicates that humor effects may be subtle and indirect.

Furthermore, this study reaffirmed previous work (Mukherjee and Dubé 2012) that demonstrated that the use of humor can be an effective messaging

strategy to mitigate the fear individuals often associate with prevention behaviors. As such, humor may be a particularly effective messaging strategy
for contexts where individuals who most need to take action to prevent future
health problems (e.g., those afraid of the dentist and who have not had a teeth
cleaning for many years) are already anxious. In these contexts, a humorous
message may help alleviate chronic fear or anxiety that has been a barrier to
action.

Another area of research on the use of humor in prevention-focused messages is that of its effects on message sharing. Campo et al. (2013) used a
cross-sectional survey to explore the effects of a pregnancy prevention campaign called "Until You're Ready, Avoid the Stork" ©. They found that both
message exposure and finding the messages humorous were significant predictors of talking with others about the campaign as well as sharing the
campaign messages with others. Given that the action tendency of happiness
is to share (Lazarus 1991) and that positive emotions can serve social bonding functions (Fredrickson 1998), this finding fits with emotion theory and
should promote additional research on the role of message-relevant humor
and preventative health behaviors.

Moderators of Humor Effects

Other research suggests that there are moderators of humor appeal effects in
health contexts. Lee (2010) analyzed the effects of efficacy components in
humorous anti-alcohol abuse messages targeting college students. Her experiment found that rebellious college students who viewed the humorous
anti-drinking message that also included a self-efficacy statement (i.e., "You
are in control of the situation") reported higher risk perceptions and higher
intentions to change their drinking behaviors than did those rebellious students who saw a humorous anti-drinking message that did not include the
affirmation of self-efficacy.

Individual differences may also moderate audience responses to humorous health messages. In another study on the effects of anti-alcohol abuse
messages, Lee and Shin (2011) compared the effects of fear- and humor-
evoking messages on audiences. They found that fear messages generated
more interest and perceived danger of excessive drinking—regardless of sensation-seeking tendencies—than did humorous messages. However, participants rated humorous messages as more likeable than fear messages, and
likability of the messages was moderated by sensation-seeking tendencies.
That is, low sensation seekers found humorous messages far more likeable
than fear messages, whereas the gap between liking of humor and fear messages was smaller for high sensation seekers. Although it did not investigate
health-related messages, another study found that individuals low in need for
cognition responded more favorably to humorous advertisements (i.e., they

reported more positive attitudes and stronger purchase intentions) than did those high in need for cognition (Zhang 1996). Additional work is needed to test if this effect replicates in a prevention context where the outcomes may have longer-term and/or more serious ramifications than the purchasing of consumer products.

The aforementioned studies suggest that, given particular audiences and particular contexts, humor can effectively promote prevention-focused health behaviors. However, if various contextual, individual difference, and/or message factors are not considered, then the use of humor may fall flat or even hurt attempts to persuade audiences. Future research could test which particular message features make a health situation appear too serious or too threatening for humor to be effective. Additionally, software for tailoring messages in electronic environments may be able to target humorous messages to people with more masculine characteristics (perhaps judged by social media output) or who identify with certain cultures that may be more apt to appreciate the humor in the message. More work to identify other moderators of humor's effects on the audiences for health messages would also advance the effective use of humor in prevention messages.

Functions of Humor in a Health Context

Meyer's (2000) four functions of humorous communication have important implications for health messages. As discussed above, humor can unite individuals through shared identification and/or clarification of values, while it can divide people by enforcing norms and/or clarifying acceptable versus unacceptable people or behaviors. These functions imply that humorous messages might be able to move previously harmful social boundaries, such as the stigma associated with certain illnesses like sexually transmitted infections, for example. However, used improperly, humorous health messages might further delineate social boundaries in ways that are harmful for promoting prevention behaviors. Research examining the role of these functions in various health contexts would help test these propositions and could uncover important mediators and/or moderators of humor's communicative effects in various health communication contexts.

As discussed previously, one emotional outcome of humor and laughter is happiness. At first glance, given the core relational theme of happiness as a sense of pleasure and security, one might assume that happiness may be less likely to motivate audiences to take action to prevent a health threat because they may already feel safe without taking additional action. However, the difference between a happy mood and happiness as a discrete emotion has yet to be fully tested and contrasted, and may provide insights as to the particular contexts where happiness may be a useful messaging strategy for motivating action to prevent illness and promote well-being. Considering the many psychological and physiological benefits of experiencing positive emotions, this is a promising area for future research into the intricacies of preventative health communication.

Additionally, preventative health researchers may consider what exactly audiences may need to feel happy *about* before taking action. For instance, if a reassuring message leads Internet users to feel as if they have met their goal of finding a reliable, trustworthy source of online health information, then these users may feel happy about that achievement while still retaining a necessary level of caution toward health threats such that they are motivated to take preventative actions. As this hypothetical situation demonstrates, it is important for researchers to gain deeper insight into message-relevant humor-provoked happiness and how it may be directed toward certain aspects or players mentioned in a health message before the emotion can be most effectively leveraged to improve preventative health messages.

HUMOR AND ENGAGEMENT WITH PUBLIC HEALTH POLICIES

Humorous messages may also be used to promote support for and adoption of health policies that encourage prevention. Considering that policy advocacy messages related to health and prevention are often serious in tone, humorous messages may be a novel approach and help gain the public's attention amid a cacophony of other policy and political messaging. Given that political communication scholars have begun to address the role of humor in political outcomes, the logical next step is to see if those outcomes apply to public support for health policies.

The research on the impact of humor in political communication, outlined above, finds that multiple processes, such as processing depth, counter-arguing, and message discounting, help determine how effective a humorous political message may be. If a humorous message about a health policy takes these same processes into consideration, it may reach wide audiences through social sharing, too. Additionally, those hoping to use humor to gain public support for preventive health policies should keep in mind that time can serve as a moderator of political humor effects, with greater passage of time after exposure to a humorous message leading to greater persuasion.

To the extent that public health policies become political in nature, such as the discourse surrounding the Affordable Care Act, taxes on sugar-sweetened beverages, or smoking bans, for example, then those advocating for such policies might want to consider crafting funny messages using well-liked spokespeople and also working to reduce message discounting via other communication channels. Furthermore, they might attempt to disseminate these messages earlier rather than later in a policy promotion campaign so that any sleeper effect of the humorous messages would have time to take shape.

CONCLUSION

Existing research points to circumstances where humorous health messages can capture attention, result in positive attitudes, and foster social sharing of health-related messages. And while the mechanisms of humor effects are not entirely clear and call for further scholarly analysis, some evidence indicates that humor's ability to reduce anxiety about a health behavior may be one of the ways in which funny messages can spur behavior change. The body of research on humor and health communication also provides guidance as to which specific circumstances may foster the success, or failure, of a humorous health message. That is, when the context is less serious and there are not strong pre-existing emotionally charged attitudes toward a health issue, humor can be a successful messaging strategy. Individual differences also play a role in determining who will be moved by a humor appeal and who will not. In particular, those with a high humor orientation or high levels of masculinity might be more prone to accept a humorous message. The amount of time after message exposure also influences how effective a humorous message is, with humorous messages gaining in effectiveness as the time after message exposure increases.

The use of humor in health messages can evoke positive emotions in audiences as well as general positive affect. Positive emotions have many physical and psychosocial benefits for those who experience them. The broaden-and-build theory posits that positive emotions, like happiness, are particularly important as individuals attempt to build resources for the future. In a health message context, evoking positive emotions can help message designers gain the attention of audiences as well as encourage audiences to associate positive feelings with preventative health behaviors and/or sources of health information. Furthermore, research indicates that combining humor with fear appeals may help reduce maladaptive response to the fear evoked by the featured threatening information in messages.

Humor is also strongly associated with the universal behavior of laughter. Because laughter is more likely in social than in isolated settings, health message designers would be wise to place humorous messages in shared spaces, like placement in a movie or film festival, concerts, or even on social media or in virtual worlds where people feel as though they are surrounded by others. More research is needed in the realm of health communication to better understand how exactly this behavior relates to the effectiveness of preventative health messages. Work on identification and communication (e.g., Comello 2009; 2013a; 2013b) may provide insights as to when socially oriented humorous health messages are effective or not, especially considering that identification is one of the uniting functions of humor described by Meyer (2000).

In conclusion, humor appeals may be attractive alternatives to message designers wanting to avoid the use of negative emotions in the prevention-focused health messages. For instance, the NFL's Play 60 campaign promotes physical activity for youth in a video featuring NFL quarterback Cam Newton (NFL.com 2014). In the video, Newton talks to a young boy about the importance of playing for 60 minutes every day The scrawny kid then tells Newton that by playing every day, he will become so good that he will make Panthers' fans forget about Newton; he'll even become Newton's mom's favorite player. The expression on Newton's face and the small boy's confidence in his future prowess make it hard for viewers not to smile. News outlets called the advertisement "adorable" (Zaldivar 2012), "amazing," and "the best thing ever" (Fogarty 2012). This is yet another example of how humor in messages can be used to promote a preventative health behavior (in this case, the need for kids to exercise every day).

People like a good joke, and if it is situation appropriate and reaches the right audience, that joke may even promote behavior change. Additional research on the role of humor in fostering health message acceptance will help increase the precision with which message designers can use humor for such positive ends and with which media effects researchers can predict how a humor-evoking health message will impact audiences.

REFERENCES

Ahrens, K., C. K. Kent, J. A. Montoya, H. Rotblatt, J. McCright, P. Kerndt, and J. D. Klausner. 2006. Healthy Penis: San Francisco's social marketing campaign to increase syphilis testing among gay and bisexual men. *PLoS Med* 3(12):e474. doi: 10.1371/journal.pmed.0030474.

Alden, D. L., W. D. Hoyer, and C. Lee. 1993. Identifying global and culture-specific dimensions of humor in advertising: A multinational analysis. *Journal of Marketing* 57(2):64–75. doi: 10.2307/1252027.

Alden, D. L., A. Mukherjee, and W. D. Hoyer. 2000. The effects of incongruity, surprise and positive moderators on perceived humor in television advertising. *Journal of Advertising* 29(2):1–15. doi: 10.1080/00913367.2000.10673605.

American Heart Association. 2014. Video: Just a little heart attack—go red for women. Retrieved February 1, 2014, from https://http://www.goredforwomen.org/about-heart-disease/symptoms_of_heart_disease_in_women/just-a-little-heart-attack/.

Bagozzi, R. P., M. Gopinath, and P. U. Nyer. 1999. The role of emotions in marketing. *Journal of the Academy of Marketing Science* 27(2):184–206. doi: 10.1177/0092070399272005.

Baumgartner, J. C. 2007. Humor on the next frontier: Youth, online political humor, and the JibJab effect. *Social Science Computer Review* 25(3):319–38. doi: 10.1177/0894439306295395.

Blanc, N., and E. Brigaud. 2013. Humor in print health advertisements: Enhanced attention, privileged recognition, and persuasiveness of preventive messages. *Health Communication*, 1–9. doi: 10.1080/10410236.2013.769832.

Booth-Butterfield, M., S. Booth-Butterfield, and M. Wanzer. 2007. Funny students cope better: Patterns of humor enactment and coping effectiveness. *Communication Quarterly* 55(3):299–315. doi: 10.1080/01463370701490232.

Bryant, J., and D. Zillmann. 1989. Using humor to promote learning in the classroom. In P. E. McGhee (Ed.), *Humor and children's development: A guide to practical applications* (pp. 49–78). New York: Haworth Press.

Cacioppo, J. T., W. L. Gardner, and G. G. Berntson. 1999. The affect system has parallel and integrative processing components: Form follows function. *Journal of Personality and Social Psychology* 76(5):839–55. doi: 10.1037/0022-3514.76.5.839.

Campo, S., N. M. Askelson, E. L. Spies, C. Boxer, K. M. Scharp, and M. E. Losch. 2013. "Wow, that was funny": The value of exposure and humor in fostering campaign message sharing. *Social Marketing Quarterly* 19(2):84–96. doi: 10.1177/1524500413483456.

Catalino, L. I., and B. L. Fredrickson. 2011. A Tuesday in the life of a flourisher: The role of positive emotional reactivity in optimal mental health. *Emotion* 11(4):938–50. doi: 10.1037/a0024889.

Christie, W., and C. Moore. 2005. The impact of humor on patients with cancer. *Clinical Journal of Oncology Nursing* 9(2):211–18. doi: 10.1188/05.CJON.211-218.

Comello, M. L. G. 2009. William James on "possible selves": Implications for studying identity in communication contexts. *Communication Theory* 19(3):337–50. doi: 10.1111/j.1468-2885.2009.01346.x.

———. 2013a. Activated self-concept as a mechanism underlying prevention message effects. *Media Psychology* 16(2):177–98. doi: 10.1080/15213269.2012.742359.

———. 2013b. Comparing effects of "My Anti-Drug" and "Above the Influence" on campaign evaluations and marijuana-related perceptions. *Health Marketing Quarterly* 30(1):35–46. doi: 10.1080/07359683.2013.758014.

Conway, M., and L. Dubé. 2002. Humor in persuasion on threatening topics: Effectiveness is a function of audience sex role orientation. *Personality and Social Psychology Bulletin* 28(7):863–73. doi: 10.1177/014616720202800701.

Danner, D. D., D. A. Snowdon, and W. V. Friesen. 2001. Positive emotions in early life and longevity: Findings from the nun study. *Journal of Personality and Social Psychology* 80(5):804–13. doi: 10.1037/0022-3514.80.5.804.

Diener, E., and C. Diener. 1996. Most people are happy. *Psychological Science* 7(3):181–85. doi: 10.1111/j.1467-9280.1996.tb00354.x.

Eisend, M. 2009. A meta-analysis of humor in advertising. *Journal of the Academy of Marketing Science* 37(2):191–203. doi: 10.1007/s11747-008-0096-y.

———. 2011. How humor in advertising works: A meta-analytic test of alternative models. *Marketing Letters* 22(2):115–32. doi: 10.1007/s11002-010-9116-z.

Fogarty, D. 2012, November 23. The "NFL Play 60" commercial with Cam Newton and the little kid is the best thing ever. Retrieved February 9, 2014, from http://www.sportsgrid.com/nfl/cam-newton-play-60/.

Fox, J. R., Koloen, G., and Sahin, V. (2007). No joke: A comparison of substance in *The Daily Show with Jon Stewart* and broadcast network television coverage of the 2004 presidential election campaign. *Journal of Broadcasting and Electronic Media, 51*(2), 213–27. doi: 10.1080/08838150701304621.

Fredrickson, B. L. 1998. What good are positive emotions? *Review of General Psychology* 2(3):300–319. doi: 10.1037/1089-2680.2.3.300.

———. 2000. Cultivating positive emotions to optimize health and well-being. *Prevention and Treatment* 3(1):No Pagination Specified. doi: 10.1037/1522-3736.3.1.31a.

———. 2001. The role of positive emotions in positive psychology: The broaden-and-build theory of positive emotions. *American Psychologist* 56(3):218–26. doi: 10.1037/0003-066X.56.3.218.

Fredrickson, B. L., and C. Branigan. 2005. Positive emotions broaden the scope of attention and thought-action repertoires. *Cognition and Emotion* 19(3):313–32.

Fredrickson, B. L., and M. F. Losada. 2005. Positive affect and the complex dynamics of human flourishing. *American Psychologist* 60(7):678–86. doi: 10.1037/0003-066X.60.7.678.

Fredrickson, B. L., R. A. Mancuso, C. Branigan, and M. M. Tugade. 2000. The undoing effect of positive emotion. *Motivation and Emotion* 24(4):237–58. doi: 10.1023/A:1010796329158.

Frijda, N. H. 1986. *The emotions*. Cambridge, England: Cambridge University Press.

Garland, E. L., B. L. Fredrickson, A. M. King, D. P. Johnson, P. S. Meyer, and D. L. Penn. 2010. Upward spirals of positive emotions counter downward spirals of negativity: Insights from the broaden-and-build theory and affective neuroscience on the treatment of emotion dysfunctions and deficits in psychopathology. *Clinical Psychology Review* 30:849–64.

Gervais, M., and D. S. Wilson. 2005. The evolution and functions of laughter and humor: A synthetic approach. *Quarterly Review of Biology* 80(4):395–430. doi: 10.1086/498281.

Goodson, F. E. 2003. *The evolution and function of cognition*. Mahwah, NJ: Erlbaum.

Gruner, C. R. 1985. Advice to the beginning speaker on using humor—what the research tells us. *Communication Education* 34(2):142–47. doi: 10.1080/03634528509378596.

Healthy Penis. 2014. Healthy Penis—SF—The campaign. Retrieved February 9, 2014, from http://healthypenis.org/sf/campaign/index.html.

Hmielowski, J. D., R. L. Holbert, and J. Lee. 2011. Predicting the consumption of political TV satire: Affinity for political humor, *The Daily Show*, and *The Colbert Report*. *Communication Monographs* 78(1):96–114. doi: 10.1080/03637751.2010.542579.

Huffington Post. 2012, February 22. "Just a little heart attack": PSA sheds light on the number one killer of women. Retrieved February 1, 2014, from http://www.huffingtonpost.com/2012/02/21/heart-attack-women-elizabeth-banks_n_1290773.html.

Isen, A. M., T. E. Shalker, M. Clark, and L. Karp. 1978. Affect, accessibility of material in memory, and behavior: A cognitive loop? *Journal of Personality and Social Psychology* 36(1):1–12. doi: 10.1037/0022-3514.36.1.1.

Johnson, P. 2002. The use of humor and its influences on spirituality and coping in breast cancer survivors. *Oncology Nursing Forum* 29(4):691–95. doi: 10.1188/02.ONF.691-695.

Kaplan, R. M., and G. C. Pascoe. 1977. Humorous lectures and humorous examples: Some effects upon comprehension and retention. *Journal of Educational Psychology* 69(1):61–65. doi: 10.1037/0022-0663.69.1.61.

Keltner, D., and G. A. Bonanno. 1997. A study of laughter and dissociation: Distinct correlates of laughter and smiling during bereavement. *Journal of Personality and Social Psychology* 73(4):687–702. doi: 10.1037/0022-3514.73.4.687.

LaMarre, H. L., K. D. Landreville, and M. A. Beam. 2009. The irony of satire: Political ideology and the motivation to see what you want to see in *The Colbert Report*. *The International Journal of Press/Politics* 14(2):212–31. doi: 10.1177/1940161208330904.

Lazarus, R. S. 1991. *Emotion and adaptation*. New York: Oxford University Press.

Lee, M. J. 2010. The effects of self-efficacy statements in humorous anti-alcohol abuse messages targeting college students: Who is in charge? *Health Communication* 25(8):638–46. doi: 10.1080/10410236.2010.521908.

Lee, M. J., and M. Shin. 2011. Fear versus humor: The impact of sensation seeking on physiological, cognitive, and emotional responses to antialcohol abuse messages. *The Journal of Psychology* 145(2):73–92. doi: 10.1080/00223980.2010.532519.

Levy, B. R., M. D. Slade, S. R. Kunkel, and S. V. Kasl. 2002. Longevity increased by positive self-perceptions of aging. *Journal of Personality and Social Psychology* 83(2):261–70. doi: 10.1037/0022-3514.83.2.261.

Lewis, I. M., B. Watson, and K. M. White. 2008. An examination of message-relevant affect in road safety messages: Should road safety advertisements aim to make us feel good or bad? *Transportation Research Part F: Traffic Psychology and Behaviour* 11(6):403–17. doi: http://dx.doi.org/10.1016/j.trf.2008.03.003.

Lewis, I. M., B. Watson, K. M. White, and R. Tay. 2007. Promoting public health messages: Should we move beyond fear-evoking appeals in road safety? *Qualitative Health Research* 17(1):61–74. doi: 10.1177/1049732306296395.

Lunsford, S. L., K. S. Simpson, K. D. Chavin, L. G. Hildebrand, L. G. Miles, L. M. Shilling, . . . P. K. Baliga. 2006. Racial differences in coping with the need for kidney transplantation and willingness to ask for live organ donation. *American Journal of Kidney Diseases* 47(2):324–31. doi: http://dx.doi.org/10.1053/j.ajkd.2005.10.018.

Markiewicz, D. 1974. Effects of humor on persuasion. *Sociometry* 37(3):407–22.

Martin, R. A. 2006. *Psychology of humor: An integrative approach.* Amsterdam: Elsevier Academic Press.

Martin, R. A., and N. A. Kuiper. 1999. Daily occurrence of laughter: Relationships with age, gender, and Type A personality. *Humor: International Journal of Humor Research* 12(4):355–84. doi: 10.1515/humr.1999.12.4.355.

McGhee, P. E. 1979. *Humor: Its origin and development.* San Francisco, CA: W H Freeman and Company.

Meyer, J. C. 2000. Humor as a double-edged sword: Four functions of humor in communication. *Communication Theory* 10(3):310–31. doi: 10.1111/j.1468-2885.2000.tb00194.x.

Monahan, J. L. 1995. Thinking positively: Using positive affect when designing health messages. In E. W. Maibach and R. Parrott (Eds.), *Designing health messages: Approaches from communication theory and public health practice* (pp. 81–98). Thousand Oaks, CA: SAGE.

Moyer-Gusé, E., C. Mahood, and S. Brookes. 2011. Entertainment-education in the context of humor: Effects on safer sex intentions and risk perceptions. *Health Communication* 26(8):765–74. doi: 10.1080/10410236.2011.566832.

Mukherjee, A., and L. Dubé. 2012. Mixing emotions: The use of humor in fear advertising. *Journal of Consumer Behaviour* 11(2):147–61. doi: 10.1002/cb.389.

Nabi, R. L. In press. Laughng in the face of fear (of disease detection): Using humor to promote cancer self-examination behavior. *Health Communication.*

Nabi, R. L., E. Moyer-Gusé, and S. Byrne. 2007. All joking aside: A serious investigation into the persuasive effect of funny social issue messages. *Communication Monographs* 74(1):29–54. doi: 10.1080/03637750701196896.

Neuhoff, C. C., and C. Schaefer. 2002. Effects of laughing, smiling, and howling on mood. *Psychological Reports* 91(3f):1079–80. doi: 10.2466/pr0.2002.91.3f.1079.

NFL.com. 2014. NFL.com—Play60. Retrieved February 3, 2014, from http://www.nfl.com/play60.

Olson, L. C. 1987. Benjamin Franklin's pictorial representations of the British colonies in America: A study in rhetorical iconology. *Quarterly Journal of Speech* 73(1):18–42. doi: 10.1080/00335638709383792.

Ostir, G. V., K. S. Markides, M. K. Peek, and J. S. Goodwin. 2001. The association between emotional well-being and the incidence of stroke in older adults. *Psychosomatic Medicine* 63(2):210–15.

Polk, J., D. G. Young, and R. L. Holbert. 2009. Humor complexity and political influence: An elaboration likelihood approach to the effects of humor type in *The Daily Show with Jon Stewart. Atlantic Journal of Communication* 17(4):202–19. doi: 10.1080/15456870903210055.

Provine, R. R. 1992. Contagious laughter: Laughter is a sufficient stimulus for laughs and smiles. *Bulletin of the Psychonomic Society* 30(1):1–4.

———. 2000. *Laughter: A scientific investigation.* New York: Viking.

Provine, R. R., and K. R. Fischer. 1989. Laughing, smiling, and talking: Relation to sleeping and social context in humans. *Ethology* 83(4):295–305. doi: 10.1111/j.1439-0310.1989.tb00536.x.

Rosner, F. 2002. Therapeutic efficacy of laughter in medicine. *Cancer Investigation* 20(3):434–36. doi: 10.1081/CNV-120001187.

Seligman, M. E. P., and M. Csikszentmihalyi. 2000. Positive psychology: An introduction. *American Psychologist* 55(1):5–14. doi: 10.1037/0003-066X.55.1.5.

Shiota, M. N., B. Campos, D. Keltner, and M. J. Hertenstein. 2004. Positive emotion and the regulation of interpersonal relationships. In P. Philippot and R. S. Feldman (Eds.), *The regulation of emotion* (pp. 129–58). Mahwah, New Jersey: Lawrence Erlbaum Associates.

Sroufe, L. A., and E. Waters. 1976. The ontogenesis of smiling and laughter: A perspective on the organization of development in infancy. *Psychological Review* 83(3):173–89. doi: 10.1037/0033-295X.83.3.173.

Sternthal, B., and C. S. Craig. 1973. Humor in advertising. *Journal of Marketing* 37(4):12–18.

Thorson, E., and M. Friestad. 1989. The effects of emotion on episodic memory for television commercials. In P. Cafferata and A. M. Tybout (Eds.), *Cognitive and affective responses to advertising* (pp. 305–26). Lexington, MA: Lexington Books.

Tugade, M. M., and B. L. Fredrickson. 2004. Resilient individuals use positive emotions to bounce back from negative emotional experiences. *Journal of Personality and Social Psychology* 86(2):320–33.

Turner, M. M. 2012. Using emotional appeals in health messages. In H. Cho (Ed.), *Health communication message design: Theory and practice* (pp. 59–72). Los Angeles: Sage.

Vega, M. Y., and E. L. Roland. 2005. Social marketing techniques for public health communication: A review of syphilis awareness campaigns in 8 US cities. *Sexually Transmitted Diseases* 32:S30–S36. doi: 10.1097/1001.olq.0000180461.0000130725.f0000180464.

Wanzer, M., M. Booth-Butterfield, and S. Booth-Butterfield. 1996. Are funny people popular? An examination of humor orientation, loneliness, and social attraction. *Communication Quarterly* 44(1):42–52. doi: 10.1080/01463379609369999.

———. 2005. "If we didn't use humor, we'd cry": Humorous coping communication in health care settings. *Journal of Health Communication* 10(2):105–25. doi: 10.1080/10810730590915092.

Weinberger, M. G., and C. S. Gulas. 1992. The impact of humor in advertising: A review. *Journal of Advertising* 21(4):35–59. doi: 10.1080/00913367.1992.10673384.

Wild, B., F. A. Rodden, W. Grodd, and W. Ruch. 2003. Neural correlates of laughter and humour. *Brain* 126(10):2121–38. doi: 10.1093/brain/awg226.

Zaldivar, G. 2012, November 23. Little kid makes Cam Newton worry about job in adorable "Play 60" NFL ad. Retrieved February 9, 2014, from http://bleacherreport.com/articles/1419672-little-kid-makes-cam-newton-worry-about-job-in-adorable-play-60-nfl-ad.

Zhang, Y. 1996. Responses to humorous advertising: The moderating effect of need for cognition. *Journal of Advertising* 25(1):15–32. doi: 10.1080/00913367.1996.10673493.

Chapter Seven

Pride

Imagine a television commercial featuring a middle-aged office manager named Joe. After decades of watching his figure expand in the mirror, Joe has had enough. He starts packing a lunch full of fruits, vegetables, and lean protein instead of eating at the burger joint near his office every day. He concocts a standing desk out of two old bookshelves and goes on a 20-minute walk during part of his lunch hour. As the pounds melt away, Joe receives many compliments from his coworkers. His doctor pats him on the back at his latest checkup and commends him for lowering his risk of heart disease, diabetes, and cancer thanks to his active lifestyle and improved diet. When his friends ask how he feels about his accomplishments, Joe utters a single word: proud.

As this example demonstrates, pride can be linked to preventative health behaviors. Preventative health behaviors often require difficult and sustained efforts, and individuals who succeed in improving their well-being are likely to feel pride for their achievements. As such, health messages that evoke this emotion could be an effective way to motivate audiences to take preventative actions. Given its applicability to a health prevention context as well as its motivational aspects, pride is a promising emotion to examine in the realm of preventative health messages. However, little empirical work has directly analyzed the role of pride in health message effects.

This chapter describes the psychological qualities and functions of pride before delving into the connections between communication research and pride. Next, it discusses existing research on the role of pride in health messaging before suggesting areas for further investigation. It then discusses the role that pride can play in messages promoting public health policies before offering concluding thoughts on the aforementioned topics. The information presented in this chapter aims to be a starting-off point to fill the current gap in empirical work about the role of pride in prevention-focused health media.

PSYCHOLOGICAL QUALITIES OF PRIDE

Pride occurs when an individual feels responsible for a socially respected and positive outcome (Lazarus 1991). According to Lazarus, the core relational theme of pride is "enhancement of one's ego-identity by taking credit for a valued object or achievement, either our own or that of someone or group with whom we identify" (271). The action tendency of pride is not entirely clear, but Lazarus hypothesizes that it is an "expressive impulse," (272) one that prompts a desire to communicate about the pride-evoking action with others. Williams and DeSteno (2008) report experimental evidence that pride motivates individuals to persevere in order to achieve long-term goals, even in the face of short-term displeasure. Although some cultures believe extreme pride to be a sin, research indicates that the emotion can serve adaptive social functions by motivating individuals to assist with group problems (Williams and DeSteno 2009) and by fostering creativity (Damian and Robins 2013).

Pride belongs to the family of self-conscious emotions, along with shame, guilt, and embarrassment (Tangney 1999). Each member of this group of emotions involves some form of self-reflection and self-evaluation. This self-reflection/evaluation does not have to be conscious and effortful—it may be implicit and occur below the level of conscious awareness. Researchers note that pride relates to an individual's evaluation of "the global features of the event—the broad and distal implications of what he or she has done" (Karsh and Eyal 2015, 28). As such, pride is associated with broad social expectations and long-term objectives (Tangney, Stuewig, and Mashek 2007; Tracy and Robins 2007; Williams and DeSteno 2009).

Because of its self-relevant nature, pride is closely linked with self-esteem, or one's feelings of self-worth. The experience of pride, a positively valenced emotion, can enhance self-worth, self-esteem, even social esteem, unlike other positive emotions that do not generally result in ego enhancement (Lazarus 1991). Self-esteem, in turn, has many beneficial psychological and interpersonal benefits (Brown and Marshall 2001).

The focus on the self that corresponds with feelings of pride does not mean pride is devoid of social influences. In fact, an individual's self-reflection as having done something that should lead to a positive or negative self-evaluation often hinges on that individual's beliefs about how others will perceive her. The self-conscious emotions are also closely linked with notions of morality, which are shaped by social settings, community norms, and culture. Pride can result from acting in ways perceived by the actor as morally correct: "When we 'do the right thing,' positive feelings of pride and self-approval are likely to result" (Tangney et al. 2007, 348). If one meets or exceeds morality standards set by society and accepted by the individual, then that individual will likely experience pride.

Feelings of pride can reinforce behaviors and motivate habit formation and long-term behavior change (Tangney et al. 2007). Tangney and colleagues point out that even the *anticipation* of a moral emotion (versus the present experience of it) can likewise also affect behavior. For instance, an individual imagining the prospect of feeling prideful may take up and then continue an action valued by society (e.g., exercising, healthy eating, etc.). Conversely, imagining the prospect of feeling guilty may motivate an individual to stop an action that is devalued by society (e.g., smoking, excessive drinking). These anticipated emotional reactions are based on previous experiences and memories of the consequences of those previous actions. Therefore, if a new situation can be linked to a previous experience of pride, individuals may act in accordance with past pride-eliciting behavior based on expectations of feeling pride again (and avoiding feelings of guilt, shame, or embarrassment). An example would be seeing a delicious slice of cake at a bakery and wanting to eat it, but then recalling a past experience of avoiding a morning donut at work and later feeling proud for remaining alert in the afternoon when other colleagues who ate the donuts experienced a sugar crash. That memory of past pride could help motivate the bakery onlooker to pass by this similar dessert.

Pride can be further subcategorized based on the locus of responsibility for the pride-inducing action. Researchers have found a difference between hubris, which is a general arrogance similar to narcissism, and feelings of pride that are, instead, directly connected to a particular action (Lewis 1992). Similarly, Tracy and Robins (2004; 2007) posit there is a distinction between hubris and achievement-oriented pride, which the authors call authentic pride. They found in their research that these two types of pride are equally common emotional experiences. However, authentic pride is more strongly associated with individuals who have adaptive, prosocial, achievement-oriented personality profiles. Additionally, hubris and authentic pride have different influences on social judgments. Experiments indicate that hubristic pride promotes prejudice and discrimination against others while authentic pride is associated with positive attitudes toward outgroups and stigmatized individuals (Ashton-James and Tracy 2012).

While there is empirical support for this categorization of pride as either authentic or hubristic, Williams and DeSteno (2010) argue that these are actually just different points on the same continuum. The authors note that differences in pride may mirror the nuances of expression of other emotions: "Much like other emotions that can be thus experienced (e.g., sadness as tied to an event or as overgeneralized to depression, fear as tied to an eliciting

object or as debilitating phobia or anxiety), pride likely has adaptive outcomes when appropriately tied to a valid eliciting situation, but potentially
maladaptive ones when overgeneralized or overblown" (181). Given that
there is little differentiation between authentic and hubristic pride in facial
expressions or psychophysiological measures, Williams and DeSteno point
out that the parsimony to be gained by conceptualizing pride as one emotion
likely outweighs the complexity of arguing the two are categorically different, natural kinds of affective states.

PRIDE AND COMMUNICATION

Pride is a common topic of interest in the interpersonal communication literature, particularly in relation to conflict and intercultural communication
(e.g., Butt, Choi, and Jaeger 2005; Mongrain and Vettese 2003; Oetzel and
Ting-Toomey 2003). For instance, Zammuner (1996) found that participants'
felt emotions of pride and pride-related states (i.e., triumph, self-satisfaction,
and excitement) were de-emphasized in interpersonal communication with
others, whereas other positive emotions of joy, satisfaction, happiness and
surprise were intensified in these interpersonal conversations. This work implies that social norms may influence when pride is *expressed* but do not
necessarily prevent individuals from feeling such an emotion.

Even in cultures that differ on the social acceptability of explicitly expressing pride, research indicates that implicit subconscious expressions of
the emotion are still able to communicate high status to others (Tracy, Shariff, Zhao, and Henrich 2013). The expression of pride is a tool humans have
for communicating and negotiating status within members of a society. Giv-
en the ease with which individuals can communicate feelings of pride (toward themselves or toward others or groups with whom they associate) via
social media posts, there are many opportunities for investigating the role of
pride in communication (and preventative health communication) via online
social networks, too (e.g., Bond et al. 2012).

Unlike its presence in the interpersonal communication literature, pride is
barely visible in the mass communication literature. However, various studies have touched on implications of their findings for understanding how
pride operates in a mass media setting. For instance, research in consumer
behavior has found that proud consumers are more likely to generate positive
word of mouth about a product (Soscia 2007). This finding suggests that
advertisements or branding initiatives that evoke pride may be particularly
successful at fostering conversations (perhaps even social media posts) about
a product or campaign. In a sports communication context, Decrop and Derbaix (2010) found that pride is an important aspect of sports marketing and is
often contagious when favored sports teams are successful. The implication

of this study is that high-achieving teams should benefit from pride-inducing strategic messaging strategies.

A recent study on behavioral decision making made explicit the connections between feelings of pride and persuasion, with findings that could easily be integrated into the study of media effects. Using a discrete emotional framework, Karsh and Eyal (2015) tested the different effects of feelings of joy versus feelings of pride on persuasion-related outcomes. Based on research indicating that joy focuses individuals on concrete-level events that resulted in a happy moment, but that pride is elicited by the recognition of more global social values and long-term goals, the researchers posited that when target requests are more abstract (i.e., construed at a higher level), emphasizing the pride to be had by accepting the message's argument will be more persuasive than will be emphasizing the potential for joy. Across three studies of various persuasion contexts (i.e., participating in a cross-cultural gathering or willingness to donate money to a sick child), Karsh and Eyal found support for this hypothesis.

The implication of this finding for media effects research is that the level of abstraction of a target behavior in a persuasive message will likely correspond to which type of emotion elicitation is more persuasive. For example, if there is a testimonial in the message about a man feeling pride for his accomplishments related to his long-term (i.e., abstract) goal of achieving inner peace through mediation, that may be more persuasive than showing the man expressing great joy and momentary happiness for this achievement. Future work is needed to test these suppositions and define which message components and features can evoke pride in audiences.

PRIDE AND PREVENTION MESSAGES

The psychology of pride points to numerous ways in which health messages may elicit and take advantage of pride in order to promote preventative health behaviors. One obvious connection between pride and health communication is that an individual can experience and express pride about his or her own health-related accomplishments, much like the hypothetical office manager described in the introduction to this chapter. Health messages that communicate to individuals who have taken preliminary steps to improve or protect their health that they should feel pride for their achievements is one way media could foster feelings of pride and perhaps motivate individuals to take action.

The topic of a prevention-focused health message could also influence the role of pride in determining message effects on audiences. Messages about health behaviors that are generally valued by a society, such as eating healthy food or exercising, would be more likely to elicit pride in audience members who are already performing those behaviors and could therefore promote maintenance of this often difficult yet effective prevention behavior. On the other hand, health messages discussing behaviors that are associated with societal taboos, such as condom use in conservative communities or abstaining from alcohol in societies where drinking is a commonplace social bonding activity, may fail to illicit pride in audiences and could instead evoke feelings of guilt or even shame. What these hypothetical messaging scenarios make apparent is the necessity of understanding the normative nature of the target behavior before crafting effective prevention messages.

Nonetheless, evoking pride in audiences may also be an effective way to subtly alter norms that may promote unhealthy or harmful behaviors, such as cultures that regularly drink to excess. For instance, Frank et al. (2012) found that a campaign to normalize condom use among Indian men generated interpersonal communication about the topic. This occurred in a society where discussing condoms and sexual relations is typically taboo. Those men in the study who reported having positive conversations with others about condom use also reported more positive attitudes toward condom use, higher self-efficacy for condom use, more positive subjective and descriptive norms, and higher intentions to use condoms in the future. Although feelings of pride were not measured in the study, it is possible that repeated exposure to the campaign message and subsequent discussions about condoms helped to both lessen the taboo and increase pride for taking steps to prevent disease. Campaigns such as this point to the ability of messages, particularly when combined with positively valenced interpersonal conversation, to shift norms in such a way that may help motivate individuals to perform the target behavior.

Furthermore, because the likely action tendency of pride is to communicate with others, health messages that elicit feelings of pride in audiences may be effective for promoting social sharing of preventative health information. Interpersonal conversations are an important dissemination component of health campaigns, one that can help spread message effects across a wider swatch of the population than media exposure alone could (Southwell and Yzer 2007; Southwell and Yzer 2009; van den Putte, Yzer, Southwell, de Bruijn, and Willemsen 2011). Given that budgets for public health campaigns are often limited (and therefore, the messages only reach a limited-size audience directly), any message strategy that can possibly promote the viral spreading or sharing of health information is of interest for health communication efforts. As mentioned above, feelings of pride also have the potential to encourage the building of social relationships in order to overcome problems (Williams and DeSteno 2009), which not only helps spread health information but could also help improve the well-being of the entire community (Fredrickson 2000; 2001). Much additional research is needed to test these ideas in multiple health contexts, but pride is a promising area for expanding the scope of mass media health campaigns.

Another important aspect of how pride may influence health communication outcomes is based on the concept of group pride and the ways in which identification with a particular group can foster pride. Ethnic pride, for instance, has been shown to influence health. A large-scale study of an ethnic minority group in the United States found that a strong sense of ethnic pride was directly associated with fewer symptoms of depression (Mossakowski 2003). A recognition of cultural factors is a key component of developing effective health messages, particularly for those messages that target minority or marginalized segments of the population (Kreuter and McClure 2004). To start, an individual's culture, including ethnic, racial, gender, and other identities, can set standards for what type of behavior will result in feelings of pride. This means that messages meant to evoke pride may need to emphasize different behaviors depending on the norms of one's group. Secondly, certain individuals may feel less pride toward their in-group than others, meaning that appeals to pride aimed at such groups would be more effective when there is a strong group identity across most group members than a weak one.

Similar to ethnic pride, racial identity can evoke feelings of pride and may also be a variable upon which to tailor pride-eliciting health messages. Based on a study of African American women and breast cancer–related messages, Lukwago and colleagues suggest that "[p]ublic health practitioners working to promote mammography might consider integrating present time orientation and racial pride into their approaches for African American women" (Lukwago et al. 2003, 1273). However, other work found that when cancer prevention materials were tailored solely on cultural constructs, including religiosity, collectivism, racial pride, and time orientation, these messages were not as effective at promoting prevention behaviors as were messages tailored on both cultural variables and psychosocial variables taken from theories of health behavior (e.g., self-efficacy, perceived barriers, etc.) (Kreuter et al. 2005). Therefore, group pride alone may not be enough to spur health behavior change without also considering other important psychosocial motivations for behavior change.

Health message designers should use caution when utilizing ethnic, racial, or even national pride in preventative health messages because not all cultures share an inclination to experience feelings of pride. Kitayama, Mesquita, and Karasawa (2006) found across multiple studies that Americans reported feeling stronger feelings of pride than did Japanese participants. The authors posit that a cultural focus on independence and autonomy of the self might make pride a more frequently and intensely experienced emotion in the United States than in Japan, a country that has cultural roots in interdependence and collective engagement.

In an individualistic culture like the United States, health messages that inspire feelings of pride may be more likely to be shared with others than will those that evoke shame, which in turn may be more effective in collectivist or honor-bound cultures. One could imagine the use of social media badges stating "I wore sunscreen at the beach" or "I received my flu vaccine today" might help foster a sense of pride in members of individualist cultures and both foster future adherence to those prevention behaviors as well as encourage others in the individual's social network to consider behaving similarly. Work in political communication research supports this notion. A field experiment testing the effects of Facebook users being encouraged to post an "I voted" message on Facebook found this action actually increased voting behavior among Facebook friends of those who posted the message (Bond et al. 2012). Future work could apply this strategy to health messages and measure self-conscious emotional responses to seeing, posting, and sharing such messages on social media.

Furthermore, the emphasis one's culture places on honor can influence the evocation of feelings of pride and shame. That is, an focus on the importance of honor can promote pride for those who act in accordance with a society's values, while the loss of honor can foster intense feelings of shame in more honor-bound societies (Mosquera, Manstead, and Fischer 2000). Researchers have found that pride has more negative social repercussions, whereas shame has more positive social repercussions in cultures that value honor than in cultures that value individualism. These cultural differences can impact whether individuals openly share feelings of pride (more likely to be shared in an individualistic culture) or shame (more likely to be shared in an honor culture) with others (Mosquera et al. 2000). Given the previous discussion of pride and sharing information via social media, message designers should also consider cultural orientations around honor before trying to invoke pride to foster message-sharing health behavior change.

However, message designers should also be cautious with using pride appeals in individualistic cultures as certain factors may moderate the effectiveness of matching culture-based emotional tendencies with the emotional tone of messages. Aaker and Williams (1998) found that a pride appeal was actually more persuasive for members of a collectivist society than for members of an individualistic culture. The authors identified the mechanism of this effect as the perceived novelty of thinking about oneself instead of others for members of the collectivist culture. The authors point out that novel stimuli can capture attention and increase elaboration, both precursors to persuasion.

While Aaker and Williams (1998) studied the effects and mechanisms of pride appeals in a consumer behavior context (they used advertisements for beer and color film as stimuli), additional research is needed to test if these effects transfer to a health context where the potential target behaviors have more meaningful ramifications for the self and others. Nonetheless, this study points to the importance of considering the novelty of a health threat and/or prevention behavior in applying pride appeals to prevention methods. If there is a relatively new or unusual virus spreading in a population (e.g., Ebola outside of sub-Saharan Africa), then the novelty of the context may suggest the use of pride-evoking messages targeted toward members of collectivist cultures and empathetic, social concern messages toward members of individualistic cultures.

Anticipated Pride and Prevention Messages

The above discussion focused on how feelings of pride experienced in the present moment can motivate preventative health behaviors. However, the ways in which preventative health messages, particularly those that focus on future outcomes, cue audiences to consider future or *anticipated* pride is another important area of research. Existing work clearly denotes the ability of anticipated pride to motivate preventative health actions. For instance, research on smoking cessation has found that anticipated pride (as well as anticipated hope) added a significant and substantial amount of variance to a model predicting intentions to quit smoking in the near future (Cappella, Romantan, and Lerman 2002; Cappella, Romantan, Patterson, and Lerman 2006). The additional predictive power of anticipated pride and hope explained greater variance in smoking cessation beyond what traditional cognitive health behavior variables (e.g., self-efficacy, perceived social norms, behavioral beliefs, etc.) explained in statistical models. These findings should motivate media effects researchers to ask target audiences about what emotions they imagine they would feel if they were to undertake the target behavior in order to be better able to predict message compliance.

Additionally, researchers might consider studying which specific message features lead audiences to anticipate feeling pride. Appraisal theory provides initial guidance for examining links between message content and audiences responding to the message with pride. Feelings of pride result from appraisals that a situation is positive and goal relevant and the outcome would be socially valued and credited to the individual (Lazarus 1991). Therefore, messages that ask audiences to imagine a positive outcome caused by their own behavior would be likely to elicit pride or anticipated pride (depending on if audiences have already or would intend to perform the target behavior).

Anticipated pride may also foster changes in social cognitive variables that are linked to health behavior change. In Bandura's social cognitive theory, two cognitive appraisals are particularly important predictions of positive health behavior change: positive outcome expectations (i.e., beliefs that performing a behavior will result in positive outcomes) and self-efficacy (i.e., a belief that one has the ability to perform the behavior). When an individual sees a message that makes clear a health behavior is socially valued and the individual likewise believes the behavior is a worthy one, then the anticipation of pride from performing that behavior may carry over into a stronger belief in the likelihood of a positive outcome, as well as greater confidence to achieve that outcome. As Bandura (2004) states, "[b]ehavior patterns are most firmly established when social and self-sanctions are compatible. Under such conditions, socially approvable behavior is a source of self-pride, and socially disapprovable behavior is self-censured" (274).

Social cognitive theory also predicts that model performing a target health behavior in a message can influence the audience's intentions to take up the behavior. If an audience member watches a model who is similar to her in life circumstances and aspirations perform a desired health behavior, then narrative involvement (i.e., transportation) and/or character involvement (i.e., identification) processes could lead audience members to imagine themselves feeling prideful if they were to take similar action. Additional research is needed to test these ideas and find potential moderators in the ability of pride to social cognitive variables.

While conceptual considerations suggest that eliciting pride via mediated modeling may be an effective way to communicate preventative health messages, researchers might also consider the potential backlash that would occur if audiences perceived the model as *too* prideful. That is, if a character meant to serve as a model comes across to audiences as overly boastful or lacking in humility, then audiences may be alienated and the message will not likely have its intended effect. Careful message pretesting with members of the target audience would help avoid this potential pitfall of portraying too much pride in this context.

Another example where message features might evoke anticipated pride is through playing with video games and using avatars (i.e., video game characters meant to represent the player, see chapter 14 about eHealth, this volume). Virtual technology allows for individually crafted mediated experiences where an avatar can be created based on a user's likeness and facial features (Bailenson 2012; Bailenson, Blascovich, and Guadagno 2008; Fox and Bailenson 2009). If viewing a self-inspired avatar act in a virtual world in a way that would evoke pride in that individual if she were to actually act that way, then perhaps the anticipated pride from the experience would motivate the user to take action. As can be imagined, anticipated pride would not occur if the individual did not imagine positive societal reactions to the health behavior.

These virtual and nonvirtual ways of constructing a health message may not be effective in eliciting pride if the health behavior is stigmatized, as discussed above. However, additional research could investigate ways to use virtual simulations of an action to demonstrate to the users that actual social reactions to a taboo health behavior (like using condoms or avoiding alcohol in an alcohol-centric culture) might not be as bad as the user imagines. Such a simulation could simultaneously help reduce anticipated shame and increase anticipated pride in taking steps to protect one's health, and help promote preventative health behaviors.

PRIDE AND ENGAGEMENT WITH PUBLIC HEALTH POLICIES

While pride can influence individual behaviors, its connections with societal value and the approval of others also make it an interesting emotional response to study in the context of health policy messages. For example, being a part of a movement that helps improve public health on a larger scale could be a source of pride for individuals who support public health policies. Pride in a locality or municipality that must combat particular public health challenges can also serve as an impetus for civic involvement in public health policies and actions. In the mid-1980s, European citizens' identification with their local cities and their corresponding levels of civic pride were touted as cornerstones of the World Health Organization's "Healthy Cities" initiative (Ashton, Grey, and Barnard 1986). Even local parks, which when used for such prevention-oriented activities as exercise, stress reduction, and making or improving social connections, can be a source of pride and social capital for those who identify as part of a community (Moore, Graefe, Citelson, and Porter 1992). Policy makers and health communication experts can think creatively about the various ways that using messaging strategies to instill pride in one's community could help promote public action to support prevention-related health policies.

Another situation where pride might impact public health policy support is in the context of the currently low levels of participation in health-related government programs (e.g., nutritional aid for poor families, free and low-cost health clinics, etc.). These programs are often stigmatized as being used only by lazy or incompetent individuals. However, they cannot help prevent disease if the individuals who most need their services do not utilize them. It is possible that anticipated shame, and a noticeable lack of pride, contributes to the low participation rates. Therefore, creating messages that aim to increase the amount of pride individuals feel when they take action to assure their own or their family's health may be a possible avenue for increasing enrollment in such programs. A social marketing campaign for the Texas Special Supplemental Nutrition Program for Women, Infants, and Children (WIC) was able to change families' perceptions of the program as merely a welfare program by increasing pride and self-esteem in program users (Bryant et al. 2001). If similar campaigns can help stimulate pride in individuals who need services from government programs, then public support for continued funding of these programs may follow.

A word of caution is necessary, of course, when thinking about the applications of pride-eliciting message components for motivating engagement with public health policies. Research indicates that self-focused motivations for civic engagement are not as effective as other-focused motivations in promoting political activity. That is, if an individual wants to earn individual pride, then supporting policy or political actions may not be the most attractive outcome. In fact, Omoto, Snyder, and Hackett (2010) found that other-focused motivation better predicted AIDS activism and civic engagement than did self-focused motivation. So if pride is to be effectively employed in policy campaigns that hope to garner public support, then perhaps group-level or ethnic pride appeals may be more effective than those focused on individual pride-producing behaviors. Future research could test these propositions as well as any possible differences in effects between different types of pride reactions at play in policy-related messages.

CONCLUSION

In summary, pride is a positive, self-conscious emotion that motivates individuals to talk about the pride-inducing event with others and take action toward long-term goals. Pride can enhance self-worth, self-esteem, and social esteem, all factors associated with mental health as well as the ability to perform important preventative health behaviors. Despite the potential of pride to motivate positive behavior change, there is a paucity of research on the role of pride and anticipated pride in health communication contexts.

Given the many links between psychological well-being and social relationships, a certain amount of pride may provide an incentive for individuals to tackle the often difficult (e.g., starting an exercise routine), anxiety-inducing (e.g., getting a shot), or long-term (e.g., improved eating habits) behaviors that are required to effectively prevent disease. Many avenues exist for future research tackling the nuances of how pride can be utilized to potentially improve preventative health messages, promote prevention-oriented public policy, and motivate long-term behavior change.

REFERENCES

Aaker, J. L., and P. Williams. 1998. Empathy versus pride: The influence of emotional appeals across cultures. *Journal of Consumer Research* 25(3):241–61. doi: http://www.jstor.org/stable/10.1086/209537.

Ashton, J., P. Grey, and K. Barnard. 1986. Healthy cities—WHO's new public health initiative. *Health Promotion International* 1(3):319–24. doi: 10.1093/heapro/1.3.319.

Ashton-James, C. E., and J. L. Tracy. 2012. Pride and prejudice: How feelings about the self influence judgments of others. *Personality and Social Psychology Bulletin* 38(4):466–76. doi: 10.1177/0146167211429449.

Bailenson, J. N. 2012. Doppelgängers—a new form of self? *Psychologist* 25(1):36–38.

Bailenson, J. N., J. Blascovich, and R. E. Guadagno. 2008. Self-representations in immersive virtual environments. *Journal of Applied Social Psychology* 38(11):2673–90. doi: 10.1111/j.1559-1816.2008.00409.x.

Bandura, A. 2004. Health promotion by social cognitive means. *Health Education and Behavior* 31(2):143–64. doi: 10.1177/1090198104263660.

Bond, R. M., C. J. Fariss, J. J. Jones, A. D. I. Kramer, C. Marlow, J. E. Settle, and J. H. Fowler. 2012. A 61-million-person experiment in social influence and political mobilization. *Nature* 489(7415):295–98. doi: http://www.nature.com/nature/journal/v489/n7415/abs/nature11421.html - supplementary-information.

Brown, J. D., and M. A. Marshall. 2001. Self-esteem and emotion: Some thoughts about feelings. *Personality and Social Psychology Bulletin* 27(5):575–84. doi: 10.1177/0146167201275006.

Bryant, C., J. Lindenberger, C. Brown, E. Kent, J. M. Schreiber, M. Bustillo, and M. W. Canright. 2001. A social marketing approach to increasing enrollment in a public health program: A case study of the Texas WIC program. *Human Organization* 60(3):234–46.

Butt, A. N., J. N. Choi, and A. M. Jaeger. 2005. The effects of self-emotion, counterpart emotion, and counterpart behavior on negotiator behavior: A comparison of individual-level and dyad-level dynamics. *Journal of Organizational Behavior* 26(6):681–704. doi: 10.1002/job.328.

Cappella, J. N., A. Romantan, and C. Lerman. 2002. *Emotional bases for quitting smoking: Extending the integrated theory of behavior change.* Annenberg Public Policy Center, University of Pennsylvania. Philadelphia, PA.

Cappella, J. N., A. Romantan, F. Patterson, and C. Lerman. 2006. *The emotional basis for quitting smoking: Anticipated emotions as predictors of intention and behavior.* [Unplublished manuscript]. Philadelphia.

Damian, R. I., and R. W. Robins. 2013. Aristotle's virtue or Dante's deadliest sin? The influence of authentic and hubristic pride on creative achievement. *Learning and Individual Differences* 26(0):156–60. doi: http://dx.doi.org/10.1016/j.lindif.2012.06.001.

Decrop, A., and C. Derbaix. 2010. Pride in contemporary sport consumption: A marketing perspective. *Journal of the Academy of Marketing Science* 38(5):586–603. doi: 10.1007/s11747-009-0167-8.

Fox, J., and J. N. Bailenson. 2009. Virtual self-modeling: The effects of vicarious reinforcement and identification on exercise behaviors. *Media Psychology* 12(1):1–25. doi: 10.1080/15213260802669474.

Frank, L. B., J. S. Chatterjee, S. T. Chaudhuri, C. Lapsansky, A. Bhanot, and S. T. Murphy. 2012. Conversation and compliance: Role of interpersonal discussion and social norms in public communication campaigns. *Journal of Health Communication* 17(9):1050–67. doi: 10.1080/10810730.2012.665426.

Fredrickson, B. L. 2000. Cultivating positive emotions to optimize health and well-being. *Prevention and Treatment* 3(1):No Pagination Specified. doi: 10.1037/1522-3736.3.1.31a.

———. 2001. The role of positive emotions in positive psychology: The broaden-and-build theory of positive emotions. *American Psychologist* 56(3):218–26. doi: 10.1037/0003-066X.56.3.218.

Karsh, N., and T. Eyal. 2015. How the consideration of positive emotions influences persuasion: The differential effect of pride versus joy. *Journal of Behavioral Decision Making* 28(1):27–35. doi: 10.1002/bdm.1826.

Kitayama, S., B. Mesquita, and M. Karasawa. 2006. Cultural affordances and emotional experience: Socially engaging and disengaging emotions in Japan and the United States. *Journal of Personality and Social Psychology* 91(5):890–903. doi: 10.1037/0022-3514.91.5.890.

Kreuter, M. W., and S. M. McClure. 2004. The role of culture in health communication. *Annual Review of Public Health* 25(1):439–55. doi: 10.1146/annurev.publhealth.25.101802.123000.

Kreuter, M. W., C. Sugg-Skinner, C. L. Holt, E. M. Clark, D. Haire-Joshu, Q. Fu, . . . D. Bucholtz. 2005. Cultural tailoring for mammography and fruit and vegetable intake among low-income African-American women in urban public health centers. *Preventive Medicine* 41(1):53–62. doi: http://dx.doi.org/10.1016/j.ypmed.2004.10.013.

Lazarus, R. S. 1991. *Emotion and adaptation.* New York: Oxford University Press.

Lewis, M. 1992. *Shame: The exposed self.* New York: The Free Press.

Lukwago, S. N., M. W. Kreuter, C. L. Holt, K. Steger-May, D. C. Bucholtz, and C. S. Skinner. 2003. Sociocultural correlates of breast cancer knowledge and screening in urban African American women. *American Journal of Public Health* 93(8):1271–74. doi: 10.2105/AJPH.93.8.1271.

Mongrain, M., and L. C. Vettese. 2003. Conflict over emotional expression: Implications for interpersonal communication. *Personality and Social Psychology Bulletin* 29(4):545–55. doi: 10.1177/0146167202250924.

Moore, R., A. Graefe, R. Citelson, and E. Porter. 1992. *The impacts of rail-trails: A study of users and property owners from three trails.* Washington, DC.

Mosquera, P. M. R., A. S. R. Manstead, and A. H. Fischer. 2000. The role of honor-related values in the elicitation, experience, and communication of pride, shame, and anger: Spain and the Netherlands compared. *Personality and Social Psychology Bulletin* 26(7):833–44. doi: 10.1177/0146167200269008.

Mossakowski, K. N. 2003. Coping with perceived discrimination: Does ethnic identity protect mental health? *Journal of Health and Social Behavior* 44(3):318–31. doi: 10.2307/1519782.

Oetzel, J. G., and S. Ting-Toomey. 2003. Face concerns in interpersonal conflict: A cross-cultural empirical test of the face negotiation theory. *Communication Research* 30(6):599–624. doi: 10.1177/0093650203257841.

Omoto, A. M., M. Snyder, and J. D. Hackett. 2010. Personality and motivational antecedents of activism and civic engagement. *Journal of Personality* 78(6):1703–34. doi: 10.1111/j.1467-6494.2010.00667.x.

Soscia, I. 2007. Gratitude, delight, or guilt: The role of consumers' emotions in predicting postconsumption behaviors. *Psychology and Marketing* 24(10):871–94. doi: 10.1002/mar.20188.

Southwell, B. G., and M. Yzer. 2007. The roles of interpersonal communication in mass media campaigns. In C. Beck (Ed.), *Communication Yearbook* (Vol. 31, pp. 420–62). New York: Lawrence Erlbaum.

———. 2009. When (and why) interpersonal talk matters for campaigns. *Communication Theory* 19(1):1–8. doi: 10.1111/j.1468-2885.2008.01329.x.

Tangney, J. P. 1999. The self-conscious emotions: Shame, guilt, embarrassment and pride. In T. Dalgleish and M. J. Power (Eds.), *Handbook of cognition and emotion* (pp. 541–68). New York, NY: John Wiley and Sons Ltd.

Tangney, J. P., J. Stuewig, and D. J. Mashek. 2007. Moral emotions and moral behavior. *Annual Review of Psychology* 58:345–72. doi: 10.1146/annurev.psych.56.091103.070145.

Tracy, J. L., and R. W. Robins. 2004. Show your pride: Evidence for a discrete emotion expression. *Psychological Science* 15(3):194–97. doi: 10.1111/j.0956-7976.2004.01503008.x.

———. 2007. The psychological structure of pride: A tale of two facets. *Journal of Personality and Social Psychology* 92(3):506–25. doi: 10.1037/0022-3514.92.3.506.

Tracy, J. L., A. F. Shariff, W. Zhao, and J. Henrich. 2013. Cross-cultural evidence that the nonverbal expression of pride is an automatic status signal. *Journal of Experimental Psychology* 142(1):163–80. doi: 10.1037/a0028412.

van den Putte, B., M. Yzer, B. G. Southwell, G.-J. de Bruijn, and M. C. Willemsen. 2011. Interpersonal communication as an indirect pathway for the effect of antismoking media content on smoking cessation. *Journal of Health Communication* 16(5):470–85. doi: 10.1080/10810730.2010.546487.

Williams, L. A., and D. DeSteno. 2008. Pride and perseverance: The motivational role of pride. *Journal of Personality and Social Psychology* 94(6):1007–17. doi: 10.1037/0022-3514.94.6.1007.

———. 2009. Pride: Adaptive social emotion or seventh sin? *Psychological Science* 20(3):284–88. doi: 10.1111/j.1467-9280.2009.02292.x.

———. 2010. Pride in parsimony. *Emotion Review* 2(2):180–81. doi: 10.1177/1754073909355015.

Zammuner, V. L. 1996. Felt emotions, and verbally communicated emotions: The case of pride. *European Journal of Social Psychology* 26(2):233–45. doi: 10.1002/(SICI)1099-0992(199603)26:2***l233::AID-EJSP748***r3.0.CO;2-#.

Chapter Eight

Interest

If you are reading this book, chances are you have an interest in the concepts of emotions, media, or health (if not in all three). However, what is interesting to one person may be dull and tedious to another. Many aspects of our environment can provoke interest. For instance, media coverage of a new medical study may provoke momentary interest in a topic that one had not previously found to be as fascinating. Understanding what message features could evoke interest in preventative health topics as well as analyzing the downstream effects of feelings of interest spurred by preventative health messages would be of huge benefit to health communication researchers. However, little research currently exists examining the role of interest, a so-called knowledge emotion, impacts media processes and effects.

Interest is a positive emotion that can influence a number of communication processes, from selective exposure and subsequent message processing and memory for message content, as well as motivation to take actions post-message exposure. This chapter outlines the psychological qualities of interest, which underscore why the study of interest is a promising area of emotion-based research for preventative health communication. Next, the chapter addresses extant research linking interest to communication processes. Then it explores the role of interest in prevention messages as well as in fostering increased public engagement with health-related policies. Additionally, this chapter provides ideas for future research about feelings of interest in the realm of health message effects.

PSYCHOLOGICAL QUALITIES OF INTEREST

Interest is an approach-oriented positive emotion linked with the concepts of curiosity, exploration, and information seeking (Fredrickson 1998; Silvia

2006). It is an emotion that belongs to the knowledge family of emotions, along with confusion, surprise, and awe. Charles Darwin described these knowledge emotions as central to the processes of learning, thinking, and exploring (Darwin 2009), underscoring the strong relationship between the experience of a knowledge emotion and subsequent cognitions about one's environment. There has been some debate over interest's qualifications to be an emotional state. However, Silvia (2005; 2006; 2008) makes a compelling case that interest contains all the components required by Lazarus (1991) to qualify as an emotion: physiological changes, facial and vocal expressions, cognitive appraisals, subjective feelings, and an adaptive function.

Feelings of interest arise when individuals appraise a situation as goal relevant, goal congruent, and containing both novelty and complexity (Silvia 2005). Additionally, interest occurs when individuals appraise their situation as one they can cope with (i.e., coping potential is high). When interest arises, an individual perceives the "ability to understand the new, complex, surprising thing" (Silvia 2006, 80). That is, an individual can only feel interest if she believes she has the intellectual ability to deal with this new and complex object or idea. Feelings of interest are also associated with appraisals of uncertainty and of incongruity with expectations (Berlyne 1960).

Izard (1977) describes the experience of interest as "the feeling of being engaged, caught-up, fascinated, curious. There is a feeling of wanting to investigate, become involved, or extend or expand the self by incorporating new information and having new experiences with the person or object that has stimulated the interest. In intense interest or excitement the person feels animated and enlivened. It is this enlivenment that guarantees the association between interest and cognitive or motor activity. Even when relatively immobile the interested or excited person has the feeling that he is 'alive and active'" (216). This description makes the connection between interest and both cognition and action quite apparent.

The main psychological function of interest is to motivate people to explore and engage with the environment around them (Izard 1977; Silvia 2006). Fredrickson's (1998; 2001) broaden-and-build model of positive emotions suggests another potential function of interest, which is its utility for long-term resource building. Unlike some positive emotions that provide short-term comfort, feelings of interest can help an individual accumulate life experiences and knowledge to later buffer against or help overcome future challenges. More research is needed to empirically confirm this secondary function of interest (i.e., long-term resource building thanks to diverse previous experiences) and its impact on human psychology and behavior (Silvia 2006). However, by orienting people to unfamiliar events, people, objects, or ideas, interest may aid in the development of well-rounded individuals who can cope well when placed in novel situations.

Feelings of interest can also motivate individuals to attend to what might otherwise be boring, mundane, or tedious tasks. This is a useful function for people who must engage in any number of routine tasks in order to prosper (e.g., find resources for oneself and one's family, prepare meals, raise children, etc.). Using interest-enhancing strategies (e.g., fostering competition, introducing aesthetic aspects to a task, or even cognitively restructuring a task to make it more novel) can help turn the tedium necessary for a long and meaningful life into an enjoyable experience (Sansone and Smith 2000).

In addition to experiencing interest in the moment, there are also certain personality traits associated with greater tendencies to experience interest than are others. One such personality trait is sensation seeking, which Zuckerman (1994) defined as the tendency to seek novel, complex, and intense experiences, despite any type of risk those experiences might bring with them (27). Given its link with a desire for the novel, high-sensation seekers are likely to find new and unfamiliar circumstances very interesting.

Another personality trait associated with feelings of interest is openness to experience, which is one of the big five personality traits frequently described in the psychology literature as the fundamental dimensions of personality (Digman 1990; McCrae and Costa 1987). Being more open to experiences increases one's chances of coming into contact with novel and complex situations, which are, in turn, likely to induce a state of interest. Conversely, being prone to boredom is another personality trait that may be associated with lower levels of interest arousal, although more research is needed to understand the impact of boredom proneness on emotional reactions and behavior (Melton and Schulenberg 2009; Silvia 2006).

INTEREST AND COMMUNICATION

Interest has a long association with educating, learning, and communicating, especially in the context of written texts (Arnold 1910; Dewey 1913). According to Silvia (2006), existing research suggests that more than a dozen different message factors can affect how interesting a written text is to the reader. Higher interest levels can subsequently have a positive impact on learning, memory, and message comprehension (Schiefele 1999; Schiefele and Krapp 1996).

Message factors that foster interest include coherence, ease of comprehension, prior knowledge, concreteness, vividness, and the element of surprise, among others (Schraw and Lehman 2001; Silvia 2006; Wade, Buxton, and Kelly 1999). Silvia points out that these message elements are all linked to appraisals of novelty or to one's ability to understand the new information being presented, both of which are vital to the elicitation of interest. Silvia (2006) also argues that the following message factors linked to interest are based on appraisals of novelty-complexity: vividness, surprising-ness, unex-pectedness, suspense, engaging themes (e.g., death, power, sex), emotive-ness, imagery, and author voice. Message factors that evoke interest that are based on appraisals of the ability to comprehend include coherence, ease of comprehension, prior knowledge, concreteness, readers' connection, mean-ingfulness, simple vocabulary, and character identification (83–84).

Three mechanisms familiar to communication researchers help explain interest's positive impact on learning. First, interest can increase attention paid toward a message. Second, interest can lead individuals to more deeply elaborate a message. And lastly, interest can lead readers to adopt various helpful reading strategies like rereading, changing one's reading rate, or rehearsing specific points to remember (Silvia 2006, 68). Of these three possible mechanisms of interest's impact on learning, Silvia points out that the empirical research on the link between interest and greater attention is mixed, while there is more and stronger support for the depth of processing and reading strategy mechanisms.

Additionally, research that distinguishes interest from happiness may in-form research on messages that evoke positive emotions. Although the two emotions are commonly grouped together, interest is distinct from happiness in many ways. Appraisals of complexity and novelty lead to feelings of interest, whereas happiness is derived from simplicity and familiarity (Silvia 2006). In a communication context, interest corresponds with uncertainty about a message or a narrative (e.g., a surprise ending to a story), regardless of whether the story ending is happy or sad, while a happy response to a message is largely conditioned upon a happy ending (Iran-Nejad 1987). These findings indicate that feelings of interest can persist even in the face of negative emotional content in messages, whereas happiness is perhaps a less hardy emotion that can easily dissipate if the communication is not positive enough for the intended audience.

Another study found that participants' interest in a piece of music was the best predictor of how long they chose to listen to the music (Crozier 1974). Interest was a better predictor of listening time than even enjoyment of the music, with enjoyment akin to feelings of happiness. These findings suggest that interest may be able to sustain attention to a message longer than other positive, approach-oriented emotions such as happiness. In short, the body of work on the effects of interest on attention, processing, and learning make interest a promising emotion for inclusion in communication studies, particu-larly those related to message exposure and knowledge gain.

INTEREST AND PREVENTION MESSAGES

As discussed above, feelings of interest can lead to information seeking, longer duration of media use, and improved learning outcomes for the content. All of these outcomes have direct and important implications for prevention-focused health messages. Because the action tendency of interest is to explore one's environment and seek information, perhaps the clearest application of interest to health communication is in the context of health information seeking (see chapter 13 about health information seeking, this volume). Health information seeking is associated with a number of beneficial outcomes such as increased health knowledge and new sources of social support (Galarce, Ramanadhan, and Viswanath 2011).

However, individuals may also avoid seeking out important health information in certain situations, despite the potential benefits. For instance, some people have a "blunter" personality type where they prefer to know as little about potential threats as possible, as opposed to individuals who are "monitors" and want to know as much as possible about threats, including health threats (Miller 1987). Therefore, the ability of interest to increase the likelihood of health information seeking may be particularly important when messages are targeted at those who are, in general, less likely to seek health information on their own.

The connection between feelings of interest and deeper message processing is also an important item for health communication researchers to recognize and explore. Dual-process models of persuasion, such as the Elaboration Likelihood Model (Petty and Cacioppo 1986a) or the Heuristic-Systematic Model (Chaiken 1980), state that messages that are elaborated more deeply usually result in stronger and more persistent attitudes. If preventative health messages can attract the audiences' attention and then provide novel and complex information to audiences, then the added motivation from the emotional state of interest could help promote central or systematic message processing of that information. Then, if the arguments for prevention provided by the message are strong, then the combination of effortful message processing and motivation from the feelings of interest to explore may result in attitude change and motivation to actually perform the target behavior.

Furthermore, a number of important preventative health behaviors require a great deal of motivation and learning on behalf of the target population. Taking care of oneself and one's loved ones in the modern world requires diligence and sustained effort, and health-preserving or disease-preventing behaviors are not always simple or straightforward. For example, learning how to purchase and prepare healthy snacks and meals and then actually following through for (hopefully) the rest of one's life to permanently change one's eating behaviors is not a one-step, short-term action. Instead, this type of task requires individuals to learn where to find affordable food, learn which foods are healthy, learn how to prepare them in a healthy manner, and then those individuals must be motivated to use their acquired information to start and maintain a healthy diet. Eliciting higher levels of interest via health messages may be just the extra push one needs to get over the proverbial hump at the beginning of a lengthy health behavior change process.

MAKING PREVENTION MESSAGES MORE INTERESTING

The potential practical applications for utilizing interest in preventative health communication design are quite promising, despite the lack of existing research on the role of interest in audience reactions to prevention-focused health messages. How, exactly, might health message creators craft more interesting prevention-oriented messages for audiences? The basic formula may be to apply the message factors discussed above (e.g., coherence, character identification, etc.) in order to present preventable health conditions and applicable prevention behaviors as novel and complex yet manageable. The final component of that formula—ensuring that audiences perceive the health threat as manageable—would require message designers to be sure to provide the target audience members with information about the effectiveness of the behavior (response-efficacy) as well as reassurance as to the audiences' own coping potential (i.e., efficacy).

While it is often an effective strategy to keep health messages simple and straightforward, appraisals of complexity are necessary to evoke interest. An over-simplified health message may, in some situations and with certain target populations, unintentionally mislead audiences into thinking a preventative health behavior is so simple they will easily be able to comply. But later, when they attempt the behavior and it is not as simple or easy as they thought, they may get frustrated and stop trying. However, message creators should also be cautious about trying to make a message more interesting without making it confusing or without overwhelming audience members. Some balance is likely required between message simplicity and complexity in order to evoke interest in audiences. In such a situation, if minimal levels of complexity were activated, then feelings of interest may provide the motivation to process a message, while some elements of simplicity may foster the ability to process a message, thereby leading to conditions ripe for elaboration and reflection on the message's arguments, based on tenets of the ELM (Petty and Cacioppo 1986b). Additional research studying the effects of various intensities of interest would help elucidate the situations under which feelings of interest can be the most helpful in fostering behavior change.

Perhaps one way to balance having enough complexity to evoke interest yet clear enough information to prevent frustration or misunderstandings is to segment the prevention message. The part of a preventative health message that discusses the target behavior (e.g., "call the quit hotline," "wear sunscreen," "eat five servings of fruits and vegetables a day," etc.) can remain as simple as possible, but the other components of the message (e.g., describing the threat, showing an exemplar's personal experience with the threat) could present complexity in ways that engage audiences. For instance, a web video encouraging smokers to quit could keep the quit line number and website (simple pieces of information to grasp) on the bottom of the screen at all times, but it could use a more visually complex animation of the physiological changes that occur in the body as soon as someone stops smoking as the central message component. This type of audio-visual and dynamic presentation of human physiology would be complex and novel, yet comprehendible enough for most audiences, especially if it were largely visual and avoided medical jargon. In this way, the message could spur interest in learning more about smoking cessation without making the target behavior seem confusing or overwhelming.

Another potential way to add novelty and complexity (and therefore, interest) to preventative health messages would be to incorporate elements of gaming and virtual reality (see chapter 14 about eHealth, this volume). A growing body of research demonstrates that games can significantly improve players' health prevention and self-care behaviors, which in turn lead to better health outcomes (Lieberman 2012). So-called serious games are video games for education and positive behavior change (McCallum 2012), and have been shown to be effective in promoting many types of health-related behaviors (Baranowski, Buday, Thompson, and Baranowski 2008). For example, serious games have been used to motivate individuals to exercise (Lieberman et al. 2011), an application often called exergaming (McCallum 2012). Virtual reality simulations that use avatars created by using an individual's actual image can also be effective ways to motivate individuals to exercise (Fox and Bailenson 2009).

By presenting stimulating and/or complex tasks to users, games and virtual reality can evoke and hold players' interest more easily than non-interactive, non-game media content. However, empirical testing of this hypothesis is necessary before applying it in the field. Future work in this area could analyze which game elements are the most likely to evoke interest in prevention behaviors and how well game-induced interest carries over into actual behavior and/or sustained behavior changes. Additionally, caution is needed to ensure that overly complex or difficult game activities do not lead to frustration (Ryan, Rigby, and Przybylski 2006), which would likely prevent engagement with the target health topic and/or behavior.

INTEREST AND ENGAGEMENT

WITH PUBLIC HEALTH POLICIES

Because interest arises when individuals appraise a situation as novel and complex, proposing novel policy-related approaches for improving public health may be one way to garner more public interest for prevention-oriented health policies. Given that public policy exists in an environment where federal legislation and regulations can be extremely complicated, policy issues can easily meet the threshold for stirring appraisals of complexity. Therefore, novel-yet-comprehendible approaches to changing health policy may be able to garner more interest from the public than are old, long-debated over approaches. While federal policy is slow to change, states and localities can serve as laboratories to test new health policies before advocates start a campaign to push for these changes on a larger scale (Boeckelman 1992). As such, local campaigns to try to institute novel prevention policies may benefit from including message components that foster feelings of interest.

One municipality that has been at the forefront of proposing novel public health policies is New York City. The Big Apple has pioneered multiple regulations aimed at preventing obesity, from banning trans fats in fast food (Angell, Cobb, Curtis, Konty, and Silver 2012) to requiring restaurants to post the caloric content of their food on the menus (Dumanovsky, Huang, Bassett, and Silver 2010) to banning large sizes of sugar-sweetened beverages (Fairchild 2013). These policy-based approaches to preventing obesity and diseases related to it have attracted copious media attention (McBeth, Clemons, Husmann, Kusko, and Gaarden 2013). The momentary public interest in these policies could be used a springboard by public health advocates in other municipalities, states, or even federal entities to push for similar policy changes.

Moreover, when famous public figures, such as former New York City mayor Michael Bloomberg or famous chef Jamie Oliver, push for such prevention-focused policy changes, their presence can also increase the public's attention to and interest in these usually mundane policy debates (Shickle et al. 2014). Research indicates that celebrity illnesses can attract attention to particular health issues (Basil 1996; Brown and Basil 2010; Myrick, Noar, Willoughby, and Brown 2014; Myrick, Willoughby, Noar, and Brown 2013). Likewise, celebrity status could increase public interest in policy debates by using these attention-grabbing celebrities to educate the public about novel policy approaches.

CONCLUSION

Interest is a positively valenced feeling and a member of the knowledge family of emotions. It arises when an individual appraises a situation as novel and complex, yet also comprehendible. The action tendency of interest is to explore and pursue whatever is eliciting the interest, making it a promising emotion for use in messages that ask individuals to invest attention and energy into preventative health behaviors and/or policies. Additionally, interest is associated with deeper message processing and increased learning. The existing literature on interest suggests a number of potential approaches for making prevention health messages more interesting, and possibly more persuasive. However, little empirical work has directly tested the role of interest in persuasion or preventative health messaging contexts. Future work in these areas would be wise to include analyses of this positively valenced and highly motivating emotional state.

REFERENCES

Angell, S. Y., L. K. Cobb, C. J. Curtis, K. J. Konty, and L. D. Silver. 2012. Change in trans fatty acid content of fast-food purchases associated with New York City's restaurant regulation: A pre–post study. *Annals of Internal Medicine* 157(2):81–86. doi: 10.7326/0003-4819-157-2-201207170-00004.

Arnold, F. 1910. *Attention and interest: A study in psychology and education.* New York: Macmillan.

Baranowski, T., R. Buday, D. I. Thompson, and J. Baranowski. 2008. Playing for real. *American Journal of Preventive Medicine* 34(1):74–82.e10. doi: 10.1016/j.amepre.2007.09.027.

Basil, M. D. 1996. Identification as a mediator of celebrity effects. *Journal of Broadcasting and Electronic Media* 40(4):478–95. doi: 10.1080/08838159609364370.

Berlyne, D. E. 1960. *Conflict, arousal, and curiosity.* New York: McGraw-Hill.

Boeckelman, K. 1992. The influence of states on federal policy adoptions. *Policy Studies Journal* 20(3):365–75. doi: 10.1111/j.1541-0072.1992.tb00164.x.

Brown, W. J., and M. D. Basil. 2010. Parasocial interaction and identification: Social change processes for effective health interventions. *Health Communication* 25(6/7):601–2. doi: 10.1080/10410236.2010.496830.

Chaiken, S. 1980. Heuristic versus systematic information processing and the use of source versus message cues in persuasion. *Journal of Personality and Social Psychology* 39(5):752–66.

Crozier, J. B. 1974. Verbal and exploratory responses to sound sequences varying in uncertainty level. In D. E. Berlyne (Ed.), *Studies in the new experimental aesthetics* (pp. 27–90). Washington, DC: Hemisphere.

Darwin, C. 2009. *The expression of the emotions in man and animals.* London; New York: Penguin.

Dewey, J. 1913. *Interest and effort in education.* Boston: Riverside.

Digman, J. M. 1990. Personality structure: Emergence of the five-factor model. *Annual Review of Psychology* 41(1):417–40. doi: doi:10.1146/annurev.ps.41.020190.002221.

Dumanovsky, T., C. Y. Huang, M. T. Bassett, and L. D. Silver. 2010. Consumer awareness of fast-food calorie information in New York City after implementation of a menu labeling regulation. *American Journal of Public Health* 100(12):2520. doi: 0.2105/AJPH.2010.191908.

Fairchild, A. L. 2013. Half empty or half full? New York's soda rule in historical perspective. *New England Journal of Medicine* 368(19):1765–67. doi: doi:10.1056/NEJMp1303698.

Fox, J., and J. N. Bailenson. 2009. Virtual self-modeling: The effects of vicarious reinforcement and identification on exercise behaviors. *Media Psychology* 12(1):1–25. doi: 10.1080/15213260802669474.

Fredrickson, B. L. 1998. What good are positive emotions? *Review of General Psychology* 2(3):300–319. doi: 10.1037/1089-2680.2.3.300.

———. 2001. The role of positive emotions in positive psychology: The broaden-and-build theory of positive emotions. *American Psychologist* 56(3):218–26. doi: 10.1037/0003-066X.56.3.218.

Galarce, E. M., S. Ramanadhan, and K. Viswanath. 2011. Health information seeking. In T. L. Thompson, R. Parrott, and J. F. Nussbaum (Eds.), *The Routledge handbook of health communication* (Second ed., pp. 167–80). New York: Routledge.

Iran-Nejad, A. 1987. Cognitive and affective causes of interest and liking. *Journal of Educational Psychology* 79(2):120–30. doi: 10.1037/0022-0663.79.2.120.

Izard, C. E. 1977. *Human emotions*. New York: Plenum.

Lazarus, R. S. 1991. *Emotion and adaptation*. New York: Oxford University Press.

Lieberman, D. A. 2012. Digital games for health behavior change: Research, design, and future directions. In S. M. Noar and N. G. Harrington (Eds.), *eHealth applications: Promising strategies for behavior change* (pp. 110–27). New York: Routledge.

Lieberman, D. A., B. Chamberlin, E. Medina, B. A. Franklin, B. M. Sanner, and D. K. Vafiadis. 2011. The power of play: Innovations in getting active summit 2011: A science panel proceedings report from the American Heart Association. *Circulation* 123(21):2507–16. doi: 10.1161/CIR.0b013e318219661d.

McBeth, M. K., R. S. Clemons, M. A. Husmann, E. Kusko, and A. Gaarden. 2013. The social construction of a crisis: Policy narratives and contemporary U.S. obesity policy. *Risk, Hazards and Crisis in Public Policy* 4(3):135–63. doi: 10.1002/rhc3.12042.

McCallum, S. 2012. Gamification and serious games for personalized health. *Studies in health technology and informatics* 177:85–96. doi: 10.3233/978-1-61499-069-7-85.

McCrae, R. R., and P. T. Costa. 1987. Validation of the five-factor model of personality across instruments and observers. *Journal of Personality and Social Psychology* 52(1):81–90. doi: 10.1037/0022-3514.52.1.81.

Melton, A. M. A., and S. E. Schulenberg. 2009. A confirmatory factor analysis of the boredom proneness scale. *The Journal of Psychology* 143(5):493–508. doi: 10.3200/JRL.143.5.493-508.

Miller, S. M. 1987. Monitoring and blunting: Validation of a questionnaire to assess styles of information seeking under threat. *Journal of Personality and Social Psychology* 52(2):345–53. doi: 10.1037/0022-3514.52.2.345.

Myrick, J. G., S. M. Noar, J. F. Willoughby, and J. Brown. 2014. Public reaction to the death of Steve Jobs: Implications for cancer communication. *Journal of Health Communication*, 1–18. doi: 10.1080/10810730.2013.872729.

Myrick, J. G., J. F. Willoughby, S. M. Noar, and J. Brown. 2013. Reactions of young adults to the death of Apple CEO Steve Jobs: Implications for cancer communication. *Communication Research Reports* 30(2):115–26. doi: 10.1080/08824096.2012.762906.

Petty, R. E., and J. T. Cacioppo. 1986a. *Communicaiton and persuasion: Central and peripheral routes to attitude change*. New York: Springer-Verlag.

———. 1986b. The elaboration likelihood model of persuasion. *Advances in Experimental Social Psychology* 19:123–205.

Ryan, R. M., C. S. Rigby, and A. Przybylski. 2006. The motivational pull of video games: A self-determination theory approach. *Motivation and Emotion* 30(4):344–60. doi: 10.1007/s11031-006-9051-8.

Sansone, C., and J. L. Smith. 2000. Interest and self-regulation: The relation between having to and wanting to. In C. Sansone and J. M. Harackiewicz (Eds.), *Intrinsic and extrinsic motivation* (pp. 341–72). San Diego, CA: Academic.

Schiefele, U. 1999. Interest and learning from text. *Scientific Studies of Reading* 3(3):257–79. doi: 10.1207/s1532799xssr0303_4.

Schiefele, U., and A. Krapp. 1996. Topic interest and free recall of expository text. *Learning and Individual Differences* 8(2):141–60. doi: http://dx.doi.org/10.1016/S1041-6080(96)90030-8.

Schraw, G., and S. Lehman. 2001. Situational interest: A review of the literature and directions for future research. *Educational Psychology Review* 13(1):23–52. doi: 10.1023/A:1009004801455.

Shickle, D., M. Day, K. Smith, K. Zakariasen, J. Moskol, and T. Oliver. 2014. Mind the public health leadership gap: The opportunities and challenges of engaging high-profile individuals in the public health agenda. *Journal of Public Health*. doi: 10.1093/pubmed/fdu003.

Silvia, P. J. 2005. What is interesting? Exploring the appraisal structure of interest. *Emotion* 5(1):89–102. doi: 10.1037/1528-3542.5.1.89.

———. 2006. *Exploring the psychology of interest*. New York: Oxford University Press.

———. 2008. Interest—The curious emotion. *Current Directions in Psychological Science* 17(1):57–60. doi: 10.1111/j.1467-8721.2008.00548.x.

Wade, S. E., W. M. Buxton, and M. Kelly. 1999. Using think-alouds to examine reader-text interest. *Reading Research Quarterly* 34(2):194–216. doi: 10.1598/RRQ.34.2.4.

Zuckerman, M. 1994. *Behavioral expressions and biosocial bases of sensation seeking*. New York: Cambridge University Press.

Chapter Nine

Hope

The links between hope and health are many. Those who are ill hope to soon feel better, and those who are healthy hope to stay that way. Feelings of hope even influence physical health. For instance, individuals who report feeling hopeful have a lower likelihood of developing hypertension, diabetes, and respiratory infections (Richman et al. 2005). However, the existing literature on hope in health communication focuses largely on patients and survivors, especially in an interpersonal context. Meanwhile, relatively little empirical work has examined hope in a prevention-related media context. Nonetheless, work in psychology and communication informs possibilities for applying research on hope to this arena, a logical step in the literature given the aforementioned connections between hope and health. Moreover, news stories about health-related breakthroughs can inspire hope in audiences that their own well-being will be better, while hope for the public good could likewise motivate collective action aimed at prevention-oriented public health policies.

This chapter starts with an exploration of the psychological qualities of hope as well as research on hope in various communication fields before addressing the preventative health communication context. The ways in which hope may influence public support for prevention-related policies are also explored. Additionally, possible directions for future research on the role of hope in prevention-focused health messages are provided.

PSYCHOLOGICAL QUALITIES OF HOPE

According to Lazarus (1999), "[t]o hope is to believe that something positive, which does not presently apply to one's life, could still materialize, and so we yearn for it" (653). The core relational theme of hope is a yearning for a positive outcome despite the real possibility of a negative outcome (Lazarus 1991). When a situation is personally relevant but uncertain, and an individual has high problem-focused coping potential and positive future expectancies, she is likely to experience feelings of hope (Lazarus 1991; C. A. Smith and Lazarus 1993). Hope is a prospect-based emotion, along with fear, satisfaction, and disappointment (Ortony, Clore, and Collins 1988). Prospect-based emotions are "affective reactions to anticipated events that have relevant consequences for the self" (Bagozzi, Baumgartner, and Pieters 1998, 8). These types of emotions are typically event based in that they are reactions to desirable (positively valenced event-based emotions) and undesirable (negatively valenced event-based emotions) incidents.

Unlike other positive emotions such as happiness or pride, hope is associated with appraisals of less personal control over a situation. This is because hope typically occurs in the midst of a negative situational context (Roseman, Spindel, and Jose 1990). If everything were perfect and all of one's goals had been obtained, there would be no need to hope. It is the perception that the future could be positive—even in the face of uncertainty and the possibility of a negative outcome—that is the hallmark of hope.

The action tendency of hope is similar to that of other positive emotions, though. Positive emotions drive individuals to approach whatever will help them achieve a hoped-for outcome or goal (Roseman 2011; C. A. Smith and Ellsworth 1985). Roseman and Evdokas (2004) argue that hope also promotes a motivational goal to plan for the future. In short, feeling hopeful encourages people to move toward their goals by taking action and/or planning for the future.

Averill and colleagues (1990) posit that four rules define when individuals will experience feelings of hope. First, the *prudential rule* states that hope can occur only when an individual appraises the probability of attainment of a desired outcome as realistic. Second, the *moralistic rule* states that people generally hope for outcomes they believe are personally and/or socially acceptable. Third, the *priority rule* argues that outcomes appraised as important will be hoped for by an individual. And fourth, the *action rule* states that people who feel hopeful are usually willing to take action to achieve their goals, if any action is possible.

In some situations certain rules of hope can outweigh others (Averill et al. 1990). For instance, if the hoped-for outcome is extremely important to an individual, then the prudential and moralistic rules may be of less consequence and the individual will experience hope against the odds. In fact, hope can also serve as a coping resource individuals use to fight off despair when those important outcomes, such as health and well-being, are at stake (Lazarus 1999). For example, research shows that cancer patients, even those in the advanced stages of the disease, maintain high levels of hope, with feelings of hope related to better coping abilities (Felder 2004).

Being hopeful is a momentary state, one that can change as individuals regulate their emotions or their surroundings change. Additionally, some individuals are more inclined to experience hope during uncertain times than others (Snyder et al. 1991). Hope is also conceptually different from the construct of optimism. Hope is an emotion, whereas optimism is not (Averill et al. 1990). Optimism, on the other hand, is the general expectation that the future will be positive, more akin to an outcome expectancy or belief than an emotion (Carver, Scheier, and Segerstrom 2010). Additionally, hope is often felt in response to more important goals than are optimistic thoughts, while the perceived likelihood of an event occurring is often higher when one is in an optimistic state than in a hopeful state (Bruininks and Malle 2005).

HOPE AND COMMUNICATION

Researchers have paid less attention to hope than to some other positive emotions in the psychology literature (e.g., happiness), and it meets the same fate in the communication literature where less attention has been paid to it than to other discrete emotions. However, more studies are addressing the role of this common emotion in various communication and media contexts. In the realm of political communication, for instance, hope as a campaign platform has drawn much scholarly attention (Finn and Glaser 2010; Kloppenberg 2012), and feelings of hope associated with particular candidates has been shown to positively influence voter preferences and behavior (Finn and Glaser 2010; Glaser and Salovey 1998).

The marketing literature has also begun addressing the potential effects of message-relevant hope. MacInnis and de Mello (2005) developed a list of marketing tactics specifically aimed at evoking hope. These tactics include promoting innovations and product customization, appealing to personal control, encouraging anticipatory imagery/fantasy, and showing consumers comparisons with ideal others or an ideal past self. Another hope-evoking marketing tactic is suggesting a resolution to audiences, one that will help consumers avoid a conflict, such as "Eat all you want and still lose weight" (MacInnis and de Mello 2005, 3).

These tactics are effective at evoking hope, the authors argue, because they rely on principles closely associated with hope's core relational theme and cognitive appraisals. This line of reasoning could encourage the creation of messages that turn impossibility into possibility, which turns a certain and negative outcome into an uncertain yet possibly positive one. Moreover, it supports the notion that persuasive messages that enhance yearning (thereby reinforcing the core relational theme of hope) will likely be better at evoking hope than those that do not leave the audience hankering for something more.

MacInnis and de Mello (2005) also explain how hope can act as a moderator of the relationship between involvement and brand attitudes. While hope results from appraisals of personal relevance, and personal relevance increases involvement with a product or message, feelings of hope can alter the impact of involvement on product evaluations. High involvement with a product promotes systematic processing and scrutiny of argument strength (Eagly and Chaiken 1993; Petty and Cacioppo 1986); however, feelings of hope bias processing toward any message component that promotes a goal-congruent positive outcome as a real possibility. The authors argue "when hope is strong, attitude favorability is based less on the strength of message arguments than on the extent to which the arguments suggest that the goal-congruent outcome is possible. Rather than engaging in objective and systematic processing, consumers engage in motivated reasoning, another form of high-involvement processing" (6).

Some research on message-relevant hope can also been found in the entertainment psychology literature. For instance, Prestin (2013) studied how underdog narratives can evoke hope in audiences. She found that those who viewed videos with underdog characters in them felt more hopeful and were more motivated to pursue their own personal goals than were those who saw a comedic video, a nature video, or were in a control condition. This study indicates that media fare that evokes hope, even if it is fictional in nature, can foster the action tendencies associated with it and lead to changes in individual goal pursuits, even if the specific plot of the hope-evoking narrative differs semantically from the individual's own goals or desired outcomes.

In another entertainment study, Oliver and Hartmann (2010) investigated the ways in which movie viewers respond to meaningful films (i.e., films that provide insight or spark consideration and reflection on the purpose of life and are not necessarily hedonically pleasing, see chapter 10 about elevation). The researchers found that these viewers took away lessons from the films such as the idea that although life is finite, one should be hopeful and recognize how precious life is, as well as the idea that "human endurance often prevails, thereby highlighting the importance of having faith in one's hopes and convictions" (142). The robust undertones of hopefulness in response to meaningful media indicate that messages that provide insight into life and what it means to be human can have a strong impact on media consumers.

What is a Hope Appeal?

Little work has ventured to define what exactly makes a persuasive message hopeful. However, Lazarus's (1991; 1999) propositions about the nature of hope provide a starting point for thinking about which message features might evoke hope in audiences. If a message portrays a future situation as uncertain but feasible and the viewer perceives the target outcome as positive and goal relevant, then this viewer will likely experience at least some degree of hope. Chadwick (2015) labeled persuasive messages that aim to evoke hope by embodying its appraisal components (i.e., importance, goal congruence, future expectation, and possibility of a positive outcome) hope appeals. Using an experimental design, she found evidence that messages about the environment that emphasized these appraisals could, in fact, evoke hope in participants. More work is needed to replicate these findings in multiple communication contexts.

HOPE AND PREVENTION MESSAGES

A large amount of research exists related to the nature and influence of hope for individuals already diagnosed with an illness. From social support conversations to messages about treatment, research indicates that those with a serious condition often depend on feelings of hope to cope with their situation (e.g., Chi 2007; Folkman and Greer 2000; Thorne, Hislop, Armstrong, and Oglov 2008). However, media research has yet to closely examine the role of hope in understanding audience reactions to prevention-focused health messages.

One realm of health-related media where hope is likely to impact is that of narratives. Narratives, or stories, are powerful tools for conveying health messages, and individuals often respond to narratives with strong emotional reactions to the plot as well as strong affective bonds with the narrative's characters (Green 2006; Kreuter et al. 2007; Murphy, Frank, Moran, and Patnoe-Woodley 2011). Because of the ability of narratives to reduce counter arguing (Green and Brock 2000), health-related stories may be able to evoke more hope than non-narrative messages that would more easily allow viewers to argue against possible positive outcomes. However, it should be noted that health-related narratives could also evoke fear in audiences when they contain vivid depictions of potential negative outcomes and/or a not-so-happy ending.

In a study of awareness of breast cancer messages, S. W. Smith et al. (2010) asked women to recall any messages about breast cancer they had seen or heard (in the media or from interpersonal sources), as well as what emotions those memorable breast cancer messages evoked. Hope was one of the feelings the participants recalled feeling in response to such messages. The participants also reported feeling fear, anger, sadness, and relief after seeing breast cancer messages. However, hope was the emotion most often recalled as being associated with treatment messages, while hope was not associated with the recollection of either prevention or detection behavior messages. The prevention-focused hopeful messages the women did recall were entirely from media, and not interpersonal, sources. This indicates that media-based appeals to hope may be a memorable way to present preventative breast cancer messages. However, additional work is needed to test this idea across multiple health contexts.

Beyond a potential impact on audience memory for health messages, feelings of hope arising from such messages have been shown to impact behavioral intentions. Volkman and Parrott (2012) tested how narratives about osteoporosis that expressed either positive or negative emotions, and that varied in the narrator's perspective, shaped reader responses to stories about osteoporosis. They found that positively toned stories were more likely to elicit feelings of happiness, hope, and relief than were negatively toned stories. Additionally, hope was directly and positively related to perceived message effectiveness, which in turn was a positive predictor of intentions to take calcium and vitamin D supplements and to perform weight-bearing exercise (behaviors that help prevent osteoporosis).

Research also indicates that feelings of hope may be tied to self-control. Although their study did not take place in a media context, Winterich and Haws (2011) tested the impact of various positive emotions on self-control related to health behaviors. They found that participants in their experiment who felt hopeful consumed less unhealthy food and had lower preferences for unhealthy snacks than did those participants feeling prideful or happy. The authors argue that this finding is likely due to hope's future orientation, whereas pride is focused on the past and happiness on the present. Because unhealthy food consumption would not have (much of) an immediate impact, the ability of hope to promote a forward-thinking mindset makes the negative long-range effects of unhealthy food more salient.

Winterich and Haws (2011) also found that a future-focused negative emotion, fear, did *not* promote self-control in the face of tempting yet unhealthy food. This finding suggests that the approach tendencies of hope may motivate both forward thinking and actions that move an individual closer to a relevant goal. While this study did not explicitly test mediated messages, it implies that when the target prevention behavior requires delayed gratification and self-control, hope appeals may be an effective messaging strategy. In particular, these findings suggest that hope appeals might be efficacious in obesity prevention and tobacco cessation, behaviors that require long-term commitments. Psychological research has already found a strong link between an individual's ability to focus on the future and the ability to exercise self-control (Fujita, Trope, Liberman, and Levin-Sagi 2006; Trope and Liberman 2010). Hope's ability to foster a focus on the future and subsequent self-control is an important one for prevention-focused health message designers to recognize and investigate in order to understand how it can most effectively be integrated into messages.

MacInnis and de Mello (2005) also advocate for using themes related to hope in persuasive health messages, particularly those targeting behaviors that require copious amounts of self-regulation. The researchers explain that "enhancement of hope may also increase a critical predictor of intentions to stop consumption: self-efficacy. Consumers may be more likely to believe that they can stop a behavior if they are made to understand that stopping is possible. Hope may also enhance another critical predictor of intentions to stop: Beliefs about the consequences of stopping. The yearning component of hope may enhance beliefs that the consequences of quitting are positive" (12). Connecting hope to efficacy is a promising avenue for crafting effective prevention-oriented health appeals.

The fact that hope ties directly into self-regulatory and social cognitive processes indicates that communication and health behavior theories should also consider adding hope into those models. For instance, both the health belief model (Rosenstock 1974) and social cognitive theory (Bandura 1986) rely on the premise that cognitive appraisals of self-efficacy (i.e., an individual's confidence in her ability to do the target behavior) are positively related to the likelihood that an individual will engage in that behavior. If feelings of hope improve expectations about the future and motivation to tackle goal-relevant actions, then these feelings likely also help improve self-efficacy and would help expand the amount of variance explained by these popular theories.

Feelings of hope can also influence the effects of preventative health messages on audiences by shaping how motivated those audiences are to elaborate on the message. Motivated reasoning, as defined by Kunda (1990), is the process of looking for and then evaluating information and forming judgments with the purpose of supporting or reaffirming a belief or a goal. This type of reasoning can have a direct impact on how consumers evaluate products when they are experiencing feelings of hope. De Mello, MacInnis, and Stewart (2007) found that when feelings of hope are threatened, individuals engage in motivated reasoning related to products that promise they can help those individuals achieve their goals. The authors identified five processes underlying this effect: 1) Individuals selectively search for information from sources that are likely to be favorable toward the product; 2) They believe the information from those sources to be more credible; 3) They are less likely to discriminate any low-credibility messages from those sources; 4) They require more negative information before they feel that they are able to evaluate a product's effectiveness; and 5) They are more likely to judge the product as effective for goal pursuit.

As de Mello et al. (2007) note, these findings have ramifications for prevention-oriented health message design. Hopeful individuals, utilizing motivated reasoning, may be less likely to give credence to small print on warning labels on tobacco products, for instance, that do not align with the individuals' goals. However, if the warning labels are too drastic or frightening, then unintended defensive reactions and/or decreased self-efficacy could ensue, and the warnings would backfire (see Hastings, Stead, and Webb 2004; Ruiter, Abraham, and Kok 2001).

In considering the role of hope in prevention-focused health messages, researchers should keep in mind that even messages promoting well-being could prime notions of disease and illness that evoke feelings of fear. For example, in an experiment on reactions to a popular PSA about skin cancer prevention, Myrick and Oliver (2014) found that the version of the PSA edited to only have uplifting content (e.g., smiling, laughter, discussion of prevention and good outcomes) resulted in greater feelings of post-message fear than did the verison that included negatively valenced content. Hope and fear are, conceptually, very closely related due to their bases in appraisals of uncertainty and a future orientation. Therefore, it is easy for individuals to experience both emotions in near proximity, even simultaneously. The task of health message designers who want to utilize a hope appeal is to recognize the likely co-existence of at least some amount of fear. Therefore, a persuasive health message needs to contain enough information about how to achieve a health goal (and avoid a health threat) so that audiences are both confident in the prevention strategy's effectiveness and in their own ability to follow the strategy (Witte, Meyer, and Martell 2000).

Another consideration for studying the ways in which hope might play a role in prevention-focused health communication is the regulatory focus. Regulatory focus is a psychological concept that deals with the extent to which an individual is motivated either to 1) realize achievements and goals, which is a promotion orientation; or, 2) to avoid threats and hazards, which is a prevention orientation (Higgins 1997). When focused on promotion, accomplishments and aspirations comprise an individual's focus, whereas a prevention orientation results in a focus on safety and responsibilities.

Holding hope for the future is one part of having a promotion focus (Higgins, Shah, and Friedman 1997). In the realm of health communication, Zhao and Pechmann (2007) found that for viewers with a stronger promotion focus, antismoking advertisements were more persuasive if they reflected a promotion tone (i.e., emphasizing the achievement of social approval if one did not smoke) than if the messages employed a prevention focus (i.e., emphasizing the threat of social disapproval for smoking). This study indicates health messages that aim to evoke hope may be more successful when targeted toward individuals with a chronic promotion focus. Hope-inducing prevention messages may also be more successful if the messages first prime or cue audiences to adopt a situational promotion focus. For instance, a message could show visuals of common societal goals (a happy and healthy family) and then move on to the main portion of the message. These suppositions require empirical analysis but provide promising areas of future research and message design for public health advocates.

Nabi (2015) also notes that the location within a health message where audiences experience hope matters for how they will respond to it. She argues that traditional fear appeals, which include a threat message component followed by an efficacy message component (Witte 1992), would be more appropriately labeled fear-hope appeals; efficacy information that provides audiences with a possible escape from the threat fits well with the core relational theme of hope of yearning for relief from a negative situation (Lazarus 1999).

Nabi (2015) further points out that previous experimental work on the effects of diabetes advertisements found that when these advertisements ended with positive efficacy information participants reported greater feelings of hope than when they saw advertisements that ended with negative information (Douglas Olsen and Pracejus 2004). Additional work is needed to empirically test hope as a potential mediator between efficacy message components and prevention-oriented outcomes. This future work could explore if both self- and response-efficacy information elicit feelings of hope in audiences, and if one type of efficacy is associated with greater hope evocation that the other.

HOPE AND ENGAGEMENT WITH PUBLIC HEALTH POLICIES

Because hope has been studied in the political communication and social movements literatures, researchers and message designers have available to them some insights as to how the evocation of hope might motivate people to support policies that aim to prevent illness. In the realm of political communication, a long line of research shows that political messages are capable of evoking emotions, including hope, in audiences. Roseman, Abelson, and Ewing (1986) were interested in how the emotional tone of political messages would resonate with voters, particularly if voters were already experiencing certain emotions in relation to political issues. The researchers found that individuals already experiencing anger or pity responded more positively to political pamphlets that matched their present pitiful or angry state. That is, people feeling anger about a political or social topic responded best to political appeals that were also angry in their tone. However, people experiencing fear and hope did not respond in such a congruent fashion. Instead, the fearful participants responded most favorably to the pamphlets that used hope appeals. There was no significant relationship between participants who were already feeling hopeful and which emotional tone in the pamphlets resonated with them.

These findings suggest that health-related policies could possibly be promoted using hopeful overtones in messages, but these messages may need to be tailored to individuals already predisposed to feel fearful about a health issue. For instance, those with a family history of cancer may respond more favorably to hope appeals about increasing funding levels for cancer research. More research is needed to see if these effects in traditional political communication contexts transfer over to a health policy support context.

Researchers have also found that hope can influence individual-level responses to political candidates. In fact, emotional responses, including feelings of hope, to candidates are frequently better predictors of voter choice and other political preferences than are cognitive factors, like policy stances or party identification (e.g., Brader 2005; 2006; Finn and Glaser 2010; Marcus 2000; Neuman, Marcus, Crigler, and MacKuen 2007; Valentino, Brader, Groenendyk, Gregorowicz, and Hutchings 2011). In these studies, hope predicts candidate support. And because these candidates can shape public health policy, feeling hopeful about them can indirectly impact these policies.

A recent test of the role of hope in shaping political support and behavior comes from Finn and Glaser (2010). The researchers used data from the 2008 American National Election Study to test the ways in which pre-election emotions toward candidates influenced support for Barack Obama and John McCain. They found that self-reported emotional responses of hope, pride, and fear predicted reported vote choice above and beyond party identification, ideology, and other predictors. Hope and pride positively predicted voting choice while fear was a negative predictor. In particular, the extent to which respondents reported that Obama made them feel hopeful served as a strong and reliable predictor of voting for Obama. If politicians are intimately connected to health-related policies, such as health care reform, then the amount of hope they inspire can indirectly influence if these policies are instigated, depending on the effectiveness of that candidate's campaign.

Although the use of hope in political messages has gained recent notoriety in national political campaigns (Finn and Glaser 2010; Kloppenberg 2012), the use of hope to motivate citizens to promote policy change often begins at the community level. Foster-Fishman, Pierce, and Van Egeren (2009) argue that engaging residents in urban and low-income neighborhoods is an important part of building healthier communities. The researchers found that both neighborhood capacity (i.e., a sense of community among the residents) and neighborhood readiness (i.e., hope for change and collective efficacy) determine norms for activism and eventual participation in movements to improve the health of a community. They defined hope as the belief that a better future is possible, which can in turn convince residents that it is worthwhile to engage in community-oriented projects and movements. While hope for change can promote individual self-efficacy, hope for a collective change can also increase collective self-efficacy, which is the idea that the entire group can enact change (Perkins and Long 2002). Both types of efficacy are important for promoting change at a community or societal level.

Hope, however, is not a straightforward guarantee of a successful push for changes in politics, policy, community, or society. As Freire argued: "The idea that hope alone will transform the world, and action undertaken in that kind of naïveté, is an excellent route to hopelessness, pessimism, and fatalism. But the attempt to do without hope, in the struggle to improve the world, as if that struggle could be reduced to calculated acts alone, or a purely scientific approach, is a frivolous illusion" (Freire 1997, 8). This quote underscores the dual realities of hope as a tool to engage citizens in the world around them. Hope is needed for motivation and persistence—it can be a long process to realize distant goals, including improved public health. However, hope alone is not enough to ensure policy change. Moreover, accidentally raising false hope can be psychologically damaging, although more research is needed to understand the effects of inducing false hope in message audiences (Nabi 2002).

CONCLUSION

Hope is a future-oriented emotion rooted in uncertainty as well as yearning for a positive outcome. Feelings of hope are associated with future-orientation, perseverance, and greater self-control than are negative feelings. In short, feelings of hope can motivate individuals to pursue prevention behaviors. Health messages that embody the appraisal components of hope with the intent of persuading audiences to take action are known as hope appeals. Hope is also important in prevention messages because the efficacy information often provided in such messages, based on health behavior theories that point out the positive link between efficacy and behavior, is likely to evoke hope in audiences. However, message designers may also consider the potential downside of invoking hope at the cost of downplaying the severity of the health threat to the point where the audience might dismiss the condition.

The politics of health care and civic engagement with health policy are also influenced by the hopefulness of citizens and the health policy–related messages they encounter. A comprehensive approach to understanding the role of hope in preventative health communication includes looking at health behavior messages as well as the best ways to communicate with and encourage citizens to engage with health policy changes that could have a drastic impact on the health of the populace.

While it is clear that feeling hopeful can influence health outcomes, what is less clear is exactly how a health message can provoke hope in various segments of the population. More empirical work and conceptual models displaying the processes behind effective hope appeals and hope-evoking messages are needed to pinpoint the various content and structural message features that arouse hope in audiences. Moreover, work is needed to determine the consequences of raising false hope. In a health context, nothing is for certain, and witnessing others who took recommended preventative actions but still suffered negative health outcomes may lead to a backlash against hope-related health messages.

Although it is intimately connected with physical health and post-diagnosis communication, hope is currently understudied in a prevention messaging context. Many questions remain about the exact mechanisms and potential moderators of hope-related health media effects. This area is ripe for future research and crucial for developing a more nuanced picture of the role of discrete emotions, in particular, in health communication.

REFERENCES

Averill, J. R., G. Catlin, and K. K. Chon. 1990. *Rules of hope*. New York: Springer-Verlag.

Bagozzi, R. P., H. Baumgartner, and R. Pieters. 1998. Goal-directed emotions. *Cognition and Emotion* 12(1):1–26. doi: 10.1080/026999398379754.

Bandura, A. 1986. *Social foundations of thought and action: A social cognitive theory*. Englewood Cliffs, NJ: Prentice-Hall.

Brader, T. 2005. Striking a responsive chord: How political ads motivate and persuade voters by appealing to emotions. *American Journal of Political Science* 49(2):388–405. doi: 10.1111/j.0092-5853.2005.00130.x.

Brader, T. 2006. *Campaigning for hearts and minds: How emotional appeals in political ads work*. Chicago, IL: University of Chicago Press.

Bruininks, P., and B. F. Malle. 2005. Distinguishing hope from optimism and related affective states. *Motivation and Emotion* 29(4):324–52. doi: 10.1007/s11031-006-9010-4.

Carver, C. S., M. F. Scheier, and S. C. Segerstrom. 2010. Optimism. *Clinical Psychology Review* 30(7):879–89. doi: 10.1016/j.cpr.2010.01.006.

Chadwick, A. E. 2015. Toward a theory of persuasive hope: Effects of cognitive appraisals, hope appeals, and hope in the context of climate change. *Health Communication* 30(6):598–611. doi: 10.1080/10410236.2014.916777.

Chi, G. 2007. The role of hope in patients with cancer. *Oncology Nursing Forum* 34(2):415–24. doi: 10.1188/07.ONF.415–24.

de Mello, G. E., D. J. MacInnis, and D. W. Stewart. 2007. Threats to hope: Effects on reasoning about product information. *Journal of Consumer Research* 34(2):153–61. doi: 10.1086/519144.

Douglas Olsen, G., and J. W. Pracejus. 2004. Integration of positive and negative affective stimuli. *Journal of Consumer Psychology* 14(4):374–84. doi: http://dx.doi.org/10.1207/s15327663jcp1404_7.

Eagly, A. H., and S. Chaiken. 1993. *The psychology of attitudes*. Fort Worth, TX: Harcourt Brace Jovanovich.

Felder, B. E. 2004. Hope and coping in patients with cancer diagnoses. *Cancer Nursing* 27(4):320–24.

Finn, C., and J. Glaser. 2010. Voter affect and the 2008 U.S. presidential election: Hope and race mattered. *Analyses of Social Issues and Public Policy* 10(1):262–75. doi: 10.1111/j.1530-2415.2010.01206.x.

Folkman, S., and S. Greer. 2000. Promoting psychological well-being in the face of serious illness: When theory, research and practice inform each other. *Psycho-Oncology* 9(1):11–19. doi: 10.1002/(SICI)1099-1611(200001/02)9:1***111::AID-PON424***r3.0.CO;2-Z.

Foster-Fishman, P. G., S. J. Pierce, and L. A. Van Egeren. 2009. Who participates and why: Building a process model of citizen participation. *Health Education and Behavior* 36(3):550–69. doi: 10.1177/1090198108317408.

Freire, P. 1997. *Pedagogy of hope.* New York: Continuum.

Fujita, K., Y. Trope, N. Liberman, and M. Levin-Sagi. 2006. Construal levels and self-control. *Journal of Personality and Social Psychology* 90(3):351–67. doi: 10.1037/0022-3514.90.3.351.

Glaser, J., and P. Salovey. 1998. Affect in electoral politics. *Personality and Social Psychology Review* 2(3):156–72. doi: 10.1207/s15327957pspr0203_1.

Green, M. C. 2006. Narratives and cancer communication. *Journal of Communication* 56:S163–S183. doi: 10.1111/j.1460-2466.2006.00288.x.

Green, M. C., and T. C. Brock. 2000. The role of transportation in the persuasiveness of public narratives. *Journal of Personality and Social Psychology* 79(5):701–21.

Hastings, G., M. Stead, and J. Webb. 2004. Fear appeals in social marketing: Strategic and ethical reasons for concern. *Psychology and Marketing* 21(11):961–86. doi: 10.1002/mar.20043.

Higgins, E. T. 1997. Beyond pleasure and pain. *American Psychologist* 52(12):1280–300. doi: 10.1037/0003-066X.52.12.1280.

Higgins, E. T., J. Shah, and R. Friedman. 1997. Emotional responses to goal attainment: Strength of regulatory focus as moderator. *Journal of Personality and Social Psychology* 72(3):515–25. doi: 10.1037/0022-3514.72.3.515.

Kloppenberg, J. T. 2012. *Reading Obama: Dreams, hope, and the American political tradition.* Princeton, NJ: Princeton University Press.

Kreuter, M. W., M. C. Green, J. N. Cappella, M. D. Slater, M. E. Wise, D. Storey, . . . S. Woolley. 2007. Narrative communication in cancer prevention and control: A framework to guide research and application. *Annals of Behavioral Medicine* 33(3):221–35.

Kunda, Z. 1990. The case for motivated reasoning. *Psychological Bulletin* 108(3):480–98. doi: 10.1037/0033-2909.108.3.480.

Lazarus, R. S. 1991. *Emotion and adaptation.* New York: Oxford University Press.

———. 1999. Hope: An emotion and a vital coping resource against despair. *Social Research* 66(2):653–78.

MacInnis, D. J., and G. E. de Mello. 2005. The concept of hope and its relevance to product evaluation and choice. *Journal of Marketing* 69(1):1–14. doi: 10.1509/jmkg.69.1.1.55513.

Marcus, G. E. 2000. Emotions in politics. *Annual Review of Political Science* 3(1):221–50. doi: 10.1146/annurev.polisci.3.1.221.

Murphy, S. T., L. B. Frank, M. B. Moran, and P. Patnoe-Woodley. 2011. Involved, transported, or emotional? Exploring the determinants of change in knowledge, attitudes, and behavior in entertainment-education. *Journal of Communication* 61(3):407–31. doi: 10.1111/j.1460-2466.2011.01554.x.

Myrick, J. G., and M. B. Oliver. 2014. Laughing and crying: Mixed emotions, compassion, and the effectiveness of a YouTube PSA about skin cancer. *Health Communication*, 1–10. doi: 10.1080/10410236.2013.845729.

Nabi, R. L. 2002. Discrete emotions and persuasion. In J. P. Dillard and M. Pfau (Eds.), *The persuasion handbook: Developments in theory and practice* (pp. 289–308). Thousand Oaks, CA: Sage.

———. 2015. Emotional flow in persuasive health messages. *Health Communication* 30(2):114–24. doi: 10.1080/10410236.2014.974129.

Neuman, W. R., G. E. Marcus, A. N. Crigler, and M. B. MacKuen (Eds.). 2007. *The affect effect: Dynamics of emotion in political thinking and behavior.* Chicago: University of Chicago Press.

Oliver, M. B., and T. Hartmann. 2010. Exploring the role of meaningful experiences in users' appreciation of "good movies." *Projections* 4(2):128–50. doi: 10.3167/proj.2010.040208.

Ortony, A., G. L. Clore, and A. Collins. 1988. *The cognitive structure of emotions.* New York: Cambridge University Press.

Perkins, D. D., and D. A. Long. 2002. Neighborhood sense of community and social capital: A multi-level analysis. In A. T. Fisher, C. C. Sonn, and B. J. Bishop (Eds.), *Psychological sense of community: Research, applications, and implications.* New York: Kluwer Academic/Plenum.

Petty, R. E., and J. T. Cacioppo. 1986. The elaboration likelihood model of persuasion. *Advances in Experimental Social Psychology* 19:123–205.

Prestin, A. 2013. The pursuit of hopefulness: Operationalizing hope in entertainment media narratives. *Media Psychology* 16(3):318–46. doi: 10.1080/15213269.2013.773494.

Richman, L. S., L. Kubzansky, J. Maselko, I. Kawachi, P. Choo, and M. Bauer. 2005. Positive emotion and health: Going beyond the negative. *Health Psychology* 24(4):422–29. doi: 10.1037/0278-6133.24.4.422.

Roseman, I. J. 2011. Emotional behaviors, emotivational goals, emotion strategies: Multiple levels of organization integrate variable and consistent responses. *Emotion Review* 3(4):434–43. doi: 10.1177/1754073911410744.

Roseman, I. J., R. P. Abelson, and M. F. Ewing. 1986. Emotion and political cognition: Emotional appeals in political communication. In R. R. Lau and D. O. Sears (Eds.), *Political cognition: The 19th annual Carnegie Symposium on Cognition* (pp. 279–94). Hillsdale, NJ: Lawrence Erlbaum Associates.

Roseman, I. J., and A. Evdokas. 2004. Appraisals cause experienced emotions: Experimental evidence. *Cognition and Emotion* 18(1):1–28. doi: 10.1080/02699930244000390.

Roseman, I. J., M. S. Spindel, and P. E. Jose. 1990. Appraisals of emotion-eliciting events: Testing a theory of discrete emotions. *Journal of Personality and Social Psychology* 59(5):899–915. doi: 10.1037/0022-3514.59.5.899.

Rosenstock, I. M. 1974. Historical origins of the Health Belief Model. *Health Education and Behavior* 2(4):328–35. doi: 10.1177/109019817400200403.

Ruiter, R. A. C., C. Abraham, and G. Kok. 2001. Scary warnings and rational precautions: A review of the psychology of fear appeals. *Psychology and Health* 16(6):613–30. doi: 10.1080/08870440108405863.

Smith, C. A., and P. C. Ellsworth. 1985. Patterns of cognitive appraisal in emotion. *Journal of Personality and Social Psychology* 48(4):813–38. doi: 10.1037/0022-3514.48.4.813.

Smith, C. A., and R. S. Lazarus. 1993. Appraisal components, core relational themes, and the emotions. *Cognition and Emotion* 7(3–4):233–69.

Smith, S. W., L. M. Hamel, M. R. Kotowski, S. Nazione, C. LaPlante, and C. K. Atkin. 2010. Action tendency emotions evoked by memorable breast cancer messages and their association with prevention and detection behaviors. *Health Communication* 25:737–46.

Snyder, C. R., C. Harris, J. R. Anderson, S. A. Holleran, L. M. Irving, S. T. Sigmon, . . . P. Harney. 1991. The will and the ways: Development and validation of an individual-differences measure of hope. *Journal of Personality and Social Psychology* 60(4):570–85. doi: 10.1037/0022-3514.60.4.570.

Thorne, S. E., T. G. Hislop, E. A. Armstrong, and V. Oglov. 2008. Cancer care communication: The power to harm and the power to heal? *Patient Education and Counseling* 71(1):34–40. doi: 10.1016/j.pec.2007.11.010.

Trope, Y., and N. Liberman. 2010. Construal-level theory of psychological distance. *Psychological Review* 117(2):440–63. doi: 10.1037/a0018963.

Valentino, N. A., T. Brader, E. W. Groenendyk, K. Gregorowicz, and V. L. Hutchings. 2011. Election night's alright for fighting: The role of emotions in political participation. *The Journal of Politics* 73(1):156–70. doi: 10.1017/S0022381610000939.

Volkman, J. E., and R. L. Parrott. 2012. Expressing emotions as evidence in osteoporosis narratives: Effects on message processing and intentions. *Human Communication Research* 38(4):429–58. doi: 10.1111/j.1468-2958.2012.01433.x.

Winterich, K. P., and K. L. Haws. 2011. Helpful hopefulness: The effect of future positive emotions on consumption. *Journal of Consumer Research* 38:505–24.

Witte, K. 1992. Putting the fear back into fear appeals: The extended parallel process model. *Communication Monographs* 12(4):329–49. doi: 10.1080/03637759209376276.

Witte, K., G. Meyer, and D. Martell. 2000. *Effective health risk messages: A step-by-step guide.* Thousand Oaks, CA: Sage.

Zhao, G., and C. Pechmann. 2007. The impact of regulatory focus on adolescents' response to antismoking advertising campaigns. *Journal of Marketing Research* 44(4):671–87. doi: 10.1509/jmkr.44.4.671.

Chapter Ten

Elevation

Of the emotions discussed in this book, elevation is the most recent to be conceptualized and studied by researchers in social psychology and communication. As such, it is not an emotion that the average layperson would recognize by name. However, most would recognize the feeling, once described to them, as a common and even important part of the human experience. Elevation is the feeling individuals get when they witness virtuous behavior in others, and it is synonymous to feelings of inspiration. It can occur when watching a documentary about Mother Teresa tending to the needs of the sick and the poor or when reading about volunteers leaving behind their own families to provide aid to the less fortunate in the aftermath of a natural or manmade disaster (Haidt 2003a). Elevation is an emotion that arises when individuals observe instances of moral beauty or moral excellence (Haidt 2000). The emotion is inherently social in nature: It requires the witness of another person's act of moral beauty or virtue, and what is or is not virtuous depends on social definitions.

Despite the little work to date in the communication literature on elevation, the emotion is a promising one for future work, particularly that related to health communication. Elevation inspires people to act altruistically, an action tendency that may be very helpful for public health advocates promoting prevention-oriented public health policies. Secondly, individuals with other-focused orientations (e.g., parents, caregivers) may be more likely to change their behavior if they feel like it will help individuals than if a message focuses on individual ramifications. For instance, a smoker may not worry much about her own health, but a message that emphasizes the ramifications for her family if she were to get sick (or if secondhand smoke caused health harms) may be more effective for that type of smoker. These are but a couple of the many potential paths for future work integrating the study of elevation with prevention-focused health media effects.

This chapter presents the highlights of the burgeoning psychology and communication literature dedicated to studying elevation. After describing the qualities of elevation, this chapter discusses applications to multiple prevention-focused messaging context as well as future directions for research on health communication and preventative health behavior.

PSYCHOLOGICAL QUALITIES OF ELEVATION

Haidt (2000) describes elevation as a "warm, uplifting feeling that people experience when they see unexpected acts of human goodness, kindness, and compassion" (1–2). Experiences of elevation include feelings of physical warmth and/or opening in the chest, a lump in the throat, tears, and/or goose bumps (Silvers and Haidt 2008). In addition to the physiological sensations of elevation, individuals experiencing elevation often describe feeling moved, touched, or inspired. Elevation is an emotion rooted firmly in the concept morality; it is a feeling that arises when one witnesses moral beauty in another, either directly or via media portrayals (Oliver, Hartmann et al. 2012). Morality is a complex, multifaceted concept, but at its core is the idea of having virtue, with virtue based on social norms, cultural practices, emotions, and intuition (Haidt and Joseph 2007). When individuals act in virtuous ways, those who share similar definitions of virtue and observe the behavior are likely to experience elevation.

Emotion researchers describe elevation as the opposite of disgust (Haidt 2003a; Lai, Haidt, and Nosek 2013). Feelings of disgust result from witnessing violations of moral rules and motivate people to remove themselves from the situation and to close off from others (Haidt 2000). However, elevation is an experience of viewing moral excellence, which in turn motivates people to move closer to others, open up, and help others (Haidt 2000; 2003a; 2003b).

Haidt (2000, 2003a) has found evidence of the existence of elevation in multiple cultures and countries. He depicts the emotion as one that helps individuals connect with humanity, thereby fostering the desire to help others. Elevation, therefore, serves the important function of encouraging altruistic behavior and a desire to affiliate with others. Many researchers have found experimental evidence of this action tendency of elevation to promote prosocial behavior (Freeman, Aquino, and McFerran 2009; Schnall and Roper 2012; Schnall, Roper, and Fessler 2010).

Psychologists categorize elevation as an "other-praising" emotion in the same family of emotions as gratitude and admiration (Algoe and Haidt 2009). Elevation has also been compared to feelings of happiness. Although both are positive in valence, elevation is distinct from feelings of happiness, which motivates individuals to celebrate and tell others about their good feelings, while elevation motivates individuals to do good and become a better person. Moreover, happiness has no direct social/relationship consequences. Elevation, on the other hand, results in a general openness to other people (Algoe and Haidt 2009).

Furthermore, while researchers generally describe elevation as a positive emotion, evidence exists that it can be a simultaneous mix of positive affect, such as inspiration or compassion, and negative affect like anxiety or sadness (Oliver, Hartmann, and Wooley 2012; Silvers and Haidt 2008). This mixed emotional state of elevation is akin to the feelings experienced during a bittersweet event or while watching a poignant movie with a self-sacrificing hero and a sad ending (Larsen, McGraw, and Cacioppo 2001; Larsen and Stastny 2011; Oliver 2008). Categorizing elevation as a mixed affective experience better captures the nuance of the emotion and its differentiation from feelings like happiness or joy. However, the approach orientation of its action tendency (i.e., to connect with other people) and its adaptive function to promote altruistic behaviors fit well with conceptualizations of positively valenced emotions (Fredrickson 1998; Fredrickson and Branigan 2005).

Witnessing virtuous actions is a precursor to feelings of elevations. However, the specific circumstances of the moral act and the actor can moderate the intensity of elevation felt by an observer. Thomson and Siegel (2013) found that individuals experienced higher levels of elevation viewing someone helping another person when the beneficiary of the good deed was also perceived as a person of good character. The researchers also found that the amount of effort required for individuals to perform a moral act could moderate elevation responses. The greater effort, or sacrifice, a good-doer has puts into a virtuous act, the greater the elevating response from those who witness the act.

Apart from contextual moderators, individuals differ in their general propensity to experience elevation after witnessing virtuous acts. Those for whom their moral identity is a central part of the self are more likely to experience intense elevation as well as to recall acts of moral goodness than are those individuals who place less importance on morality (Aquino, McFerran, and Laven 2011). Furthermore, Schnall et al. (2010) point out that since elevation has been linked with increased oxytocin levels in lactating women (Silvers and Haidt 2008), there may be sex differences in the influence of elevation on behavior.

In short, elevation is a mixed valence (although generally positive) emotional response to witnessing moral beauty, such as instances of kindness, charity, gratitude, fidelity, or self-sacrifice, among other virtuous actions. The action tendency of elevation is to open up and to help others as well as to emulate the moral virtue that has just been witnessed. The social nature of elevation points to its usefulness for building bonds between people and fostering good will, similar to the function of positive emotions. The links between this emotion that moves and inspires people and media processes and effects, as well as its potential role in preventative health communication, are discussed below.

ELEVATION AND COMMUNICATION

People can directly witness acts of moral beauty. However, elevation also occurs as the result of viewing mediated messages. Of note, media have been heavily relied upon in psychology experiments studying elevation as a way to evoke the emotion in participants. For instance, Haidt (2003a) used a documentary about Mother Teresa in the elevation-arousing condition of his experiment, as well as other media as stimuli for the remaining conditions (e.g., a clip from *America's Funniest Home Videos* to evoke amusement in the humor condition). Likewise, participants asked to describe a time when they felt moved reported instances of media consumption, such as viewing a scene of courage in the face of imminent death in the movie *Titanic* or reading newspaper accounts of those who volunteer to help others in the wake of a natural disaster (Haidt 2003a). The movie *Schindler's List* and the book *A Tale of Two Cities* are other examples listed by participants in a different study as media that prompted feelings of elevation (Aquino et al. 2011). Indeed, media is often intertwined with various aspects of morality, including moral emotions (Tamborini 2013).

To date, entertainment researchers have taken the lead in applying and advancing psychological findings about elevation to the realm of media research. Oliver and her colleagues have found across multiple studies that, in addition to gaining hedonic pleasure from viewing media, audiences seek out media that is meaningful, that they appreciate it because those types of media provide insight into the human experience (Oliver 2008; Oliver and Bartsch 2011; Oliver and Hartmann 2010; Oliver and Raney 2011). Oliver and Bartsch (2010) describe this sense of appreciation of media as "an experiential state that is characterized by the perception of deeper meaning, the feeling of being moved, and the motivation to elaborate on thoughts and feelings inspired by the experience" (76). Once viewing this type of non-hedonic entertainment media, meaningful reactions to media have been found to evoke feelings of elevation, which in turn motivate media audiences to strive to be better people and to help others (Oliver, Hartmann, and Wooley 2012).

In addition to fostering prosocial behaviors, the communication literature also demonstrates that feelings of elevation in response to media promote deeper information processing. While some entertainment fare can be emotionally gratifying for audiences, with little need for further cognitive elaboration of the content, meaningful media experiences can prompt deeper reflection and a quest to better understand one's emotional reactions (Cup-chik 1995; 2011). Bartsch and Oliver (2011) argue that meaningful media can lead audiences to reflect and elaborate deeply on that content. They also explain that media consumption can combine both superficial and deep levels of affective processing. Recent work supports the supposition that meaning-ful entertainment media, which can evoke feelings of elevation in audiences, is significantly more likely to lead to reflective thoughts than are less mean-ingful media portrayals (Bartsch, Kalch, and Oliver 2014). Furthermore, a greater number of reflective thoughts was positively associated with positive attitudes toward the film. Research on also demonstrates that meaningful reactions to media can increase reflective thoughts about politics, issue inter-est, and information seeking, more so than can hedonic involvement, which instead has been found to promote superficial information processing (Bartsch and Schneider 2014). If meaningful media portrayals that evoke elevation can lead to greater elaboration of media content, which in turn improves attitudes toward the content, elevation may be a promising emotion to integrate into persuasive messages.

In addition to fostering greater reflection of media content, elevating me-dia may also be a potential mechanism for reducing prejudice against margi-nalized groups. For instance, Lai et al. (2013) showed participants in their experiment either an inspiring video or a control video. Feelings of elevation prompted by the inspiring video led to a decrease in participants' implicit and explicit prejudices against gay men, whereas those who viewed the control video did not exhibit a reduction in prejudice. Researchers have also found that feelings of elevation lessened White participants' social dominance over African Americans and led to an increase in donations by the elevated partic-ipants to African American charities (Freeman et al. 2009). Additionally, narrative news stories (as opposed to policy-focused stories) have been shown to elicit in readers feelings of compassion (akin to elevation) and empathy for stigmatized groups (Oliver, Dillard, Bae, and Tamul 2012). The researchers found that these emotional reactions to the narrative news stories in turn predicted intentions to help the stigmatized groups mentioned in the news stories (prisoners, immigrants, and the elderly) as well as actual infor-mation-seeking behavior.

Another important outcome of consuming elevating media is the ability of the emotional response to motivate individuals to share information with others. Sharing information is quite easy to do in person or via communica-tion technology (especially thanks to the Internet), and it can drastically increase the breadth of media exposure. For instance, Berger and Milkman (2012) studied how users shared stories on the *New York Times* website. They found that awe-inspiring stories were the most shared, even after con-trolling for how surprising, interesting, practical, or prominently featured the content was. Awe is another positive-oriented moral emotion in the same family as elevation and points to the importance of moral emotions in fostering social sharing.

Additionally, Berger and Milkman (2012) found that strong emotional arousal, as opposed to low-arousal states, were more likely to promote sharing of news content. Another study of more than 165,000 posts on the microblogging website Twitter found that emotionally charged Twitter messages were retweeted more often and more quickly than were neutral Twitter posts (Stieglitz and Dang-Xuan 2013). The evidence cited above points to the centrality of emotion, including those similar to feelings of elevation, for fostering social sharing. Specifically, the action tendency of elevation to connect with others and help other people makes this area a promising one for future research on the role of elevation in media effects and information dissemination.

Overall, the extant research on elevation and media effects shows that mediated portrayals of virtue can evoke feelings of elevation in media consumers, and that these feelings of elevation can encourage continued reflection on the media content that elicited the emotion. Research on elevation and communication has been most robust in the entertainment literature, where preliminary work has found that individuals seek out media they think they will appreciate or that will teach them about the human experience and offer the chance to experience feelings of elevation. Given the action tendencies of elevation to foster altruistic behavior, elevating media have the potential to inspire audiences to take action, including helping others and sharing of information, and can also help lessen stereotypes and/or stigma against outgroups. These initial findings about elevation and mediated communication set a promising stage for additional research as well as applications of this work to a disease prevention context.

ELEVATION AND PREVENTION MESSAGES

Elevation is an appealing emotion to study in a health communication context for a number of reasons. The action tendencies of the emotion—wanting to be a better person and to help others—have important implications for personal, community-level, and public health. Additionally, elevation's foundation in morality links the emotion with societies that place a high value on health and well-being. Moral foundations theory (MFT) describes five domains of moral salience that influence cultural virtues (Haidt and Joseph 2007). These domains are care/harm, fairness/reciprocity, in-group/loyalty, authority/respect, and purity/sanctity. Of these, the care/harm domain is of high interest in a health communication context because preventative health behaviors can be construed as caring for oneself or for others. The inverse, a failure to take preventative health action, could also be viewed as a violation of this particular moral domain to care for individuals.

The high value society places on health and well-being make the study of elevation and moral foundations—a framework that emphasizes human values and compassion—an approach that could readily apply to audience reactions to health messages (Myrick and Oliver 2014). Imagine a PSA showcasing a child who eats spinach at his mother's request, this despite his extreme dislike of the leafy green vegetable. The kid squirms and barely manages to swallow his big bite of spinach, but once he does, he announces he did it so his mom wouldn't worry about him because he knows vegetables are important for growing boys. Audiences may view this child's act as a caring one— he cares for his mom and doesn't want her to worry—and they may also view the mother as a caring individual for looking out for the health of her child. Audiences could perceive their compliance with the care-related moral foundation as examples of moral beauty, thereby evoking feelings of elevation in audience members. This is but one of many possible examples of how moral foundations and elevation embedded in health messages may help shape preventative health-related outcomes.

Very little research exists in the health communication literature that directly tests the role of elevation in encouraging preventative health behaviors. However, work on mixed emotional reactions to health messages provides important insights to how elevation might be a useful force for encouraging preventative health behaviors. Carrera, Muñoz, and Caballero (2010) found that mixed-emotion messages were more likely to lower post-message discomfort and motivate participants to decrease their binge drinking than were negative-only emotional appeals. The researchers operationalized mixed emotions with a short text narrative that sequentially evoked sadness, fear, joy, and finally relief. This differs from the psychological research that defines mixed emotions as occurring simultaneously, not necessarily sequentially (Du, Tao, and Martinez 2014; Larsen and McGraw 2011; Larsen et al. 2001; Larsen and Stastny 2011). Instead, the sequential approach may better be described as emotional flow and may have different effects on message consumers (Lang, Sanders-Jackson, Wang, and Rubenking 2012; Nabi 2015; Nabi and Green 2014). Nonetheless, the findings that multiple emotional reactions to a health message resulted in improved health behaviors hold promise for the ability of a mixed-affective state like elevation to likewise foster positive outcomes. Future research could test the differences between the evocation of elevation, a singular mixed (i.e., positive and negative in valence; ambivalent) affective state, and the sequential evocation of various discrete emotions.

Another health communication study presents some evidence of the ability of moral emotions like elevation to promote preventative health behaviors and the dissemination of preventative health information. Researchers were interested in the mechanisms behind the popularity of a YouTube PSA about melanoma prevention and detection (Myrick and Oliver 2014). The five-minute video, called "Dear 16-year-old Me" and produced by a Canadian non-profit organization, received millions of online views and copious media coverage. The video is a first-person account of patients, family members, and dermatologists giving advice to their sixteen-year-old selves. The individuals in the video alternate between telling jokes to relaying somber tales of regret for dangerous skin-related behaviors, such as tanning or not using sunscreen.

Myrick and Oliver (2014) edited the video to isolate certain emotionally evocative segments and then experimentally tested the effects of these different versions of the video on audiences. One version was the original, which included a mix of emotional portrayals (e.g., some individuals smiling and telling jokes, other content involving sad stories and tears, etc.). Another second version of the video was edited such that all the sad moments in the video were removed, while a third version edited out the happy, frivolous moments in the video. Finally, participants in a fourth control condition watched an emotionally neutral informational video about melanoma narrated by a doctor. Statistical analyses revealed that the original (i.e., mixed affect) video and the video devoid of the happy images were the most effective at evoking feelings of compassion in participants. Compassion, an emotional state akin to elevation, in turn predicted greater perceived severity of melanoma and greater intentions to share the video PSA with others.

The researchers also measured actual sharing-related behavior and viewing of an online petition urging *Cosmopolitan* magazine to run a story about melanoma with a cover photo of a woman with a scar from a melanoma removal (and sign if they chose to do so) as well as intentions to perform skin-protective behaviors (e.g., wear sunscreen and protective clothing) (Myrick and Oliver 2014). Intentions to share "Dear-16-year-old Me" with others and perceived severity of melanoma directly predicted all three of these behavioral/behavioral-intention measures. Moreover, bootstrapping analyses revealed significant and positive indirect effects of compassionate reactions to the mixed-affective video on all three behavioral/behavioral-intention measures. These findings underscore the ability of compassion in response to a moving persuasive health message to motivate not only individual health behaviors but also social behaviors like sharing information and advocating for greater awareness.

Aside from a YouTube video featuring personal inspiring health exemplars as well as medical professionals elevation may also play an important role in audience reactions to narratives with health-related themes. Characters in narratives who demonstrate moral beauty while performing health-related behaviors (e.g., donating a kidney or bone marrow, raising money for a health-related cause, volunteering at a community clinic, etc.) could inspire audience members to act similarly. The purposeful inclusion of health les-sons in entertainment narratives is known as entertainment-education (EE). According to Singhal and Rogers (1999), EE "is the process of purposely designing and implementing a media message to both entertain and educate, in order to increase audience knowledge about an educational issue, create favorable attitudes, and change overt behavior" (xii). The health communica-tion community has embraced EE as one way to use popular media narratives to increase exposure to accurate health information and to promote health behavior change (Piotrow and de Fossard 2004).

A common conceptual framework for understanding the ability of EE to induce health behavior changes is social cognitive theory (Bandura 1986; 2004). Social cognitive theory posits that individuals learn through observa-tion and then model behaviors that are rewarded while avoiding behaviors for which they witness others receiving punishment. Research indicates that watching a model take a preventative health action and end up the better for it can increase the observer's self-efficacy for doing the behavior, another important predictor of behavior (Bandura 1993; Strecher, McEvoy DeVellis, Becker, and Rosenstock 1986).

Emotional arousal is also linked to important social cognitive variables (e.g., self-efficacy and outcome expectations), and subsequently to behavior change. For instance, high self-efficacy is associated with the hope of being able to take action while low self-efficacy can encourage feelings of anxiety (Bandura 1993; Bandura, Caprara, Barbaranelli, Gerbino, and Pastorelli 2003; Robinson and Snipes 2009). Moreover, SCT posits that four processes allow individuals to learn via behavioral modeling: attention, retention, pro-duction, and motivation (Bandura 1986; 2001; 2004). Emotions can influ-ence each one of these processes (Lang et al. 2012; Lazarus 1991; Levine and Pizarro 2004; Roseman 2011). Because elevation has only recently attracted the attention of emotion and communication researchers, more work is nec-essary to see if and how elevating entertainment narratives of individuals who model preventative health behaviors influence audience behaviors. However, it is likely that viewing a model act altruistically by helping others with an illness or by helping others take preventive action may result in audiences expecting similar positive outcomes if they were to take on those behaviors and foster increased confidence that they, too, can take these ac-tions.

Existing research on elevation suggests that emotional reactions to EE narratives could encourage audiences to imitate protagonists' behaviors, above and beyond behaviors predicted by cognitive-based effects alone. Schnall et al. (2010) induced elevation by showing participants a video from *The Oprah Winfrey Show* about people who mentored underprivileged youth. However, the researchers did not ask participants if they were willing to model the same behavior. Instead, the researchers asked if they would be willing to participate in an additional unpaid study, an unrelated yet still altruistic task. This finding indicates that feelings of elevation "inspired help-ing in spirit, not in kind" (319). Although this study did not take place in a traditionally EE context, it did feature media content (talk show) that em-ployed aspects of narrative storytelling similar to many used in an EE setting (e.g., moving music, a plot structure). Because elevation can motivate audi-ences to behave in a prosocial, altruistic manner, and not necessarily the semantically identical featured in the media content that evoked elevation, the motivational aspect of the emotion may be able to overcome resistance to persuasion.

While much of the research in EE analyzes the impact of media processes with emotional implications, like identification, parasocial interaction, empa-thy, and transportation, little work has looked at emotional reactions, specifi-cally, as drivers of EE effects. An exception is a study by Murphy, Frank, Moran, and Patnoe-Woodley (2011) comparing emotions, involvement, and transportation as potential mechanisms of EE effects in reaction to a storyline about lymphoma in a popular television drama, *Desperate Housewives*. The researchers found that transportation into and involvement with the narrative were the best predictors of change in cancer-related knowledge, attitudes, and behavior. However, they also found through structural equation model-ing that character-specific involvement increased transportation into the nar-rative as well as emotional reactions to the narrative, which in turn shaped these same outcomes (knowledge, attitudes, and behavior).

It is important to note, though, that the researchers grouped positive and negative emotional reactions together in their study, which leads to a less nuanced understanding of the potential mediating role of discrete emotional reactions to EE, each with different action tendencies (Dillard and Seo 2013). Future work in EE could attempt to parse out the influences of discrete emotional activation from previously measured factors such as audience in-volvement processes and more cognitive-oriented variables like self-efficacy and risk perception. EE storylines that feature altruistic health-related/caring behaviors, in particular, may have distinct effects than those featuring self-involved preventative health actions given elevation's unique action tenden-cies to motivate a desire to be a better person and help others. Furthermore, the increase in reflective thoughts associated with feelings of elevation may make EE storylines that feature health-related moral beauty be particularly effective for promoting prevention behaviors that require sustained thought and engagement, such as lifestyle changes to exercise and diet (versus one-time actions, like getting a vaccine).

ELEVATION AND ENGAGEMENT WITH
PUBLIC HEALTH POLICIES

Elevation's aforementioned action tendency—to help others and become a better person—has clear implications for message designers who hope to motivate audiences to participate in communal efforts to promote public health and disease prevention, even if they will not personally benefit directly from the action. Feelings of compassion after viewing a moving PSA about melanoma motivated individuals to advocate for disease prevention by signing an online petition (Myrick and Oliver 2014). Oliver et al.'s (2012) study of compassionate reactions to news stories of stigmatized groups also demonstrated that meaningful emotions could spur action on behalf of others. Additional research is needed to test this link between elevation and civic engagement in preventative health contexts and with various types of messages beyond video PSAs.

Another important moderator of elevation evocation to consider in this context of prevention-focused policy messages is political ideology. Morality and political ideology are linked as conservatives and liberals place different amounts of weight on different sets of moral foundations (Graham, Haidt, and Nosek 2009; Haidt, Graham, and Joseph 2009). Researchers have found that liberals often base their moral judgments on the harm/care and fairness/reciprocity foundations instead of on in-group/loyalty, authority/respect, or purity/sanctity foundations; meanwhile, conservatives are more likely to endorse the five foundations more equally (Graham et al. 2009). If political actors or ideologies become tied to messages about prevention policies, then feelings of elevation in response to policy messages may depend on audience members' political ideology and/or party affiliation.

This line of research on moral foundations suggests that such elevating messages related to the care/harm foundation may resonate more strongly with liberals. Therefore, certain health policy messages that aim to evoke elevation may be more persuasive if targeted at liberals. Health policy message creators might instead consider crafting messages that better encapsulate all five moral foundations and accompanying moral emotions (e.g., awe, disgust, and/or shame) to better connect with conservative audiences. More research is needed to more fully understand the effects of moral emotions, such as elevation, and moral foundations in a health and policy communication context on civic engagement.

CONCLUSION

Research on moral emotions finds that witnessing examples of moral beauty can evoke feelings of elevation in observers. Individuals who feel elevated describe the experience as being moved, touched, or inspired. Experiencing this moral emotion subsequently motivates people to connect with others, help others, and attempt to become a better person. Although the study of elevation is in its infancy, research in psychology and communication point to its propensity to promote altruistic behaviors and positive attitudes toward outgroup members. The implications for health communication are many, including the ability to motivate individuals to change their own behavior as well as help others prevent illness. Feelings of elevation resulting from eleva- tion-inducing health policy messages may also inspire individuals to advo- cate for policies that could improve public health on a larger scale.

Researchers who strive to create theoretical models that help explain the processes behind elevation effects in a health media context should consider both the motivational ability of elevation as well as elevation's ability to promote reflective thinking and message elaboration. Applying concepts from dual-process models of information processing such as the elaboration likelihood model (Petty and Cacioppo 1986) to future theorizing on elevation effects would provide greater insight in this area. The cognitive-functional model (Nabi 1999; 2002) could possibly be amended to accommodate posi- tive and/or mixed emotions to also help explain elevation effects on health message processing and persuasion. Additionally, the mood-as-resource par- adigm (Das and Fennis 2008; Trope and Neter 1994; Trope and Pomerantz 1998), which argues that positive emotions help buffer against self-threaten- ing information and promotes attention to negative information that benefits the individual in the long term (e.g., information about health threats), is another conceptual framework with implications for explaining the effects of post-message exposure elevation or compassion (Myrick and Oliver 2014). Integrating these conceptual frameworks into a model of elevation effects is a promising route for advancing the study and application of elevation in a heath media context.

The practical implications of integrating elevation into health messages are many. Given the ethical questions associated with using fear appeals, preventative health appeals aiming to elevate audiences are a promising alter- native to using scare tactics to motivate audiences to take action. Additional- ly, the altruistic tendencies associated with the emotion make it a particularly attractive one to include in messages aimed at increasing civic engagement with public health issues. However, the dearth of research on the role of elevation in preventative health communication leaves many conceptual and practical questions unanswered and begs for further research and theory de- velopment.

REFERENCES

Algoe, S. B., and J. Haidt. 2009. Witnessing excellence in action: The "other-praising" emotions of elevation, gratitude, and admiration. *The Journal of Positive Psychology* 4(2):105–27. doi: 10.1080/17439760802650519.

Aquino, K., B. McFerran, and M. Laven. 2011. Moral identity and the experience of moral elevation in response to acts of uncommon goodness. *Journal of Personality and Social Psychology* 100(4):703–18. doi: 10.1037/a0022540.

Bandura, A. 1986. *Social foundations of thought and action: A social cognitive theory*. Englewood Cliffs, NJ: Prentice-Hall.

———. 1993. Perceived self-efficacy in cognitive development and functioning. *Educational Psychologist* 28(2):117–48. doi: 10.1207/s15326985ep2802_3.

———. 2001. Social cognitive theory of mass communication. *Media Psychology* 3(3):265–99. doi: 10.1207/s1532785xmep0303_03.

———. 2004. Health promotion by social cognitive means. *Health Education and Behavior* 31(2):143–64. doi: 10.1177/1090198104263660.

Bandura, A., G. V. Caprara, C. Barbaranelli, M. Gerbino, and C. Pastorelli. 2003. Role of affective self-regulatory efficacy in diverse spheres of psychosocial functioning. *Child Development* 74(3):769–82. doi: 10.1111/1467-8624.00567.

Bartsch, A., A. Kalch, and M. B. Oliver. 2014. Moved to think: The role of emotional media experiences in stimulating reflective thoughts. *Journal of Media Psychology: Theories, Methods, and Applications* 26(3):125–40. doi: 10.1027/1864-1105/a000118.

Bartsch, A., and M. B. Oliver. 2011. Making sense of entertainment: On the interplay of emotion and cognition in entertainment experience. *Journal of Media Psychology: Theories, Methods, and Applications* 23(1):12–17. doi: 10.1027/1864-1105/a000026.

Bartsch, A., and F. M. Schneider. 2014. Entertainment and politics revisited: How non-escapist forms of entertainment can stimulate political interest and information seeking. *Journal of Communication*, n/a-n/a. doi: 10.1111/jcom.12095.

Berger, J., and K. L. Milkman. 2012. What makes online content viral? *Journal of Marketing Research* 49(2):192–205. doi: 10.1509/jmr.10.0353.

Carrera, P., D. Muñoz, and A. Caballero. 2010. Mixed emotional appeals in emotional and danger control processes. *Health Communication* 25:726–36.

Cupchik, G. C. 1995. Emotion in aesthetics: Reactive and reflective models. *Poetics* 23(1–2):177–88. doi: http://dx.doi.org/10.1016/0304-422X(94)00014-W.

———. 2011. The role of feeling in the entertainment=emotion formula. *Journal of Media Psychology: Theories, Methods, and Applications* 23(1):6–11. doi: 10.1027/1864-1105/a000025.

Das, E., and B. M. Fennis. 2008. In the mood to face the facts: When a positive mood promotes systematic processing of self-threatening information. *Motivation and Emotion* 32(3):221–30.

Dillard, J. P., and K. Seo. 2013. Affect and persuasion. In J. P. Dillard and L. Shen (Eds.), *The SAGE handbook of persuasion: Developments in theory and practice* (Second ed., pp. 150–66). Thousand Oaks, CA: SAGE.

Du, S., Y. Tao, and A. M. Martinez. 2014. Compound facial expressions of emotion. *Proceedings of the National Academy of Sciences* 111(15):E1454–E1462. doi: 10.1073/pnas.1322355111.

Fredrickson, B. L. 1998. What good are positive emotions? *Review of General Psychology* 2(3):300–319. doi: 10.1037/1089-2680.2.3.300.

———. 2001. The role of positive emotions in positive psychology: The broaden-and-build theory of positive emotions. *American Psychologist* 56(3):218–26. doi: 10.1037/0003-066X.56.3.218.

Fredrickson, B. L., and C. Branigan. 2005. Positive emotions broaden the scope of attention and thought-action repertoires. *Cognition and Emotion* 19(3):313–32.

Freeman, D., K. Aquino, and B. McFerran. 2009. Overcoming beneficiary race as an impediment to charitable donations: Social dominance orientation, the experience of moral elevation, and donation behavior. *Personality and Social Psychology Bulletin* 35(1):72–84. doi: 10.1177/0146167208325415.

Graham, J., J. Haidt, and B. A. Nosek. 2009. Liberals and conservatives rely on different sets of moral foundations. *Journal of Personality and Social Psychology* 96(5):1029–46. doi: 10.1037/a0015141

Haidt, J. 2000. The positive emotion of elevation. *Prevention and Treatment* 3(1):1–5. doi: 10.1037/1522-3736.3.1.33c.

———. 2003a. Elevation and the positive psychology of morality. In C. L. M. Keyes and J. Haidt (Eds.), *Flourishing: Positive pscyhology and the life well-lived* (pp. 275–89). Washington, DC: American Psychological Association.

———. 2003b. The moral emotions. In R. J. Davidson, K. R. Scherer, and H. H. Goldsmith (Eds.), *Handbook of affective sciences* (pp. 852–70). Oxford: Oxford University Press.

Haidt, J., J. Graham, and C. Joseph. 2009. Above and below left–right: Ideological narratives and moral foundations. *Psychological Inquiry* 20(2–3):110–19. doi: 10.1080/10478400903028573.

Haidt, J., and C. Joseph. 2007. The moral mind: How five sets of innate intuitions guide the development of many culture-specific virtues, and perhaps even modules. In P. Carruthers, S. Laurence, and S. Stich (Eds.), *The innate mind* (Vol. 3, pp. 367–91). New York: Oxford University Press.

Lai, C. K., J. Haidt, and B. A. Nosek. 2013. Moral elevation reduces prejudice against gay men. *Cognition and Emotion* 28(5):781–94. doi: 10.1080/02699931.2013.861342.

Lang, A., A. Sanders-Jackson, Z. Wang, and B. Rubenking. 2012. Motivated message processing: How motivational activation influences resource allocation, encoding, and storage of TV messages. *Motivation and Emotion*, 1–10. doi: 10.1007/s11031-012-9329-y.

Larsen, J. T., and A. P. McGraw. 2011. Further evidence for mixed emotions. *Personality Processes and Individual Differences* 100(6):1095–110.

Larsen, J. T., A. P. McGraw, and J. T. Cacioppo. 2001. Can people feel happy and sad at the same time? *Journal of Personality and Social Psychology* 81(4):684–96. doi: 10.1037/0022-3514.81.4.684.

Larsen, J. T., and B. J. Stastny. 2011. It's a bittersweet symphony: Simultaneously mixed emotional responses to music with conflicting cues. *Emotion* 11(6):1469–73.

Lazarus, R. S. 1991. *Emotion and adaptation.* New York: Oxford University Press.

Levine, L. J., and D. A. Pizarro. 2004. Emotion and memory research: A grumpy overview. *Social Cognition* 22(5):530–54.

Murphy, S. T., L. B. Frank, M. B. Moran, and P. Patnoe-Woodley. 2011. Involved, transported, or emotional? Exploring the determinants of change in knowledge, attitudes, and behavior in entertainment-education. *Journal of Communication* 61(3):407–31. doi: 10.1111/j.1460-2466.2011.01554.x.

Myrick, J. G., and M. B. Oliver. 2014. Laughing and crying: Mixed emotions, compassion, and the effectiveness of a YouTube PSA about skin cancer. *Health Communication*, 1–10. doi: 10.1080/10410236.2013.845729.

Nabi, R. L. 1999. A cognitive-functional model for the effects of discrete negative emotions on information processing, attitude change, and recall. *Communication Theory* 9(3):292–320. doi: 10.1111/j.1468-2885.1999.tb00172.x.

———. 2002. Anger, fear, uncertainty, and attitudes: A test of the cognitive-functional model. *Communication Monographs* 69(3):204–16.

———. 2015. Emotional flow in persuasive health messages. *Health Communication* 30(2):114–24. doi: 10.1080/10410236.2014.974129.

Nabi, R. L., and M. C. Green. 2014. The role of a narrative's emotional flow in promoting persuasive outcomes. *Media Psychology*, 1–26. doi: 10.1080/15213269.2014.912585.

Oliver, M. B. 2008. Tender affective states as predictors of entertainment preference. *Journal of Communication* 58(1):40–61. doi: 10.1111/j.1460-2466.2007.00373.x.

Oliver, M. B., and A. Bartsch. 2010. Appreciation as audience response: Exploring entertainment gratifications beyond hedonism. *Human Communication Research* 36(1):53–81. doi: 10.1111/j.1468-2958.2009.01368.x.

————. 2011. Appreciation of entertainment: The importance of meaningfulness via virtue and wisdom. *Journal of Media Psychology: Theories, Methods, and Applications* 23(1):29–33. doi: 10.1027/1864-1105/a000029.

Oliver, M. B., J. P. Dillard, K. Bae, and D. Tamul. 2012. The effect of narrative news format on empathy for stigmatized groups. *Journalism and Mass Communication Quarterly* 89(2):205–24. doi: 10.1177/1077699012439020.

Oliver, M. B., and T. Hartmann. 2010. Exploring the role of meaningful experiences in users' appreciation of "good movies." *Projections* 4(2):128–50. doi: 10.3167/proj.2010.040208.

Oliver, M. B., T. Hartmann, and J. K. Woolley. 2012. Elevation in response to entertainment portrayals of moral virtue. *Human Communication Research* 38(3):360–78. doi: 10.1111/j.1468-2958.2012.01427.x.

Oliver, M. E., and A. A. Raney. 2011. Entertainment as pleasurable and meaningful: Identifying hedonic and eudaimonic motivations for entertainment consumption. *Journal of Communication* 61:984–1004. doi: 10.1111/j.1460-2466.2011.01585.x.

Petty, R. E., and J. T. Cacioppo. 1986. The elaboration likelihood model of persuasion. *Advances in Experimental Social Psychology* 19:123–205.

Piotrow, P. T., and E. de Fossard. 2004. Entertainment-education as a public health intervention. In A. Singhal, M. J. Cody, E. M. Rogers, and M. Sabido (Eds.), *Entertainment-education and social change: History, research, and practice* (pp. 41–60). Mahwah, NJ: Lawrence Erlbaum Associates.

Robinson, C., and K. Snipes. 2009. Hope, optimism and self-efficacy: A system of competence and control enhancing African American college students academic well-being. *Multiple Linear Regression Viewpoints* 35(2):16–26.

Roseman, I. J. 2011. Emotional behaviors, emotivational goals, emotion strategies: Multiple levels of organization integrate variable and consistent responses. *Emotion Review* 3(4):434–43. doi: 10.1177/1754073911410744.

Schnall, S., and J. Roper. 2012. Elevation puts moral values into action. *Social Psychological and Personality Science* 3(3):373–78. doi: 10.1177/1948550611423595.

Schnall, S., J. Roper, and D. M. T. Fessler. 2010. Elevation leads to altruistic behavior. *Psychological Science* 21(3):315–20. doi: 10.1177/0956797609359882.

Silvers, J. A., and J. Haidt. 2008. Moral elevation can induce nursing. *Emotion* 8(2):291–95. doi: 10.1037/1528-3542.8.2.291.

Singhal, A., and E. M. Rogers. 1999. *Entertainment-education: A communication strategy for social change.* Mahwah, NJ: Lawrence Erlbaum Associates.

Stieglitz, S., and L. Dang-Xuan. 2013. Emotions and information diffusion in social media: Sentiment of microblogs and sharing behavior. *Journal of Management Information Systems* 29(4):217–48. doi: 10.2753/MIS0742-1222290408.

Strecher, V. J., B. McEvoy DeVellis, M. H. Becker, and I. M. Rosenstock. 1986. The role of self-efficacy in achieving health behavior change. *Health Education and Behavior* 13(1):73–92. doi: 10.1177/109019818601300108.

Tamborini, R. 2013. *Media and the moral mind.* New York: Routledge.

Thomson, A. L., and J. T. Siegel. 2013. A moral act, elevation, and prosocial behavior: Moderators of morality. *The Journal of Positive Psychology* 8(1):50–64. doi: 10.1080/17439760.2012.754926.

Trope, Y., and E. Neter. 1994. Reconciling competing motives in self-evaluation: The role of self-control in feedback seeking. *Journal of Personality and Social Psychology* 66(4):646–57. doi: 10.1037/0022-3514.66.4.646.

Trope, Y., and E. M. Pomerantz. 1998. Resolving conflicts among self-evaluative motives: Positive experiences as a resource for overcoming defensiveness. *Motivation and Emotion* 22(1):53–72. doi: 10.1023/a:1023044625309.

TV by the Numbers. 2013, July 21. AMC announces Chris Hardwick as Host of 'Talking Bad.' Retrieved May 31, 2014, from http://tvbythenumbers.zap2it.com/2013/07/21/amc-announces-chris-hardwick-as-host-of-talking-bad/193046/.

Chapter Eleven

Health Campaigns

Slogans like "Friends don't let friends drive drunk" or "Just say no" are quite familiar to many American media consumers. Images from heath campaigns also permeate American pop culture: an egg hitting a hot frying pan as the narrator describes, "This is your brain on drugs" was part of an iconic anti-drug public service announcement. Health campaigns that produced these memorable phrases and images are commonplace in the American mass media landscape.

Health campaigns have their roots in the clean living movements of the nineteenth century (Engs 2000), but they have become more common in recent decades as media technology advanced and the role of the federal government in promoting health likewise expanded (Paisley and Atkin 2013). An overview of the literature supports the conclusion that mass media health campaigns can help improve public health, especially when such campaigns are combined with supplemental services and products, community-based outreach, and supportive public policies (Wakefield, Loken, and Hornik 2010).

Campaigns are inherently rooted in emotion. As Perloff (2010) describes them, "[c]ampaigns reflect this nation's cultivation of the art of persuasion. They rely on argumentation, sloganeering, and emotional appeals in an effort to mold public attitudes" (324). Perloff's portrayal of a campaign makes clear the strong link between these persuasive messages and emotional arousal. In order for campaigns to be as effective as possible in conveying health threats and their remedies, campaign designers must take into account the emotional nature of message content as well as the likely emotional reactions of audiences. Be it a frightening representation of what smoking can do to the lungs or a moving video of a father dancing with his daughter at her wedding thanks to early detection of his colon cancer, campaigns are often designed to tug at the heartstrings.

There are many vexing yet preventable public health problems that benefit from campaigns to educate and motivate the public to take preventative actions. Tobacco is the leading cause of preventable death in the United States; it kills more than five million people across the globe each year (Centers for Disease Control and Prevention 2014). Excessive alcohol consumption is a leading cause of premature death in the United States and is the cause of one in ten deaths among working-age American adults (Stahre, Roeber, Kanny, Brewer, and Zhang 2014). Additionally, the obesity epidemic continues to be the source of numerous preventable maladies, like type 2 diabetes and heart disease, that are associated with suffering, increases in health care costs, and premature death (Masters, Powers, and Link 2013).

In a preventative health context, the goal of evoking emotions in the audience is to persuade them to take action in order to improve their own lives and/or the lives of those around them. The purpose of this chapter is to outline a portion of the research that describes the links between emotions and the effects of prevention-oriented health campaigns on audiences. To further illuminate the links between emotions and prevention-oriented campaigns, this chapter also explores the use of emotional appeals in anti-tobacco campaigns as a case study of this relationship. In reviewing and discussing the existing literature on health campaigns and emotions, this chapter also offers avenues for new research and message design strategies, particularly as they pertain to the largely underexplored area of using positive and mixed emotions in health campaigns.

CAMPAIGNS AND EMOTIONS

Health campaigns have long relied on emotions to garner the attention of mass audiences and motivate behavior change. From the discrete approach, the foremost emotion to emerge from the existing literature on campaigns is fear. Fear appeals are commonplace in health campaigns aiming to prevent a variety of diseases, from anti-tobacco messages (Biener and Taylor 2002) to AIDS prevention (Freimuth, Hammond, Edgar, and Monahan 1990). In an oft-cited meta-analysis, Witte and Allen (2000) found that for experimental studies of fear appeals, greater levels of fear were associated with a relatively weak but stable positive influence on attitudes, intentions, and behavior. The meta-analysis offers many important implications for health campaign design, such as the importance of including information on severity, susceptibility, self-efficacy, and response efficacy in effective fear appeals. However, it is less clear if the finding that feelings of fear promote persuasion would hold in the nonexperimental setting of a real-world media campaign and actual behavior (Hastings, Stead, and Webb 2004). Nonetheless, many health campaigns rely on fear appeals to try to move audiences.

Fear appeals do not only scare their audiences, though. Dillard, Plotnick, Godblod, Freimuth, and Edgar (1996) found that fear appeal PSAs about AIDS evoked multiple emotions, not just fear. As Plutchik (1980) posited, emotions frequently co-occur with other emotions. Other studies confirm that health-related PSAs can evoke multiple emotions in audiences (e.g., Dillard and Peck 2000; Fishbein, Hall-Jamieson, Zimmer, von Haeften, and Nabi 2002). Dillard et al. found that most emotional responses to the PSAs shown to participants in their study were significant predictors of message acceptance. However, not all had a positive relationship with acceptance. While both fear and sadness predicted greater message acceptance, anger predicted greater rejection of the message. The authors found the effects of these different discrete emotions on message acceptance were mediated by heuristic (and not systematic) processing. In the case of those AIDS PSAs, emotional reactions to the campaign messages served as heuristic cues for audiences. That is, the participants' emotional reactions to the PSAs acted as a readily accessible source of information about the relationship between the audience member topic and behaviors discussed (Schwarz and Clore 1988).

These findings add additional nuance to the message-relevant-emotion-to-behavior link such that it may promote initial message acceptance based on heuristic persuasion, but those post-message attitudes may not be as strong as those formed by systematic processing (Chaiken 1980). However, the PSAs used in this study were visual, and the amount of information from this type of media (i.e., moving visuals and audio) may have created more cognitive load than text-based campaign messages, thus motivating heuristic processing. Future research is needed to understand how audiences' emotional reactions to mediated campaign messages impact persuasion and behavior.

Given the frequent use of emotional imagery and emotional appeals in health campaigns, it is helpful to have a conceptual framework for understanding the role of emotions in campaigns. Dunlop, Kashima, and Wakefield (2008) outlined just such a foundation. Their model examines the role of negative emotions, specifically, in mass-mediated health campaigns. The authors argue that emotional responses to health campaigns can be categorized as message-referent, plot-referent, and/or self-referent. They point out that the first two categories (message- and plot-referent) are emotional responses to the content of the message, while the final category (self-referent) are emotions triggered by "thoughts about one's life and self that are stimulated by the ad" (Dunlop et al. 2008, 55). Message- and plot-referent emotional responses can foster self-referent emotions, especially if the message content is engaging or the plot is a quality narrative that transports the audience (Green and Brock 2000) and leads to identification with characters (Cohen 2001).

Dunlop et al. (2008) posit that greater arousal of negative emotions in response to a health campaign message simultaneously leads to interpersonal discussion about the health topic and the impact of the perceived personal risk. According to their model, interpersonal discussion also impacts perceived personal risk, perceived efficacy, and social norms. Finally, their model predicts that perceived personal risk, perceived efficacy, and social norms are positive predictors of persuasive outcomes. The Dunlop et al. model argues that emotions can have a direct influence on behavior, such as when feelings alter individuals' risk perceptions and motivate action. However, emotions can also indirectly influence message reception when they shape other outcomes, such as interpersonal discussion, perceived efficacy, and social norms that, in turn, also impact risk perceptions and actions.

Individuals often talk about campaign messages with others, and this interpersonal communication is an important component of understanding a campaign's ability to change public behavior. Although the focus of a campaign is initially placed on mass communication, a growing body of research is investigating the role of interpersonal communication on campaign effects. As Southwell and Yzer (2007; 2009) describe it, the intersection of conversation and campaigns is a crucial communication space where health messages are disseminated. For instance, van den Putte, Yzer, Southwell, de Bruijn, and Willemsen (2011) found that interpersonal communication contributed significantly to the effectiveness of an anti-smoking campaign. The authors suggested that future campaigns utilize emotion-inducing mass media messages in order to foster interpersonal communication about the recommended behaviors.

Research has, in fact, connected the initiation of campaign-inspired conversation to emotional arousal. Dunlop, Kashima, and Wakefield (2010) studied female college students' responses to a radio campaign promoting the HPV vaccine. In their analysis of friendship dyads, the researchers found that participants who had stronger emotional reactions to the HPV vaccine ads were more likely to discuss the ads in the days following the initial experiment than were those who had weak emotional reactions to the HPV messages. Although emotions are short-lived phenomena, this study demonstrates that their impact can have downstream ramifications.

Conversations about emotion-evoking campaign messages operate as an agent of information diffusion for health messages, alongside mass media and other social influences. Morgan (2009) investigated the role of interpersonal conversation in organ donation campaigns under the framework of social representations theory (SRT) (Moscovici 1988). Broadly speaking, SRT posits that mass media content and interpersonal discussions both help shape the cognitions that influence social representations of an issue, which then influences the public's perceptions and ultimately their behaviors. In short, mass and interpersonal communication help individuals make sense of a situation. Morgan posits that the use of emotionally arousing content in campaigns motivates discussion and a desire to make sense of the campaign's suggested behavior. Because of the importance of emotional evocation in fostering interpersonal conversation about campaigns, she argues that relying on statistics will be less effective for organ donation and other campaigns.

In short, emotionally arousing messages are often a mainstay of health campaigns. Although fear is the most commonly employed emotional strategy, audiences frequently experience multiple emotions in response to health campaign messages. Health campaigns can influence health behaviors directly by influencing risk perceptions, motivating behavior change, and facilitating sense-making. Emotional responses to campaign messages can also indirectly shape behavior by prompting interpersonal conversation and changes in social norms and perceived efficacy. While an overarching look at the role of emotions in health campaigns is useful for understanding the breadth of their impact, a look at a specific prevention-oriented health context allows for an in-depth view of the potential effects of emotions in this domain. Below, the literature on anti-smoking campaigns provides researchers with a case study for understanding the multifaceted role of discrete emotional reactions in determining the effectiveness of health campaigns.

SMOKING PREVENTION AND CESSATION CAMPAIGNS

Globally, tobacco takes a huge toll on public health. According to the Centers for Disease Control and Prevention (2014), tobacco use causes more than five million deaths per year worldwide, with expectations for that number to rise to eight million by 2030. Domestically, tobacco is the leading cause of preventable death in the United States (Centers for Disease Control and Prevention 2014). Because of its deadly impact and addictive nature, many health campaigns have targeted tobacco use and attempted to persuade users to stop and non-users not to start. And because of the profits involved, the tobacco industry works hard in the other direction. Tobacco companies promote their products with emotional appeals that position tobacco as an effective way to fulfill the audiences' psychosocial needs like camaraderie, self-confidence, freedom, independence, pleasure, relaxation, and even social acceptability (Anderson, Glantz, and Ling 2005).

To combat the effective emotion-based marketing strategies of the tobacco industry, and to combat the highly addictive nature of their products, emotional content is also a common component of anti-tobacco campaign messages. These anti-smoking campaigns are using fire (emotional campaign messages) to fight fire (emotional tobacco ads). From graphic images of amputations and stomas caused by tobacco use to hopeful images of living a healthy life after quitting, a variety of emotional content is embedded in anti-tobacco campaign messages.

Research has examined the effects of emotional reactions to campaign messages on smoking cessation and intentions to avoid starting. Hafstad, Aarø, and Langmark (1996) studied the links between exposure to a mass media anti-smoking campaign targeting female adolescents in Norway, affective reactions to the campaign, and intentions to avoid smoking. The media messages used in the campaign were designed to create cognitive dissonance in audiences by juxtaposing societal values (i.e., being in control, being fit and attractive, and being socially responsible) with the realities of smoking (i.e., negative health impacts, unattractiveness, etc.). The researchers found that smokers had stronger emotional reactions toward the campaign messages than did non-smokers. They also found that girls had stronger emotional reactions to the messages than did boys. Moreover, positive emotional reactions to the campaign messages were the best predictor of positive behavioral outcomes (i.e., intentions to quit among smokers and intentions to never start among non-smokers). Another study by Hafstad, Stray-Pedersen, and Langmark (1997) points to the ability of emotionally evocative anti-smoking campaigns to foster interpersonal communication about the negative aspects of smoking, which in turn can facilitate behavioral outcomes. Both positive affective reactions and discussing the campaign with others were positive predictors of desired behavioral outcomes in that campaign.

In another example of the role of emotions in anti-smoking campaigns, Biener, Ji, Gilpin, and Albers (2004) found that the perceived effectiveness of anti-smoking advertisements that ran in Massachusetts during the mid-1990s depended, in part, on youths' emotional reactions to them. Members of the target audience rated a set of anti-smoking advertisements featuring serious health consequences of tobacco use as very high in negative emotion. These particular ads were the ones that participants ages twelve to fifteen rated as most effective, more so than advertisements employing humor appeals. Additionally, participants were more likely to remember the anti-smoking advertisements that evoked negative emotion than the humor appeals or advertisements featuring messages about normative behavior.

Anti-smoking campaigns that evoke emotion are also important insomuch as they foster greater discussion of the campaign's message than would less emotionally evocative messages. In a study of reactions to an emotion-based campaign targeting smokers at risk for emphysema, Durkin and Wakefield (2006) found that about a quarter of viewers of the emotional television advertisement discussed it with someone else. Those participants who discussed the advertisement with others were more likely to quit smoking than were those who did not engage in interpersonal conversation about the campaign. The connection between emotions and discussion and/or information sharing points to the dual considerations of using emotional content in health campaigns. Emotions can directly motivate individual behavior change but also indirectly motivate changes by jump-starting conversations with others that can eventually lead to behavior change.

Furthermore, socioeconomic status (SES) of audience members can result in different reactions to anti-smoking campaigns, as well as different levels of effectiveness of various campaign messaging strategies. A multiwave survey study of smoking cessation media campaigns in New York state found that smokers with low levels of education and income (i.e., low SES) were less likely than high SES smokers to recall ads that focused on how to quit (Niederdeppe, Farrelly, Nonnemaker, Davis, and Wagner 2011). The researchers also found that these low SES smokers perceived advertisements about how to quit as less effective than advertisements that relied on graphic imagery or personal testimonials. These two strategies are inherently emotion evoking as both visuals and exemplars are powerful tools for eliciting emotion (Zillmann 2006). Research also shows that use of personal emotional narratives in television news stories about social issues can help reduce political knowledge gaps between viewers with high or low education, more so than fact-based stories that only interview experts and not individuals directly impacted by an issue (Bas and Grabe 2013). This research indicates that emotional visuals and personal testimonies can be particularly promising communication strategies that help to shape policy perceptions and reduce health disparities related to tobacco use.

While different discrete emotions may be evoked by anti-tobacco campaign messages, other features of emotion can also influence audience reactions to these messages. The arousal component of emotion and individual differences in preferences for high-sensation content is also an important consideration for anti-tobacco campaigns. The intensity of the emotion evoked by an anti-smoking advertisement has been found to be an important predictor of message recall across multiple studies, with more emotional intensity leading to greater recall (Biener, Wakefield, Shiner, and Siegel 2008; Dunlop, Perez, and Cotter 2012). In other studies, researchers have found that the ability of a message to stimulate the audience (i.e., its message sensation value, or MSV) should match audiences' stable preferences for high- or low-sensation context in order to improve the effectiveness of anti-tobacco PSAs (Strasser et al. 2009).

The aforementioned studies underscore the importance of incorporating and measuring emotion and affect-related variables in research on anti-smoking campaigns. The evidence suggests that humor appeals are ineffective in promoting tobacco avoidance, while negative emotional reactions to anti-tobacco advertisements may be an effective way to promote positive outcomes. However, the answer is not so simple as to try to scare, anger, or disgust people into avoiding tobacco. Positive affective reactions can also foster behavior change, as demonstrated by the work of Hafstad et al. (1997).

These seemingly contradictory findings—negative and positive emotions have different effects in different studies—could be artifacts of a reliance on dimensional views of emotion. Future work examining the role of discrete emotions and mixed emotions could advance anti-smoking campaign message development and deployment.

In order to further explore the role of emotion in this context, two specific anti-tobacco campaigns that relied on different types of emotional appeals are discussed below. The "Tips from Former Smokers" and truth® campaigns focused on eliciting different emotional responses from audiences (fear and anger, respectively), yet both experienced success in changing attitudes and behavior. A detailed discussion of two example campaigns offers the chance to gain insight into multiple roles of various emotions in the context of anti-tobacco campaigns and also to explore future areas for future research and campaign design.

Tips

For three months in 2012, the CDC launched and ran the first federally funded anti-tobacco media campaign in the United States, a $54 million effort called "Tips from Former Smokers," "Tips" for short (Centers for Disease Control and Prevention 2012). The creators of the Tips advertisements purposefully designed them to be emotionally evocative in order to give smokers the motivation they need to attempt to overcome nicotine addiction and quit (Emery, Szczypka, Abril, Kim, and Vera 2014). The campaign relied on a combination of content elements in order to evoke an emotional response in audience members. Its messages combined moving personal testimonies with graphic images, meant to induce fear, in the hope that audiences would associate their negative reactions to the advertisements with smoking and then seek help in order to quit (Rigotti and Wakefield 2012).

Rigotti and Wakefield (2012) described some of the televised Tips advertisements: "A 31-year-old man with bilateral below-knee amputations describes losing his legs and fingertips to Buerger disease. Three people with head and neck cancer diagnosed before 50 years of age talk about daily life with a stoma ('Don't face the shower head.' and 'Be very careful with shaving.'). The mother of a young boy with severe asthma advises in English or Spanish, 'Don't be too shy to tell people not to smoke around your kids.' Three former smokers talk about how they quit and urge viewers, 'Do whatever it takes, no matter how many times it takes. We did it. You can, too'" (907).

Evaluations of the campaign suggest that Tips has been effective at drawing the attention of smokers. During the initial campaign, calls to the national smoking quitline (1-800-QUIT-NOW) increased by 132 percent, and unique visits to the National Cancer Institute's smoking cessation website increased by 428 percent (McAfee, Davis, Alexander Jr, Pechacek, and Bunnell 2013). Baseline and follow-up surveys indicated that exposure to and awareness of the Tips campaign increased cessation attempts among smokers by about 12 percent, while non-smokers who were aware of the campaign reported making slightly more recommendations to smokers to quit (Centers for Disease Control and Prevention 2012). Furthermore, the researchers found that awareness of the Tips campaign corresponded with a greater likelihood of talking with friends and family about the dangers of smoking, an important outcome given the role of interpersonal communication in facilitating positive campaign outcomes (McAfee et al. 2013).

The results from the initial 2012 campaign were promising enough that the CDC launched a new round of Tips advertisements in 2014 (Serrie 2014). This iteration of the campaign also included messages about the threat of cancer from smoking, but additionally it included ads addressing other, less-emphasized risks of smoking, like the negative impacts on oral health, on people with HIV, and on pregnant women. Although the personal testimonies used in the campaign came from different people than the messages used in the first campaign, and some of the health outcomes featured in the messages are different from the first round of the campaign, the newer messages follow the same formula of using personal testimonies and graphic images to portray the seriousness of the health threats associated with smoking.

Beyond the behavioral outcomes of Tips, research into the communication responses to the campaign also shed light on the role of emotional responses in the campaign's effects. Emery et al. (2014) studied how the public reacted to the campaign on social media by conducting a content analysis of nearly two hundred thousand tweets related to the Tips campaign. Using coding categories based on the concepts of the Extended Parallel Process Model, the researchers found that nearly nine out of ten tweets (87 percent) showed signs of message acceptance (e.g., stating that the advertisements seemed effective or made them want to quit), while 7 percent of the tweets appeared to reject the messages put forward by the campaign (e.g., stating that the ads made them want to smoke more or that the ads were a waste of tax dollars). Many of the tweets analyzed in the study explicitly expressed sentiments associated with fear, such as mentioning that the ads were scary or frightening. Although there was no data connecting the Twitter responses directly to behavioral reactions, these results indicate the campaign did evoke emotions and fostered message acceptance in the majority of social media users who viewed the advertisements.

The early evaluations of Tips point to the effectiveness of showing audiences vivid consequences of smoking in order to foster behavior change. However, so far none of the published evaluations have specifically measured fear reactions as mediators of persuasion, nor have they linked actual fear reactions to actual quitting behavior. Given that previous research shows that health messages intended to be fear appeals can evoke multiple emotions (Dillard et al. 1996; Williams-Piehota, Pizarro, Schneider, Mowad, and Salovey 2005), it is also possible the positive behavioral outcomes of the Tips campaign are not associated solely with fear reactions. Research on how smokers and their loved ones respond to the ads, including which emotional reactions best predicted conversations and behavior change, would significantly advance our understanding of why, exactly, Tips appears to be effective. Moreover, are the most frightening of the ads (e.g., ads showing amputation or stomas) associated with greatest effectiveness, or are more moderately frightening ads (ads showing asthma) more effective? How do the various emotional responses to the Tips campaign relate to depth of information processing and long-term smoking cessation behaviors? Research that answers these questions would help determine the psychosocial and emotional mechanisms behind the Tips campaigns' preliminary accomplishments.

truth®

The Florida Department of Health used funds from its settlement with the tobacco industry to create and implement the "truth"® campaign in 1998 (Hicks 2001). The campaign specifically targeted youth ages twelve to seventeen in the hopes= of preventing them from starting to smoke and convincing them to quit if they already did. Known as tobacco counter-advertising or counter-marketing, the truth® campaign used prominently placed media advertisements to emphasize the tactics used by the tobacco industry to promote their products. Furthermore, the campaign sought to make truth® its own brand, just like the strategies used by cigarette companies, and it included giveaways of branded items, such as T-shirts, in addition to keeping a consistent theme throughout its media messages (Farrelly et al. 2002).

The advertising agency hired to create the campaign found in its formative research that Florida youth were already well aware that tobacco could kill, convincing the agency that further repeating that fact would not be an effective strategy for changing youths' attitudes or behaviors (Hicks 2001). Based on their research, the campaign designers decided to instead focus on the affective connection many youth form with tobacco use: "We learned that a youth's reason for using tobacco had everything to do with emotion and nothing to do with rational decision making. Tobacco was a significant, visible, and readily available way for youth to signal that they were in control . . . what made tobacco so alluring to youth was its deadly qualities" (Hicks 2001, 4).

The campaign designers decided to "turn the tables on tobacco" and use the truth® campaign to turn anti-tobacco protest into its own form of youth rebellion, except the rebellion would be against the "duplicity and manipulation of the tobacco industry" and not against parents or teachers (Hicks 2001, 4). An example of the "truth" messaging strategy that employed what the designers called "edgy humor" was an advertisement with an old white man with balding white hair laying on the beach smoking a cigarette wearing nothing but a women's bikini and men's black work socks. The text read "No wonder tobacco executives hide behind sexy models. WARNING: Their brand is lies. Our brand is truth" (Hicks 2001, 4). Other ads in the campaign were more graphic. In a television ad titled "Body Bags," a group of teens stands outside the corporate headquarters of tobacco giant Philip Morris (now called Altria) with stacks of body bags near them, yelling into a megaphone that the body bags represent the number of people who die each day as a result of smoking (Apollonio and Malone 2009).

Youth who saw and recalled televised truth® advertisements in the Florida campaign were less likely to start smoking in the first six months of the campaign than were those who were unaware of the campaign (Hicks 2001, 4). Furthermore, research indicates that those who saw more of the advertisements (that is, they received a higher dose) reported stronger anti-tobacco industry manipulation attitudes (Sly, Hopkins, Trapido, and Ray 2001). Eventually, the truth® campaign was expanded to the national level and proved successful on that playing field, too. Exposure to the national truth® campaign proved successful in changing adolescents' attitudes, beliefs, and intentions to smoke (Sly, Trapido, and Ray 2002). Dunlop (2011) found that the campaign was able to facilitate interpersonal communication, although the benefit to behavior change depended on if those exposed to the campaign evaluated it favorably (leading to positive attitudes, beliefs, and intentions) or unfavorably (leading to negative attitudes, beliefs, and intentions).

The emotion most likely evoked by the truth® campaign is anger—anger toward tobacco companies that the campaign portrays as manipulating the public. The action tendency of anger is to seek revenge and remedy the wrongdoing. By not purchasing tobacco products, youth may have satisfied this action tendency and felt they were avenging the wrongs done to them by youth-targeted marketing practices.

Additionally, the display of body bags and other evidence of the danger of tobacco, used to show the duplicity of the tobacco industry, likely evoked at least some level of fear. This fear, as discussed above, may have contributed to the ability of the campaign ads to prevent smoking initiation. Multiple studies have found that the activation of fear and anger often accompany each other (e.g., Schwartz and Weinberger 1980; C. A. Smith and Ellsworth 1987). Despite the likelihood that both of these emotional reactions to the Tips campaign occurred and influenced important communication and health outcomes, the literature is lacking in an analysis of specific multiemotional responses to this campaign. Future work could examine these emotions, as well as others, as potential mechanisms for the campaign's effectiveness.

Another emotional reaction to explore in conjunction with a campaign like truth® would be schadenfreude, which is the experience of malicious pleasure at an another's misfortune (Leach, Spears, Branscombe, and Doosje 2003). Schadenfreude is linked with feelings of envy such that the experience is particularly likely if the misfortune befalls on an envied other (R. H. Smith et al. 1996). Whether the misfortune is deserved or undeserved also makes a difference in how much schadenfreude an individual may experience. If individuals perceive a person or entity suffering from a misfortune to be deserving of the bad luck, then feelings of schadenfreude are likely to be stronger than if the target was undeserving (van Dijk, Ouwerkerk, Goslinga, and Nieweg 2005). In the case of the truth®, the purpose of the campaign was to show that the tobacco companies purposefully deceived and manipulated the public. If audiences accepted the campaign messages, as the evaluations suggest they did, then they likely felt the tobacco companies deserved the loss of their business as well as any government sanctions that may have been placed on the industry

POSITIVE EMOTIONS AND COMBINATIONS OF EMOTIONS EVOKED BY CAMPAIGNS

Both the general discussion of research on health campaigns as well as the examinations of anti-smoking campaigns presented above heavily emphasized negative emotions. Yet health campaigns with more uplifting messages and positive emotional overtones do exist. For instance, the American Cancer Society launched a campaign with the mantra "Help Create a World with Less Cancer and More Birthdays" as a way to motivate people to seek information and take steps to prevent cancer occurrence and reoccurrence, detect it early, and help fund research for cancer treatment (PCNA: Preventive Cardiovascular Nurses Association 2012; Seffrin 2011). The campaign included social media messages with celebrities and famous musicians singing "happy birthday" as well as mass television ads with uplifting images and music. No explicit appeal to fear was involved.

Using fear may not be an effective way to maintain commitment to long-term behavior change for all types of health issues. In an opinion piece on the limitations of fear appeals in tobacco control, Hastings and MacFadyen (2002) write, "We know that smoking is emotionally involving and that quitting is a hard, often drawn out process. It cries out for relationship building that, at the very least, will make quitters feel better about themselves. . . . Fear messages do not sit easily with this thinking. If they have any relational dimension at all, it is as the hectoring parent to the erring child, rather than the adult to adult of commercial marketing" (74). The authors go on to note that fear appeals may inspire smokers to attempt to quit, but they do little to build lasting relationships and foster sustained attention to general well-being, including better diet, exercise, and other healthy behaviors, instead of only smoking cessation. Furthermore, using fear to focus audiences' attention squarely on personal risks of smoking and individual behavior change leaves little space for discussing cultural, societal, and political factors that also encourage tobacco use and other unhealthy behaviors.

Additionally, campaigns are often promoted in conjunction with community organizations that can both provide additional information and social support in order to foster positive health behaviors (Stephens, Rimal, and Flora 2004). The social support provided by such organizations often includes attempts to offer individuals some hope, inspiration, and other forms of emotional support (Uchino 2006; Uchino, Cacioppo, and Kiecolt-Glaser 1996). If these secondary sources of campaign-related information and support are grounded in more positive emotional overtones of support and hope while the original mass media message was fear inducing, then research in the persuasion literature on matching indicates that the initial messages pointing audiences to these resources may be more effective if they are likewise hopeful or inspirational in tone (e.g., DeSteno, Petty, Rucker, Wegener, and Braverman 2004; DeSteno, Petty, Wegener, and Rucker 2000).

However, the alternative possibility is that fear-inducing campaign messages may motivate individuals to seek out these local organizations that can provide relief from their anxiety, resulting in emotional shifts that promote attitude change and possibly action (Nabi and Green 2014). Future research could investigate the relationships between the emotional tone of mass media campaign messages and the emotional nature of local organizations' messages and/or interpersonal communication in order to see how inter-message emotions impact health behaviors. Of course, many individual differences and contextual factors may moderate the nature of the relationship between a campaign message and a local organization's message, and these should also be configured into more advanced campaign pretesting and evaluation designs.

While fear appeals may be effective at gaining the public's attention, particularly in an oversaturated media environment, campaign designers might also consider creating messages that include a mix of emotional appeals given the strong link between emotional arousal and effectiveness of campaigns. For instance, Biener and Taylor (2002) describe a televised anti-tobacco ad called "Cigarette Pack" in which a smoker puts a picture of his daughter on his cigarette packs to remind him why he needs to quit. Biener and Taylor describe this ad as one capable of evoking hope and empathy for those striving to kick the habit, and it ran alongside other ads that they describe as evoking emotions from sadness for family members, anger toward tobacco companies, and fear that tobacco can kill. The researchers did find the overall campaign to be effective, although they did not analyze the various effects of specific emotional responses such as hope, compassion, or fear.

Additionally, in an experiment comparing the efficacy of empathy-versus fear-arousing anti-smoking PSAs (Biener 2002; Biener, McCallum-Keeler, and Nyman 2000), the researchers found that both could be effective when compared to a control ad. However, the empathy-arousing PSAs were more effective than the fear-arousing ones, partially because feelings of fear had a negative indirect effect on persuasion because fear induced higher levels of reactance against the message. Fear may be an effective strategy for campaign designers, especially when the assessment of persuasiveness is recorded immediately after message exposure. However, evoking fear may also contribute to boomerang effects against health campaign messages, such as reactance or distrust of the source who is attempting to manipulate audience feelings in a negative direction.

While there are promising alternatives to fear appeals, researchers should keep in mind that it is often unavoidable to illicit at least some amount of fear when discussing a health threat. Therefore, it is important to understand how multiple emotions operate side by side with cognitions to shape audience reactions to campaigns. For example, Dillard and Peck (2000) tested both emotional and cognitive reactions to multiple health- and safety-related public service announcements. They found that different discrete emotions had different effects on perceived effectiveness of the PSAs. In their study, fear, sadness, and happiness all had a positive impact on perceived effectiveness, while anger and contentment had negative effects on the measure. Furthermore, the dominant cognitive response of participants to the PSAs was also a significant and positive predictor of perceived effectiveness, often more so than any one emotion. This study demonstrates that a discrete emotional approach to analyzing a variety of emotions, both negative *and* positive, can provide insights into campaign message effectiveness.

This is one example of how positive and mixed emotional messages can be an effective part of a larger campaign plan that still includes messages portraying the seriousness of health threats such as tobacco use. Because positive emotions can serve as a buffer against self-threatening information (Das and Fennis 2008; Raghunathan and Trope 2002), disseminating more positive-oriented messages at the beginning of a campaign may prevent rejection and promote engagement with more-threatening fear-inducing messages that could come later in the campaign. Future work in this area could study the role of emotional flow across the span of multiple exposures to a variety of health campaign messages (Nabi and Green 2014).

Furthermore, the dual importance of emotional *and* cognitive reactions to campaign messages deserves attention in a discussion of the role of emotions in health campaigns. Monahan (1995) points out a number of ways that positive emotional appeals, specifically, can elicit both cognitive and behavioral responses from audiences. First, positive affect can capture the public's attention because they can overcome barriers to selective perception. Especially for audiences who are not motivated to think deeply about a campaign message, positive affect may serve as a heuristic that the message is safe and they should engage with it. Then, because positive emotions result in an approach motivation, a positive emotional response to a health campaign message allows the audience to be open and receptive. Furthermore, positive emotions can facilitate recall of campaign messages as well as contribute to positive attitudes and behavior change. These cognitive and behavioral responses to positive-toned health messages described by Monahan are ones that could be utilized by future campaigns, particularly in contexts where a fear appeal may be either ineffective or unethical (Guttman and Salmon 2004; Hastings et al. 2004).

Which positive and mixed emotions might be most useful will depend on the health threat and the target audience. If the threat is specific to a certain ethnic group, then pride appeals may be effective (see chapter 7 about pride, this volume), while more general threats might benefit from some messaging evoking hope (see chapter 9 about hope, this volume). In the case where there is a novel approach to prevention (e.g., a new type of sunscreen), fostering feelings of interest may also be an effective approach for audiences who like to learn (see chapter 8 about interest, this volume).

What would make these decisions clearer would be the development of a greater theoretical base for understanding how positive emotions impact reactions to health campaign messages, akin to Dunlop et al. (2008)'s framework for understanding the role of negative emotions in health campaigns. This conceptual framework should consider the approach motivations associated with positive emotions as well as the conditions under which positive emotional reactions may foster heuristic versus systematic information processing of health risk information. Because positive affect can serve as a buffer against self-threatening information (Das and Fennis 2008; Raghunathan and Trope 2002), the juxtaposition of a health threat in a message alongside the approach motivation of positive emotions may, in certain circumstances, promote greater processing of health threat information than would positive or negative emotions on their own. Future research is needed to test these suppositions in a variety of health contexts.

Moreover, future work on the role of emotions in health campaigns would also benefit from the measurement of discrete emotions in addition to general positive and negative affect. For instance, a study of students' (grades five through twelve) perceptions of thirty anti-drug public service announcements (PSAs) found that perceived effectiveness of the PSAs was highly and positively correlated with realism, amount learned, and negative emotion, while perceived effectiveness was negatively correlated with positive emotion ($r =$ -.35, $p =$.06) (Fishbein et al. 2002). Furthermore, the researchers found that none of the three humorous PSAs in the sample were judged to be effective, with two of the three humorous PSAs rated were perceived by students as having significant negative effects. These findings are helpful in that humor appeared to be ineffective. Yet the lumping together of positive and negative emotion makes it less clear how different emotions impacted the outcomes.

As with any persuasive health message, careful planning, formative research, pretesting, and early evaluation work should be used to find the most effective strategies. For some contexts, such as contaminated food recalls or a new vaccine to thwart the quick spread of a novel strain of influenza, fear appeals may be necessary in order for campaign messages to quickly grab the public's attention and motivate them to act. However, in situations in which the public is already highly knowledgeable about the health threat and ways to overcome it, fresh approaches integrating positive and mixed emotions into health campaigns may prove useful in the toolkit of public health advocates.

CONCLUSION

Emotion-evoking media content is a vital ingredient in prevention-focused health campaigns. In particular, using fear to point the attention of audiences toward health threats and motivate them to address those threats is a common campaign tactic. Researchers have found fear appeals to be (generally) effective at shaping attitudes in experimental settings as well as in evaluations of campaigns. However, there are ethical and empirical concerns about their efficacy for fostering actual behavior change, in addition to information seeking or attitude change. Moreover, little work to date has directly compared fear-based campaigns with those that instead rely on messages promoting positive lifestyles or that aim to evoke positive emotions. Research on combining negative and positive emotion-based health campaign messages is also lacking, and may provide additional insights as to the most effective types of emotional appeals to use in mass media campaigns aimed at preventing illness.

Beyond studying the effects of evoking specific emotions in campaign audiences, campaign designers would be well served to keep in mind the emotional intensity of their messages as research indicates higher intensity is associated with greater message recall. Many preventable conditions continue to threaten the public, from tobacco, drug, and alcohol abuse to obesity-related disease and various types of cancer. Including an analysis of audiences' emotional reactions, as well as investigating what type of campaign message features foster these various emotional reactions, is an important step for advancing research on how to create more effective public health campaigns.

REFERENCES

Anderson, S. J., S. A. Glantz, and P. M. Ling. 2005. Emotions for sale: Cigarette advertising and women's psychosocial needs. *Tobacco Control* 14(2):127–35. doi: 10.1136/tc.2004.009076.

Apollonio, D. E., and R. E. Malone. 2009. Turning negative into positive: Public health mass media campaigns and negative advertising. *Health Education Research* 24(3):483–95. doi: 10.1093/her/cyn046.

Bas, O., and M. E. Grabe. 2013. Emotion-provoking personalization of news: Informing citizens and closing the knowledge gap? *Communication Research.* doi: 10.1177/0093650213514602.

Biener, L. 2002. Anti-tobacco advertisements by Massachusetts and Philip Morris: What teenagers think. *Tobacco Control* 11(suppl 2):ii43–ii46. doi: 10.1136/tc.11.suppl_2.ii43.

Biener, L., M. Ji, E. A. Gilpin, and A. B. Albers. 2004. The impact of emotional tone, message, and broadcast parameters in youth anti-smoking advertisements. *Journal of Health Communication* 9(3):259–74. doi: 10.1080/10810730490447084.

Biener, L., G. McCallum-Keeler, and A. L. Nyman. 2000. Adults' response to Massachusetts anti-tobacco television advertisements: Impact of viewer and advertisement characteristics. *Tobacco Control* 9(4):401–7. doi: 10.1136/tc.9.4.401.

Biener, L., and T. M. Taylor. 2002. The continuing importance of emotion in tobacco control media campaigns: A response to Hastings and MacFadyen. *Tobacco Control* 11(1):75–77. doi: 10.1136/tc.11.1.75.

Biener, L., M. Wakefield, C. M. Shiner, and M. Siegel. 2008. How broadcast volume and emotional content affect youth recall of anti-tobacco advertising. *American Journal of Preventive Medicine* 35(1):14–19. doi: http://dx.doi.org/10.1016/j.amepre.2008.03.018.

Centers for Disease Control and Prevention. 2012. Increases in quitline calls and smoking cessation website visitors during a national tobacco education campaign—March 19–June 10, 2012. *Morbidity and Mortality Weekly Report* 61(34):667–70.

———. 2014, April 24. Smoking and tobacco use. Retrieved June 26, 2014, from http://www.cdc.gov/tobacco/data_statistics/fact_sheets/fast_facts/.

Chaiken, S. 1980. Heuristic versus systematic information processing and the use of source versus message cues in persuasion. *Journal of Personality and Social Psychology* 39(5):752–66.

Cohen, J. 2001. Defining identification: A theoretical look at the identification of audiences with media characters. *Mass Communication and Society* 4(3):245–64. doi: 10.1207/S15327825MCS0403_01.

Das, E., and B. M. Fennis. 2008. In the mood to face the facts: When a positive mood promotes systematic processing of self-threatening information. *Motivation and Emotion* 32(3):221–30.

DeSteno, D., R. E. Petty, D. D. Rucker, D. T. Wegener, and J. Braverman. 2004. Discrete emotions and persuasion: The role of emotion-induced expectancies. *Journal of Personality and Social Psychology* 86(1):43–56. doi: 10.1037/0022-3514.86.1.43.

DeSteno, D., R. E. Petty, D. T. Wegener, and D. D. Rucker. 2000. Beyond valence in the perception of likelihood: The role of emotion specificity. *Journal of Personality and Social Psychology* 78(3):397–416. doi: 10.1037/0022-3514.78.3.397.

Dillard, J. P., and E. Peck. 2000. Affect and persuasion: Emotional responses to public service announcements. *Communication Research* 27(4):461–95. doi: 10.1177/009365000027004003.

Dillard, J. P., C. A. Plotnick, L. C. Godblod, V. S. Freimuth, and T. Edgar. 1996. The multiple affective outcomes of AIDS PSAs: Fear appeals do more than scare people. *Communication Research* 23(1):44–72. doi: 10.1177/009365096023001002.

Dunlop, S. M. 2011. Talking "truth": Predictors and consequences of conversations about a youth antismoking campaign for smokers and nonsmokers. *Journal of Health Communication* 16(7):708–25. doi: 10.1080/10810730.2011.552000.

Dunlop, S. M., Y. Kashima, and M. Wakefield. 2008. Can you feel it? Negative emotion, risk, and narrative in health communication. *Media Psychology* 11:52–75.

Dunlop, S. M., Y. Kashima, and M. Wakefield. 2010. Predictors and consequences of conversations about health promoting media messages. *Communication Monographs* 77(4):518–39. doi: 10.1080/03637751.2010.502537.

Dunlop, S. M., D. Perez, and T. Cotter. 2012. The natural history of antismoking advertising recall: The influence of broadcasting parameters, emotional intensity and executional features. *Tobacco Control*. doi: 10.1136/tobaccocontrol-2011-050256.

Durkin, S., and M. Wakefield. 2006. Maximizing the impact of emotive antitobacco advertising: Effects of interpersonal discussion and program placement. *Social Marketing Quarterly* 12(3):3–14. doi: 10.1080/15245000600851334.

Emery, S. L., G. Szczypka, E. P. Abril, Y. Kim, and L. Vera. 2014. Are you scared yet? Evaluating fear appeal messages in tweets about the Tips campaign. *Journal of Communication* 64(2):278–95. doi: 10.1111/jcom.12083.

Engs, R. C. 2000. *Clean living movements: American cycles of health reform.* Westport, CT: Praeger.

Farrelly, M. C., C. G. Healton, K. C. Davis, P. Messeri, J. C. Hersey, and M. L. Haviland. 2002. Getting to the "truth": Evaluating national tobacco countermarketing campaigns. *American Journal of Public Health* 92(6):901–7. doi: 10.2105/AJPH.92.6.901.

Fishbein, M., K. Hall-Jamieson, E. Zimmer, I. von Haeften, and R. Nabi. 2002. Avoiding the boomerang: Testing the relative effectiveness of antidrug public service announcements before a national campaign. *American Journal of Public Health* 92(2):238–45. doi: 10.2105/AJPH.92.2.238.

Freimuth, V. S., S. L. Hammond, T. Edgar, and J. L. Monahan. 1990. Reaching those at risk: A content-analytic study of AIDS PSAs. *Communication Research* 17(6):775–91. doi: 10.1177/009365029001700604.

Green, M. C., and T. C. Brock. 2000. The role of transportation in the persuasiveness of public narratives. *Journal of Personality and Social Psychology* 79(5):701–21.

Guttman, N., and C. T. Salmon. 2004. Guilt, fear, stigma and knowledge gaps: Ethical issues in public health communication interventions. *Bioethics* 18(6):531–52. doi: 10.1111/j.1467-8519.2004.00415.x.

Hafstad, A., L. E. Aarø, and F. Langmark. 1996. Evaluation of an anti-smoking mass media campaign targeting adolescents: The role of affective responses and interpersonal communication. *Health Education Research* 11(1):29–38. doi: 10.1093/her/11.1.29.

Hafstad, A., B. Stray-Pedersen, and F. Langmark. 1997. Use of provocative emotional appeals in a mass media campaign designed to prevent smoking among adolescents. *The European Journal of Public Health* 7(2):122–27. doi: 10.1093/eurpub/7.2.122.

Hastings, G., and L. MacFadyen. 2002. The limitations of fear messages. *Tobacco Control* 11(1):73–75. doi: 10.1136/tc.11.1.73.

Hastings, G., M. Stead, and J. Webb. 2004. Fear appeals in social marketing: Strategic and ethical reasons for concern. *Psychology and Marketing* 21(11):961–86. doi: 10.1002/mar.20043.

Hicks, J. J. 2001. The strategy behind Florida's "truth" campaign. *Tobacco Control* 10(1):3–5. doi: 10.1136/tc.10.1.3.

Leach, C. W., R. Spears, N. R. Branscombe, and B. Doosje. 2003. Malicious pleasure: Schadenfreude at the suffering of another group. *Journal of Personality and Social Psychology* 84(5):932–43. doi: 10.1037/0022-3514.84.5.932.

Masters, R. K., D. A. Powers, and B. G. Link. 2013. Obesity and US mortality risk over the adult life course. *American Journal of Epidemiology* 177(5):431–42. doi: 10.1093/aje/kws325.

McAfee, T., K. C. Davis, R. L. Alexander Jr, T. F. Pechacek, and R. Bunnell. 2013. Effect of the first federally funded US antismoking national media campaign. *The Lancet* 382(9909):2003–11. doi: 10.1016/S0140-6736(13)61686-4.

Monahan, J. L. 1995. Thinking positively: Using positive affect when designing health messags. In E. W. Maibach and R. Parrott (Eds.), *Designing health messages: Approaches from communication theory and public health practice* (pp. 81–98). Thousand Oaks, CA: SAGE.

Morgan, S. E. 2009. The intersection of conversation, cognitions, and campaigns: The social representation of organ donation. *Communication Theory* 19(1):29–48. doi: 10.1111/j.1468-2885.2008.01331.x.

Moscovici, S. 1988. Notes towards a description of social representations. *European Journal of Social Psychology* 18(3):211–50. doi: 10.1002/ejsp.2420180303.

Nabi, R. L., and M. C. Green. 2014. The role of a narrative's emotional flow in promoting persuasive outcomes. *Media Psychology*, 1–26. doi: 10.1080/15213269.2014.912585.

Niederdeppe, J., M. C. Farrelly, J. Nonnemaker, K. C. Davis, and L. Wagner. 2011. Socioeconomic variation in recall and perceived effectiveness of campaign advertisements to promote smoking cessation. *Social Science and Medicine* 72(5):773–80. doi: 10.1016/j.socscimed.2010.12.025.

Paisley, W., and C. K. Atkin. 2013. Public communication campaigns—the American experience. In R. E. Rice and C. K. Atkin (Eds.), *Public communication campaigns* (Fourth ed., pp. 21–34). Thousand Oaks, CA: Sage.

PCNA: Preventive Cardiovascular Nurses Association. (2012). PCNA news. *Journal of Cardiovascular Nursing* 27(6):457–60. doi: 10.1097/JCN.0b013e318272b5c0.

Perloff, R. M. 2010. *The dynamics of persuasion: Communication and attitudes in the 21st century* (4th ed.). New York: Routledge.

Plutchik, R. 1980. *Emotion: A psychoevolutionary synthesis*. New York: Harper and Row.

Raghunathan, R., and Y. Trope. 2002. Walking the tightrope between feeling good and being accurate: Mood as a resource in processing persuasive messages. *Journal of Personality and Social Psychology* 83(3):510–25. doi: 10.1037/0022-3514.83.3.510.

Rigotti, N. A., and M. Wakefield. 2012. Real people, real stories: A new mass media campaign that could help smokers quit. *Annals of Internal Medicine* 157(12):907–9. doi: 10.7326/0003-4819-156-1-201201010-00541.

Schwartz, G. E., and D. A. Weinberger. 1980. Patterns of emotional responses to affective situations: Relations among happiness, sadness, anger, fear, depression, and anxiety. *Motivation and Emotion* 4(2):175–91. doi: 10.1007/BF00995197.

Schwarz, N., and G. L. Clore. 1988. How do I feel about it? The informative function of mood. In K. Fiedler and J. P. Forgas (Eds.), *Affect, cognition and social behavior* (pp. 44–62). Toronto: C. J. Hogrefe.

Seffrin, J. R. 2011. Conquering cancer in the 21st century: Leading a movement to save more lives worldwide. *Health Education and Behavior* 38(2):111–15. doi: 10.1177/1090198111404836.

Serrie, J. 2014. CDC releases new round of anti-smoking ads featuring former smokers. *Fox News.* http://www.foxnews.com/health/2014/06/24/cdc-releases-new-round-anti-smoking-ads-featuring-former-smokers/.

Sly, D. F., R. S. Hopkins, E. Trapido, and S. Ray. 2001. Influence of a counteradvertising media campaign on initiation of smoking: the Florida "truth" campaign. *American Journal of Public Health* 91(2):233–38.

Sly, D. F., E. Trapido, and S. Ray. 2002. Evidence of the dose effects of an antitobacco counteradvertising campaign. *Preventive Medicine* 35(5):511–18. doi: http://dx.doi.org/10.1006/pmed.2002.1100.

Smith, C. A., and P. C. Ellsworth. 1987. Patterns of appraisal and emotion related to taking an exam. *Journal of Personality and Social Psychology* 52(3):475–88. doi: 10.1037/0022-3514.52.3.475.

Smith, R. H., T. J. Turner, R. Garonzik, C. W. Leach, V. Urch-Druskat, and C. M. Weston. 1996. Envy and schadenfreude. *Personality and Social Psychology Bulletin* 22(2):158–68. doi: 10.1177/0146167296222005.

Southwell, B. G., and M. C. Yzer. 2007. The roles of interpersonal communication in mass media campaigns. In C. Beck (Ed.), *Communication Yearbook* (Vol. 31, pp. 420–62). New York: Lawrence Erlbaum.

———. 2009. When (and why) interpersonal talk matters for campaigns. *Communication Theory* 19(1):1–8. doi: 10.1111/j.1468-2885.2008.01329.x.

Stahre, M., J. Roeber, D. Kanny, R. D. Brewer, and X. Zhang. 2014. Contribution of excessive alcohol consumption to deaths and years of potential life lost in the United States. *Preventing Chronic Disease* 11. doi: 10.5888/pcd11.130293.

Stephens, K. K., R. N. Rimal, and J. A. Flora. 2004. Expanding the reach of health campaigns: Community organizations as meta-channels for the dissemination of health information. *Journal of Health Communication* 9 (sup1):97–111. doi: 10.1080/10810730490271557.

Strasser, A. A., J. N. Cappella, C. Jepson, M. Fishbein, K. Z. Tang, E. Han, and C. Lerman. 2009. Experimental evaluation of antitobacco PSAs: Effects of message content and format on physiological and behavioral outcomes. *Nicotine and Tobacco Research* 11(3):293–302. doi: 10.1093/ntr/ntn026.

Uchino, B. N. 2006. Social support and health: A review of physiological processes potentially underlying links to disease outcomes. *Journal of Behavioral Medicine* 29(4):377–87. doi: 10.1007/s10865-006-9056-5.

Uchino, B. N., J. T. Cacioppo, and J. K. Kiecolt-Glaser. 1996. The relationship between social support and physiological processes: A review with emphasis on underlying mechanisms and implications for health. *Psychological Bulletin* 119(3):488–531. doi: 10.1037/0033-2909.119.3.488.

van den Putte, B., M. Yzer, B. G. Southwell, G.-L. de Bruijn, and M. C. Willemsen. 2011. Interpersonal communication as an indirect pathway for the effect of antismoking media content on smoking cessation. *Journal of Health Communication* 16(5):470–85. doi: 10.1080/10810730.2010.546487.

van Dijk, W. W., J. W. Ouwerkerk, S. Goslinga, and M. Nieweg. 2005. Deservingness and schadenfreude. *Cognition and Emotion* 19(6):933–39. doi: 10.1080/02699930541000066.

Wakefield, M. A., B. Loken, and R. C. Hornik. 2010. Use of mass media campaigns to change health behaviour. *The Lancet* 376(9748):1261–71. doi: 10.1016/S0140-6736(10)60809-4.

Williams-Piehota, P., J. Pizarro, T. R. Schneider, L. Mowad, and P. Salovey. 2005. Matching health messages to monitor-blunter coping styles to motivate screening mammography. *Health Psychology* 24(1):58–67. doi: 10.1037/0278-6133.24.1.58.

Witte, K., and M. Allen. 2000. A meta-analysis of fear appeals: Implications for effective public health campaigns. *Health Education and Behavior* 27(5):591–615.

Zillmann, D. 2006. Exemplification effects in the promotion of safety and health. *Journal of Communication* 56:S221–S237. doi: 10.1111/j.1460-2466.2006.00291.x.

Chapter Twelve

Health Journalism

Despite tales of impending doom for the journalism industry, Americans are actually spending more time consuming news content than they used to, with the Internet the fastest growing source of that content (Pew Research Center Journalism Project 2014). The Internet is an especially important medium for the dissemination of health information, including that from news websites. Meanwhile, news outlets continue to produce health-related content in print, radio, podcast, and television formats, too. Because it is so commonly a source of health information for the public and can serve to educate them on potential health threats as well as preventative behaviors to avoid such threats, emotional reactions to news stories are likewise an important area for health communication researchers to study.

Health journalism is reporting that covers issues of personal or public health (Myrick 2014). Broadly speaking, health journalism can also include reporting on medicine and other issues with medical implications, such as sports news that covers the surgery of a star athlete or celebrity coverage that discusses substance abuse and addiction. Health and medical reporting is a common beat, or news topic, covered by major international and national news outlets as well as at many local ones. The public can use information seen in the news media to take preventive actions, or not, depending on how motivated they are. Moreover, coverage of health issues in the news can also influence public support for health-related policies (Coleman, Thorson, and Wilkins 2011; Iyengar 1991; Lawrence 2004).

And despite its reputation for being coldly objective, journalism can evoke strong emotions in news consumers (Bas and Grabe 2015). News of threatening diseases or injuries could lead to feelings of fear or anxiety in audiences. Additionally, health news reports that tell the moving stories of individuals and their trials with illness can spark empathy and feelings of elevation, among other emotions, in news audiences. Pictures, videos, and other visual content in health-related news stories can amplify news consumers' emotional responses to journalistic reports on issues of health.

The purpose of this chapter is to discuss various models of health journalism and the corresponding implications for how and when discrete emotions arise from consuming health news. This topic is of particular importance for understanding media influences on prevention behaviors given that news coverage can educate audiences about potential threats, provide them with information about how to take preventative action, and even motivate them to take action to help themselves or others. Throughout this chapter, conceptual frameworks that help explain the role of emotions in health news effects are presented as tools for better understanding the many ways in which health news media may influence health behaviors and health-related policy support. Directions for future research related to emotions and health journalism are also discussed.

PROBLEMS WITH HEALTH JOURNALISM AND PROPOSED SOLUTIONS

Those who closely monitor health journalism warn that much reporting falls short of the level of quality necessary to fully inform the public about such issues or promote responsible health behaviors (Schwitzer 2014; Thorson 2006). As Schwitzer (2014) points out, many health news stories fail to describe risk in absolute (versus relative) terms, to explain the limitations of observational and/or correlational studies, to present anecdotes in adequate context, to use a multitude of sources apart from news releases, to distinguish between surrogate markers and clinical end points, to parse out both the benefits and harms of screening tests, to adequately question new medical/ health technologies, and to be more critical in their coverage of health care businesses.

These shortcomings of health news stories may distort news consumers' perceptions of threat, efficacy, and the necessity of action for addressing preventable health problems. This list of inadequacies is lengthy and has motivated researchers and public health advocates to champion different models for improving health journalism. Two of these frameworks are the public health model of journalism and behavioral journalism. Below, these models are outlined and compared. They take quite different approaches to informing the public about health issues via news media, and they likely have different implications for how news audiences will respond to health news, including to stories with implications for prevention.

The public health model of journalism calls for reporters to include information on context, risk factors, and prevention strategies in stories related to public health, broadly defined (Coleman and Thorson 2002; Dorfman, Thorson, and Stevens 2001; Dorfman, Woodruff, Chavez, and Wallack 1997). Coleman and Thorson (2002) explicate this approach to health reporting as one that "sees the causes of death and injury as preventable rather than inevitable. By studying the interaction among the victims, the agent, and the environment, the public health approach seeks to define risk factors, then develop and evaluate methods to prevent problems that threaten public health" (402). The public health model asks reporters to emphasize the wide ecology of influences on public health, ranging from individual behaviors to cultural, political, and economic factors. It argues that including the latter, societal-level factors in health news reports is of utmost importance for convincing the public that policy and community-wide changes are often needed to improve public health.

Notably, the public health model takes a broad approach to defining what is a public health issue. For example, the model includes violence and crime issues in the category of public health problems because they lead directly to bodily and mental harm. This comprehensive definition of what a public health issue is stands in contrast to how health topics are traditionally defined by many news organizations. In the typical news media environment, violence and crime are not viewed or written about as health issues but instead would be in breaking news or local news segments (Thorson 2006).

Behavioral journalism, on the other hand, calls on reporters to employ narratives about real cases of individual behavior change in their reporting on health issues (McAlister et al. 2000). McAlister and his colleagues argue that these real-life examples of overcoming health problems can serve as a catalyst for motivating others in the same target population to change their behaviors, and therefore hopefully prevent disease and illness. Behavioral journalism relies on traditional information-gathering techniques such as interviewing and acquiring extensive background information, as well as on traditional storytelling platforms, from documentaries and feature-length stories to talk show segments (McAlister and Fernandez 2002).

However, unlike traditional reporters, the behavioral journalist relies upon the tenets of behavioral science theories, primarily social cognitive theory (Bandura 1986), to present information to news audiences. Specifically, behavioral journalists report information that presents audiences with a role model they can imitate and who can help them learn vicariously in order to improve their own self-efficacy for taking action. This approach to reporting on public health issues has produced documented behavior change in multiple countries and contexts, from smoking cessation in Finland (Puska et al. 1987) to HIV prevention in cities across the United States (McAlister et al. 2000).

While the public health model calls for adding more contextual information to health reporting, behavioral journalism instead emphasizes the need to take a personalized, exemplar-based approach to health reporting, similar to feature reporting. These are contrasting approaches—one calls for a thematic, big-picture, abstract presentation style, and one argues for the use of concrete, relatable anecdotes. The differences between the models come down to the locus of control over health issues. That is, news stories under the public health model portray society as a primary influencer of health outcomes while behavioral journalism portrays individuals as having great agency over outcomes. To date, the public health model of reporting has largely been applied in the context of violence and crime where societal actions are, indeed, central for improving the situation. Meanwhile, behavioral journalism interventions have been applied primarily to contexts where individual behaviors are highly effective in preventing harm. These varying contexts can help explain the different tactics used to move toward the same goal of improving the ability of health reporting to improve public health.

Additionally, the two styles of reporting have implications for the audiences' emotional reactions to news stories, discussed in further detail below. Stories of individuals dealing with health issues are often narrative in form, and narratives are more likely to evoke strong emotions than are statistics or abstract generalities (Dunlop, Kashima, and Wakefield 2008; Oliver, Dillard, Bae, and Tamul 2012). As for their impact on specific emotions, the public health model's ability to place a health condition in greater context may help alleviate anxiety. For instance, an individual may realize that her personal risk of a health threat is actually greater than she thought after seeing statistics indicating that women her age are at high risk for skin cancer. On the other hand, seeing a news story where an exemplar is successful in preventing a health threat and models individual steps for others to use to avoid the threat may reduce anxiety and increase hope in those reading a story based on the tenets of behavior journalism. Empirical research comparing the effects of the two models on news audiences is needed to test potential theoretical explanations, from exemplification or framing theory to narrative transportation and character involvement, and to see which model of health reporting may produce the most knowledge gain and behavior change in which specific audiences.

Conflicting Headlines

Another difficulty facing health journalists, health news consumers, and media researchers are the realities of health reports that result in conflicting headlines with confusing behavioral recommendations. Conflicting headlines occur when one day, the television news anchor tells viewers that coffee can improve longevity. But a few weeks later (after a new scientific study is published), the same news anchor tells the same viewers that drinking coffee may actually be unhealthy. The back-and-forth of health advice generated by this juxtaposition of seemingly contradictory behavioral implications can make it quite difficult for news consumers to decide which health news stories to trust.

There can be small or large intervals of time between news reports providing conflicting health advice, depending on the publication of academic studies that make their way into the media coverage. For instance, the news media heavily reported the benefits of hormone replacement therapy for postmenopausal women, but longitudinal research eventually revealed that these treatment regimens could increase the risk of breast cancer, and new headlines followed (Lawton, Rose, McLeod, and Dowell 2003; Zuckerman 2003). After years of touting its benefits, the news media then had to report on the substantial drawbacks to hormone therapy. While the news coverage was dictated by the advancements in medical science, the conflicting headlines nonetheless can cause many to question the perhaps overly optimistic nature of the earlier coverage. The back-and-forth messages imbedded in health news stories have been linked to public cynicism toward health news, especially for stories related to diet and nutrition (Lupton and Chapman 1995).

Conflicting themes in the news, also called competitive frames, are commonplace in political coverage, too (Chong and Druckman 2007). One political actor states that an event implies eminent doom while another promotes it as a promising sign of improvement, and the news media display both statements for public consumption. Conflicting frames have direct implications for how audiences feel in response to news coverage. In fact, conflict-based coverage of contentious political issues, such as campaign finance reform, can produce feelings of anger and disgust in the public (Gross and Brewer 2007). Unlike political news coverage, science, health, and medical news can be riddled with conflicting information that is not necessarily due to political differences. Rather, conflicting health and science news headlines are typically related to the technical and uncertain nature of scientific findings that become oversimplified when reporters make sweeping statements about the implications of those findings (Friedman, Dunwoody, and Rogers 1999).

Such presentations of conflicting information between and among stories may cause audiences to feel uncertain and can alter those audience members' perceptions of the credibility of that information (Jensen 2008; Jensen and Hurley 2012). According to Brashers's (2001) theory of uncertainty management, "responses to uncertainty are shaped by appraisals and emotional reactions to the experience" (481). Uncertainty is a central appraisal for evoking emotional responses such as fear and hope (Lazarus 1991). Therefore, it is highly plausible that the more uncertainty these conflicting headlines generate in audiences, the stronger the audience members' uncertainty-linked emotional responses, like fear and hope, will be.

In addition to examining the effects of conflicting health news reports on news audiences from the paradigm of uncertainty management, the concept of cognitive dissonance can help explain why conflicting headlines might discourage news audiences from taking action in response to health news stories. Festinger (1957) postulated that people experience an aversive affective state known as cognitive dissonance when there is a disconnect between any of the cognitive elements of a situation (e.g. one's behavior and one's attitudes about that behavior differ). In order to decrease this unpleasant dissonance experienced when one has a negative attitude about a behavior but cannot or will not change the behavior, individuals will alter their attitudes toward the communication source. When confronted with dissonant information, those with very strong attitudes or behavioral patterns may intensify their previous beliefs instead of changing them by altering the importance or credibility of the dissonant information, or by causing the individual to focus on new beliefs that support the consonant beliefs (Festinger, Riecken, and Schachter 1956).

In a health news context, the theory of cognitive dissonance implies that if an audience member could not or would not change a health behavior, then a health story presenting information incongruent with the audience member's current behavior would cause that individual to discredit some or all of the sources of information, such as the researchers being quoted, the journalists doing the reporting, the news organization represented by the journalists, the medium of communication (e.g., "Internet health news cannot be trusted"), or even the news media in general. This discrediting could also take the form of state reactance and feelings of anger toward the discredited source(s) (Harmon-Jones 2000). Additionally, if a news viewer is aware of this pattern of conflicting headlines in health news stories, he might disregard any one news story incongruent with his current health-related behavior and wait until the next story comes out that better supports his behavior. Then, the individual could latch onto that story's conclusions and use it in his defense if any future news stories do not support it.

On the other hand, individuals without a firmly established attitude toward the health behavior discussed in the conflicting news stories may not experience much cognitive dissonance. In those cases, these individuals may instead experience anxiety (if they take part in a behavior being touted as unhealthy or if they do not take part in a prevention behavior touted as healthy) or hope (if they take part in a prevention behavior being touted as healthy or if they do not take part in a behavior touted as unhealthy) when presented with conflicting headlines. Additional research is needed to test how the experience of cognitive dissonance may moderate reactions to conflicting headlines in health news stories.

Both uncertainty management and cognitive dissonance paradigms can help researchers understand how audiences might react to conflicting health news headlines. However, a search for existing research connecting conflicting health news stories and emotional reactions of health news audiences comes up mostly blank. Holbert and Hansen (2008) stressed the need to study inter-media emotional reactions to understand media effects in a real-world environment where individuals consume media from many sources over a long period of time. In this real-world context, emotional reactions to one health news story could very likely influence how audiences respond to subsequent news stories on the same or related health topics. Holbert and Hansen found in their study of political media that emotion from one mediated event (a politically charged movie) did, in fact, carry over and influence how audiences reacted to a subsequent political message (a presidential debate). In the context of contradictory health news headlines, fear, hope, and anger, perhaps even disgust, are very plausible emotional reactions for audiences to experience and would be good starting points for future research investigating the role of emotions in health news effects.

THEORETICAL CONSIDERATIONS

In addition to the aforementioned challenges with health journalism and possible solutions, existing communication theories provide guidance in predicting how news consumers may respond to health reporting with information on potential threats and preventative actions. Below, two particularly relevant conceptual frameworks are described: exemplification and framing. These two theoretical perspectives appear repeatedly throughout the body of scholarly work on health journalism and provide a conceptual foundation for examining the role of emotions in prevention-focused health news effects.

Exemplification

One factor that facilitates emotional responses to news media is the use of personal stories about individuals directly affected by an issue (i.e., exemplars) to illustrate a specific case study to news audiences. Exemplars are commonly utilized in news stories as they can put a human face on what may be a seemingly abstract issue. Research indicates that journalists choose exemplars for health stories, in particular, in order to inform, inspire, and/or sensationalize a health issue (Hinnant, Len-Ríos, and Young 2013). However, news stories of lay exemplars battling illness can also focus news consumers' attention on rare and unusual cases at the expense of fostering an understanding of the typical case (Kreuter et al. 2007). Exemplification theory posits that the number of exemplars discussed in a news story will have stronger emotional appeal to the reader than will any type of base-rate data, or statistical representation of the frequency of the phenomenon (Zillmann and Brosius 2000). Researchers have frequently used health-related news coverage to demonstrate the existence of exemplification effects (e.g., Gibson and Zillmann 1994; Zillmann, Perkins, and Sundar 1992).

One reason exemplification effects occur is that audiences can make emotional connections with the exemplars better than they can connect with numbers. The ability of an exemplar to induce emotions in audiences is known as affective reactivity. As Zillmann (2006) explains: "In the assessment of health risks, for example, exemplars associated with affective reactivity will receive disproportional attention and thereby render overestimates of the incidence and magnitude of threats to health" (S224). This is why exemplars have a stronger influence on audience perceptions of risk than do any actual, objective risk statistics cited in the news story. Exemplars have an especially significant impact on risk perceptions for members of the news audience who are not very good at understanding numerical relationships (Gibson, Callison, and Zillmann 2011).

Research has also shown that images in news stories are capable of influencing audience perceptions about health issues by serving as visual exemplars. Zillmann (2006) argues that visual exemplars, perhaps even more so than text-based exemplars, have potent impacts on risk perceptions. Even small changes in images accompanying news stories can significantly alter audience perceptions of the problem discussed in the text. For example, when the text of the news story said nothing about race but the race of the people in images accompanying a news story about a tick-borne illness was manipulated by the researchers, Gibson and Zillmann (2000) found that participants estimated an increased risk of the illness for people of whichever ethnicity matched that of the visual exemplars in the photos versus risk for people of a different race.

While affective reactivity has been used as an explanation of exemplification effects for both in-text and visual exemplars, little research has delved into the impact of specific discrete emotional reactions to the use of exemplars versus base-rate statistics. However, there are multiple emotions that are likely evoked by both reporting devices. Exemplars who succeed could induce hope, or even relief, while those who fail or have not yet succeeded my spark fear or anxiety, or anger if the news consumer blames the individual for the inability to overcome a health barrier, even compassion if the news consumer believes the individual is not at fault. Furthermore, while less emotionally evocative than exemplars, base-rate statistics can still induce fear (if they indicate a disease is severe and the audience member is susceptible), hope (if the statistics describe a promising prevention strategy or treatment), or compassion if the health issue is severe but the audience member does not perceive herself to be susceptible. Empirical tests of the potential for discrete emotional reactions, and various combinations of them, to mediate between the use of exemplars and audience reactions to news stories may advance scholarly understandings of the mechanisms behind health news effects on audiences.

Message Framing

Framing is a multifaceted scholarly term that has been applied in multiple streams of communication research. For the purposes of this chapter, framing is the phenomenon that occurs when a message highlights some feature of an issue over others. Entman (1993) defines the act of framing as "to select some aspects of a perceived reality and make them more salient in a communicating text, in such a way as to promote a particular problem definition, causal interpretation, moral evaluation, and/or treatment recommendation for the item described" (52).

Gain and loss frames are commonly used in news media coverage and frequently appear in health news stories (e.g., Myrick, Major, and Jankowski 2014). Typically, gain-framed messages emphasize the benefits (e.g., lives saved) of choosing a particular option, whereas loss-framed messages emphasize the costs (e.g., lives lost) associated with not choosing a particular option. Ghanem (1997) referred to gain and loss frames as affective frames because they can evoke different types of affect, positive or negative, respectively. Prospect theory posits people will make different judgments and decisions depending on if the information they receive is framed as a gain or as a loss (Kahneman and Tversky 1979).

Another important component of prospect theory is the proposition that people are more inclined to avoid a loss than they are to try to obtain a gain; that is, losses loom psychologically larger than gains (Tversky and Kahneman 1991). This proposition is known as the loss aversion hypothesis, and it is one of the more robust findings of prospect theory (McDermott 2004). Media research supports the notion that negative news may be more impactful on audiences than positive information. For instance, negative news has been shown to draw greater attention and perceptions of importance from audiences (Rozin and Royzman 2001). Moreover, research shows that gain and loss frames portrayed in messages can be intensified when individuals experience an emotional reaction to the frames, with emotions increasing perceptions of losses more than they increase perceptions of gains (Druckman and McDermott 2008).

Aside from gain and loss frames, Iyengar (1991) delineated another dimension of media framing that appears commonly in news stories, including health news stories. Thematic news frames emphasize broader trends and social conditions, such as those emphasized in the public health model of reporting. Iyengar argued that news stories employing thematic frames foster a sense of shared responsibility and can promote collective action to address social issues. The episodic news frame, on the other hand, depicts public issues in terms of specific instances—a single event or case. Unlike for thematic frames, Iyengar maintained that episodic frames focus audiences' attention on individuals as the likely causes of issues, and individual behavior as the preferred solution.

Research indicates that episodic and thematic framing of media content can evoke different emotions in audiences. Gross (2008) studied reactions to differently framed opinion columns about mandatory minimum sentences for criminals. In her studies, participants were randomly assigned to read either a thematic or episodically framed column arguing against mandatory minimum sentencing. Across two studies she found that episodic frames were more emotionally engaging for participants than were thematic frames. Major (2011) presented some preliminary empirical evidence relating emotional reactions to news frames to reactions to health-related policies. Her experiment involved manipulating both gain-loss frames and episodic-thematic frames of news stories about lung cancer and obesity (resulting in four experimental conditions for each health condition). Although participants' emotional reactions to the news stories did not mediate the relationships between thematic, episodic, or loss frames and attitudes toward responsibility for health issues, she did find one emotional reaction served as a mechanism between gain frames and the attribution of responsibility for health problems. Specifically, gain frames resulted in stronger feelings of guilt, which in turn impacted audiences' attribution of responsibility for the health conditions. That is, participants who read gain-framed stories about lung cancer or obesity felt *less* guilt after reading the stories, and this decrease in guilt contributed to weaker beliefs that society was responsible for these conditions. This finding, although small in magnitude (the point estimate of the indirect effect was -.01 and the standard error was less than .01), the findings point to a potential link between health news frames, emotional responses to that news, and subsequent judgments of responsibility for health issues.

Future work is clearly needed to understand why exactly certain frames, be they gain, loss, episodic, or thematic, result in various emotional reactions (i.e., what specific message features in these frames foster emotional reactions; is it the use of exemplars or hopeful/anxious language, or what exactly?). One avenue for research in this realm is to combine visual and text frames and test their effects. Work on visual framing (Ahn, Fox, Dale, and Avant 2014; Brantner, Lobinger, and Wetzstein 2011; Grabe and Bucy 2009) is a nascent but promising area of exploration for better understanding the role of emotions in responses to differentially framed messages and could likewise be applied to work on health news effects.

It is important to note that meta-analyses show that neither gain or loss frames have been shown to be more effective for promoting prevention or detection behaviors (O'Keefe and Jensen 2007; 2009). However, most of the studies included in these two meta-analyses focused on persuasive health messages, not news media. However, the results reveal that the effects of frames in health media, be it persuasive or news based, are still not clearly understand by researchers. Further research is needed to understood the mechanisms behind framing effects on health behavior in both persuasive and news contexts (O'Keefe 2012).

Apart from analyzing how traditional message frames impact emotional and behavior responses to health news, research indicates that emotions themselves may serve a similar function to frames. Nabi (2003) argues that emotions act like frames because they privilege certain types of information over others, with emotionally relevant information is more accessible than information with no connection to emotional appraisals or action tendencies. For example, the experience of fear results in an action tendency to avoid the threat, so feeling fearful makes information about how to avoid the threat more relevant to the message consumer than other information in a message not directly related to the threat.

This bias in the accessibility of different types of information, based on the type of emotion experienced by the media consumer, can in turn impact judgments and decision making. Nabi (2003) tested the emotions-as-frames model by examining differences in reactions to the societal problems of drunk driving (a familiar topic for the sample) and gun violence (a more distant topic for the sample) between participants who either felt fearful or who felt angry. She posited that since the appraisals associated with anger (e.g., other-focused blame) and fear (e.g., threat, danger) differ, then these emotional states would operate as different frames for thinking about social issues, which in turn motivates a desire for frame-consistent information. Indeed, Nabi found that angry participants were more likely to remember individual-focused causes and retributive solutions to the problem of drunk driving, whereas fearful participants were more likely to recall societal-level causes and protective solutions for drunk driving. There were no effects of the emotional states on judgments of gun violence, likely due to the lack of schema development in her sample related to that topic (as compared to the more familiar situation of drunk driving).

Kühne and Schemer (2013) found similar effects when studying how feelings of anger and sadness may operate as frames through which individuals perceive news about road safety policies. While anger is associated with other-blame, sadness is linked with appraisals of situational influence outside of individual control (Lazarus 1991). Kühne and Schemer found that a news story framed to elicit anger in their participants increased the accessibility of information about punishment and resulted in a stronger preference for punitive measures. In the condition in which participants read a news story framed to induce sadness, information about how to help victims was more accessible to participants, who also reported a preference for remedial measures to address road safety. The resulting accessibility of information preferences for additional information were in line with the emotional tendencies of anger and sadness, respectively, providing additional support for the emotions-as-frames concept in the context of news media.

In addition to influencing information accessibility and judgments about story topics, emotional frames can affect information processing. H. J. Kim and Cameron (2011) found that an anger-inducing story about a cell phone battery explosion accident resulted in heuristic processing by participants, whereas a sadness-inducing story resulted in systematic processing of the news story. Moreover, S. J. Kim and Niederdeppe (2014) presented evidence that visuals could be used to emotionally frame anti-smoking advertisements as either sad or angry, with different persuasive outcomes for the different visually framed messages. While the visual effects did not take place in a news context, the mechanisms of effects could be applied and tested in future studies of non-persuasive content.

The findings from the aforementioned studies provide strong support for the emotions-as-frames model as an effective framework for understanding how health news might influence audiences. This is particularly important to consider in the context of online news where an Internet user can easily turn from health information presented on a news website to a search engine to find information that matches the emotional appraisals and action tendencies of the user's current emotional state. The influence of emotional frames on health news consumers may differ, though, depending on the pre-existing emotional state audiences bring to the health news story as well as on the type of discrete emotional overtones in the content itself. Future work could explore the interaction of multiple emotional frames within the same health news story as well as how positive emotions may result in different framing effects than would the negative emotions studies under this model to date.

CONCLUSION

The news media are an important source of health information for the public. Yet reports on health issues often fall short of the ideals espoused by public health advocates for educating the public about health threats and possible remedies. Two approaches to improving health reporting, the public health model and behavioral journalism, use different means (thematic reporting on a broad range of health-related topics and the use of moving exemplars, respectively) to strive toward the same end of improving health journalism. Both models of health reporting have implications for emotional arousal and emotional connections to health stories and the individuals featured in such news accounts.

Multiple theories provide researchers with a framework for understanding how health news might impact audiences. Exemplification theory, cognitive dissonance theory, research on various types of frames, and empirical work on the relationships between news content and emotions all describe various ways in which news accounts can spark fear or provide hope, anger audiences or inspire prevention behaviors. Future work is needed to test the impact of different formats of health news content on discrete emotions and blends of those emotions. Advances in understanding the effects of health news on consumers' emotional reactions, risk perceptions, and behaviors are important in an increasingly oversaturated information environment. Journalistic reports distill complicated medical science and health advice into digestible information for the masses, a valuable service in this media-rich environment. As news reports are viewed as a credible source of health information and appear frequently in the public's media diet, then these effects can have real implications for individual and public health.

REFERENCES

Ahn, S. J., J. Fox,, K. R. Dale, and J. A. Avant. 2014. Framing virtual experiences: Effects on environmental efficacy and behavior over time. *Communication Research*. doi: 10.1177/0093650214534973.

Bandura, A. 1986. *Social foundations of thought and action: A social cognitive theory.* Englewood Cliffs, NJ: Prentice-Hall.

Bas, O., and M. E. Grabe. 2015. Emotion-provoking personalization of news: Informing citizens and closing the knowledge gap? *Communication Research* 42(2):159–85. doi: 10.1177/0093650213514602.

Brantner, C., K. Lobinger, and I. Wetzstein. 2011. Effects of visual framing on emotional responses and evaluations of news stories about the Gaza Conflict 2009. *Journalism and Mass Communication Quarterly* 88(3):523–40. doi: 10.1177/107769901108800304.

Brashers, D. E. (2001). Communication and uncertainty management. *Journal of Communication* 51(3):477–97. doi: 10.1111/j.1460-2466.2001.tb02892.x

Chong, D., and J. N. Druckman. 2007. Framing public opinion in competitive democracies. *American Political Science Review* 101(04):637–55. doi: doi:10.1017/S0003055407070554.

Coleman, R., and E. Thorson. 2002. The effects of news stories that put crime and violence into context: Testing the public health model of reporting. *Journal of Health Communication* 7(5):401–25. doi: 10.1080/10810730290001783.

Coleman, R., E. Thorson, and L. Wilkins. 2011. Testing the effect of framing and sourcing in health news stories. *Journal of Health Communication* 16(9):941–54. doi: 10.1080/10810730.2011.561918.

Dorfman, L., E. Thorson, and J. E. Stevens. 2001. Reporting on violence: Bringing a public health perspective into the newsroom. *Health Education and Behavior* 28(4):402–19. doi: 10.1177/109019810102800402.

Dorfman, L., K. Woodruff, V. Chavez, and L. Wallack. 1997. Youth and violence on local television news in California. *American Journal of Public Health* 87(8):1311–16. doi: 10.2105/AJPH.87.8.1311.

Druckman, J. N., and R. McDermott. 2008. Emotion and the framing of risky choice. *Political Behavior* 30(3):297–321. doi: 10.1007/s11109-008-9056-y.

Dunlop, S. M., Y. Kashima, and M. Wakefield. 2008. Can you feel it? Negative emotion, risk, and narrative in health communication. *Media Psychology* 11:52–75.

Entman, R. M. 1993. Framing: Toward clarification of a fractured paradigm. *Journal of Communication* 43(4):51–58. doi: 10.1111/j.1460-2466.1993.tb01304.x.

Festinger, L. 1957. *A theory of cognitive dissonance.* Evenston, IL: Row.

Festinger, L., H. W. Riecken, and S. Schachter. 1956. *When prophecy fails: A social and psychological study of a modern group that predicted the destruction of the world.* Minneapolis, MN: University of Minnesota Press.

Friedman, S. M., S. Dunwoody, and C. L. Rogers. 1999. *Communicating uncertainty: Media coverage of new and controversial science.* Mahwah, NJ: Lawrence Erlbaum Associates.

Ghanem, S. 1997. Filling in the tapestry: The second level of agenda setting. In M. E. McCombs, D. L. Shaw, and D. Weaver (Eds.), *Communication and democracy: Exploring the intellectual frontiers in agenda-setting theory* (pp. 29–40). Mahwah, NJ: Lawrence Erlbaum Associates.

Gibson, R., C. Callison, and D. Zillmann. 2011. Quantitative literacy and affective reactivity in processing statistical information and case histories in the news. *Media Psychology* 14(1):96–120. doi: 10.1080/15213269.2010.547830.

Gibson, R., and D. Zillmann. 1994. Exaggerated versus representative exemplification in news reports perception of issues and personal consequences. *Communication Research* 21(5):603–24. doi: 10.1177/009365094021005003.

———. 2000. Reading between the photographs: The influence of incidental pictorial information on issue perception. *Journalism and Mass Communication Quarterly* 77(2):355–66.

Grabe, M. E., and E. P. Bucy. 2009. *Image bite politics: News and the visual framing of elections.* New York: Oxford University Press.

Gross, K. 2008. Framing persuasive appeals: Episodic and thematic framing, emotional response, and policy opinion. *Political Psychology* 29(2):169–92. doi: 10.1111/j.1467-9221.2008.00622.x.

Gross, K., and P. R. Brewer. 2007. Sore losers: News frames, policy debates, and emotions. *The Harvard International Journal of Press/Politics* 12(1):122–33. doi: 10.1177/1081180x06297231.

Harmon-Jones, E. 2000. A cognitive dissonance theory perspective on the role of emotion in the maintenance and change of beliefs and attitudes. In N. H. Frijda, A. S. R. Manstead, and S. Bem (Eds.), *Emotions and beliefs: How feelings influence thoughts* (pp. 185–211). Cambridge: Cambridge University Press.

Hinnant, A., M. E. Len-Ríos, and R. Young. 2013. Journalistic use of exemplars to humanize health news. *Journalism Studies* 14(4):539–54. doi: 10.1080/1461670X.2012.721633.

Holbert, R. L., and G. J. Hansen. 2008. Stepping beyond message specificity in the study of emotion as mediator and inter-emotion associations across attitude objects: Fahrenheit 9/11, anger, and debate superiority. *Media Psychology* 11(1):98–118. doi: 10.1080/15213260701832512.

Iyengar, S. 1991. *Is anyone responsible? How television frames political issues.* Chicago: University of Chicago Press.

Jensen, J. D. 2008. Scientific uncertainty in news coverage of cancer research: Effects of hedging on scientists' and journalists' credibility. *Human Communication Research* 34(3):347–69. doi: 10.1111/j.1468-2958.2008.00324.x.

Jensen, J. D., and R. J. Hurley. 2012. Conflicting stories about public scientific controversies: Effects of news convergence and divergence on scientists' credibility. *Public Understanding of Science* 21(6):689–704. doi: 10.1177/0963662510387759.

Kahneman, D., and A. Tversky. 1979. Prospect theory: An analysis of decision under risk. *Econometrica* 47(2):263–91. doi: 10.2307/1914185.

Kim, H. J., and G. T. Cameron. 2011. Emotions matter in crisis: The role of anger and sadness in the publics' response to crisis news framing and corporate crisis response. *Communication Research* 38(6):826–55. doi: 10.1177/0093650210385813.

Kim, S. J., and J. Niederdeppe. 2014. Emotional expressions in antismoking television advertisements: Consequences of anger and sadness framing on pathways to persuasion. *Journal of Health Communication*, 1–18. doi: 10.1080/10810730.2013.837550.

Kreuter, M. W., M. C. Green, J. N. Cappella, M. D. Slater, M. E. Wise, D. Storey, . . . S. Woolley. 2007. Narrative communication in cancer prevention and control: A framework to guide research and application. *Annals of Behavioral Medicine* 33(3):221–35.

Kühne, R., and C. Schemer. 2013. The emotional effects of news frames on information processing and opinion formation. *Communication Research.* doi: 10.1177/0093650213514599.

Lawrence, R. G. 2004. Framing obesity: The evolution of news discourse on a public health issue. *The Harvard International Journal of Press/Politics* 9(3):56–75. doi: 10.1177/1081180x04266581.

Lawton, B., S. Rose, D. McLeod, and A. Dowell. 2003. Changes in use of hormone replacement therapy after the report from the Women's Health Initiative: Cross sectional survey of users. *BMJ* 327(7419):845–46. doi: 10.1136/bmj.327.7419.845.

Lazarus, R. S. 1991. *Emotion and adaptation.* New York: Oxford University Press.

Lupton, D., and S. Chapman. 1995. "A healthy lifestyle might be the death of you": Discourses on diet, cholesterol control and heart disease in the press and among the lay public. *Sociology of Health and Illness* 17(4):477–94. doi: 10.1111/1467-9566.ep10932547.

Major, L. H. 2011. The mediating role of emotions in the relationship between frames and attribution of responsibility for health problems. *Journalism and Mass Communication Quarterly* 88(3):502–22. doi: 10.1177/1077699011088000303.

McAlister, A., and M. Fernandez. 2002. "Behavioral journalism" accelerates diffusion of healthy innovations. In R. Hornik (Ed.), *Public health communication: Evidence for behavior change* (pp. 315–26). Mahwah, NJ: Lawrence Erlbaum Associates.

McAlister, A., W. Johnson, C. Guenther-Grey, M. Fishbein, D. Higgins, and K. O'Reilly. 2000. Behavioral journalism for HIV prevention: Community newsletters influence risk-related attitudes and behavior. *Journalism and Mass Communication Quarterly* 77(1):143–59. doi: 10.1177/107769900007700111.

McDermott, R. 2004. Prospect theory in political science: Gains and losses from the first decade. *Political Psychology* 25(2):289–312. doi: 10.1111/j.1467-9221.2004.00372.x.

Myrick, J. G. 2014. Journalism and health. In T. L. Thompson (Ed.), *Encyclopedia of health communication* (pp. 605–8). Thousand Oaks, CA: Sage.

Myrick, J. G., L. H. Major, and S. M. Jankowski. 2014. The sources and frames used to tell stories about depression and anxiety: A content analysis of 18 years of national television news coverage. *Electronic News* 8(1):49–63. doi: 10.1177/1931243114523962.

Nabi, R. L. 2003. Exploring the framing effects of emotion. *Communication Research* 30(2):224–47. doi: 10.1177/0093650202250881.

O'Keefe, D. J. 2012. From psychological theory to message design: Lessons from the story of gain-framed and loss-framed persuasive messages. In H. Cho (Ed.), *Health communication message design: Theory and practice* (pp. 3–20). Los Angeles: SAGE.

O'Keefe, D. J., and J. D. Jensen. 2007. The relative persuasiveness of gain-framed loss-framed messages for encouraging disease prevention behaviors: A meta-analytic review. *Journal of Health Communication* 12(7):623–44. doi: 10.1080/10810730701615198.

———. 2009. The relative persuasiveness of gain-framed and loss-framed messages for encouraging disease detection behaviors: A meta-analytic review. *Journal of Communication* 59(2):296–316. doi: 10.1111/j.1460-2466.2009.01417.x.

Oliver, M. B., J. P. Dillard, K. Bae, and D. J. Tamul. 2012. The effect of narrative news format on empathy for stigmatized groups. *Journalism and Mass Communication Quarterly* 89(2):205–24. doi: 10.1177/1077699012439020.

Pew Research Center Journalism Project. 2014. State of the news media 2014. Retrieved July 21, 2014, from http://www.journalism.org/packages/state-of-the-news-media-2014/.

Puska, P., A. McAlister, H. Niemensivu, T. Piha, J. Wiio, and K. Koskela. 1987. A television format for national health promotion: Finland's "Keys to Health." *Public Health Report,* 102(3):263–69.

Rozin, P., and E. B. Royzman. 2001. Negativity bias, negativity dominance, and contagion. *Personality and Social Psychology Review* 5(4):296–320. doi: 10.1207/s15327957pspr0504_2.

Schwitzer, G. 2014. A guide to reading health care news stories. *JAMA Internal Medicine.* doi: 10.1001/jamainternmed.2014.1359.

Thorson, E. 2006. Print news and health psychology: Some observations. *Journal of Health Psychology* 11(2):175–82. doi: 10.1177/1359105306061178.

Tversky, A., and D. Kahneman. 1991. Loss aversion in riskless choice: A reference-dependent model. *The Quarterly Journal of Economics* 106(4):1039–61. doi: 10.2307/2937956.

Zillmann, D. 2006. Exemplification effects in the promotion of safety and health. *Journal of Communication* 56:S221–S237. doi: 10.1111/j.1460-2466.2006.00291.x.

Zillmann, D., and H.-B. Brosius. 2000. *Exemplification in communication: The influence of case reports on the perception of issues.* Mahwah, NJ: Lawrence Erlbaum Associates.

Zillmann, D., J. W. Perkins, and S. S. Sundar. 1992. Impression-formation effects of printed news varying in descriptive precision and exemplifications. *Zeitschrift für Medienpsychologie* 4(3):168–85.

Zuckerman, D. 2003. Hype in health reporting: "Checkbook science" buys distortion of medical news. *International Journal of Health Services* 33(2):383–89. doi: 10.2190/PMM9-DPUT-HN3Y-LMJQ.

Chapter Thirteen

Health Information Seeking

The desire to seek information about one's surroundings is an intuitive human drive (Panksepp 2007; Pirolli and Card 1999). Seeking health information, in particular, is directly relevant to well-being in the modern world where a number of health threats exist. Rutten, Squiers, and Hesse (2006) define health information seeking as an effort to reduce or manage the uncertainty or the stress associated with health-related concerns. Those who seek health information can benefit from gains in knowledge and improved social support as well as enhanced coping abilities and greater levels of self-efficacy (Galarce, Ramanadhan, and Viswanath 2011; Morahan-Martin 2004; Shim, Kelly, and Hornik 2006). Now, in the digital era, health information seeking is easier than ever before. More than three-quarters (80 percent) of American Internet users report searching for health information online (Fox 2013).

Kuhlthau's (1991) posits that health information seeking is an integration of the affective, cognitive, and physical aspects of the human experience. Multiple theoretical models exist to predict when people will seek health or risk information, such as Brasher's (2001) uncertainty management model, Griffin, Dunwoody, and Neuwirth (1999) risk information seeking and processing (RISP) model, or Afifi and Weiner's (2004) theory of motivated information management (for a review of these and other models, see Kahlor 2010). These theories that aim to predict health information–seeking behaviors differ in their emphasis on risk, knowledge, uncertainty, and other cognitive variables. However, one common theme emerges from the models: emotional states, particularly the negative emotions of anxiety and fear, can motivate people to seek health information.

Despite this common theme (i.e., emotions motivate people to search for more information) among theoretical perspectives and conceptual models, little scholarly work has focused directly on the ways in which specific discrete emotions, particularly those other than anxiety/fear, impact 1) motivations to search; 2) the nature of health information searches; and, 3) post-search outcomes. To date, the impact and nuances of discrete emotions have not received extensive or nuanced attention in most scholarly conceptualizations of these three phases of the health information seeking–process.

This chapter aims to explore conceptual frameworks and existing research findings related to emotions that may help advance current conceptualizations of the health information seeking process, particularly as they pertain to seeking that may benefit prevention behaviors. Evidence indicates that information seeking with a goal of preventing illness may take a different shape than searchers with a treatment focus. For instance, Tian and Robinson (2008) found that cancer victims use different media channels to seek health information than do adults who have never been diagnosed with cancer. However, literature is lacking that demonstrates more specifically how prevention-inspired motivations for searching differ from detection or treatment motivations, or how the nuances of the search process and post-search outcomes might differ between these contexts. As such, this chapter presents a wide array of research on the links between emotions and health information seeking with the hope that future research will start filling in the gaps in the literature related to the specific preventative health context.

This chapter has four main objectives: to summarize the emotions literature as it relates to the communication behavior of health information seeking; to argue that emotions other than fear and anxiety can also impact the information-seeking process; to outline how different theories of emotion could be applied to advance health information–seeking research; and, finally, to discuss methodological approaches that may enhance our understanding of health information seeking. As an overarching roadmap for achieving these aims, figure 13.1 presents a model of the different points in the health information–seeking process in which emotions may influence mechanisms and outcomes. While multiple types of health information seeking are discussed in this chapter, the focus is on information seeking involving the Internet, including searches of mass media content and of computer-mediated communication. Therefore, this model is based primarily on online health information searching. However, it could be easily adapted to additional search contexts. The model details the process as having four different steps: motivation to search, initiation of the search, nature of the search, and post-search outcomes. The model includes a feedback loop such that the last step, post-search outcomes, loops back to the first step (motivations to search). Emotions can shape any one of these steps, as the rest of this chapter discusses in detail.

WHY WE SEARCH

Why do people search for health information? Researchers posit that a desire for knowledge and to control uncertainty are strong motivations to seek health information (for a review of health information–seeking theories, see Kahlor 2010). Many scholars argue that a discrepancy between current and desired levels of knowledge or of uncertainty leads individuals to feel anxious, which further motivates the search for health information (Kahlor). Is a mole no big deal or cancerous? I know I should eat more vegetables, but how do I cook them to taste better? What is my own risk for heart disease? These are all queries that could reflect uncertainty and could drive individuals to seek information related to prevention and secondary prevention (i.e., early detection) behaviors. Multiple models of health information seeking rely on the premise that feelings of uncertainty about a health issue spark anxiety and increased risk perceptions, which in turn motivate individuals to search for more information (Afifi and Morse 2009; Afifi and Weiner 2004; Freimuth,

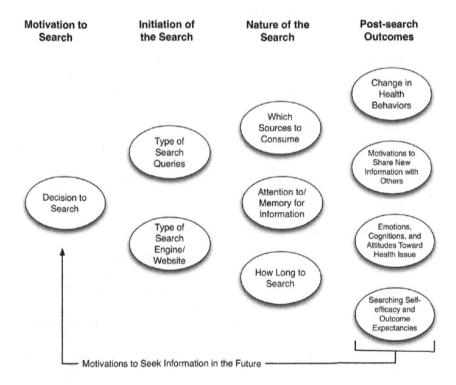

Figure 13.1. Conceptual Model of the Role of Emotions in the Health Informa-tion–Seeking Process

Stein, and Kean 1989; Griffin et al. 1999; J. D. Johnson and Meischke 1993; Kahlor 2010; Rimal and Real 2003).

According to Brashers (2001), uncertainty exists when "details of the situation are ambiguous, complex, unpredictable, or probabilistic; when information in unavailable or inconsistent; and when people feel insecure in their own state of knowledge or the state of knowledge in general" (478). When individuals have not met the threshold for desired knowledge or uncertainty, these models predict that individuals will continue to search for information until they surpass their thresholds. In the theory of motivated information management (TMIM) (Afifi and Weiner 2004), for example, uncertainty discrepancy (the difference between an individual's perceived level of uncertainty and the individual's desired level of uncertainty) serves as the motivation and first step in a process that leads to interpersonal information seeking.

A thorough review of all extant health information–seeking theories is beyond the scope of this chapter (see Galarce et al. 1999; Kahlor 2010). However, it is important to note that many existing theories focus on motivations for seeking, with health information seeking (or intentions to seek health information) as the outcome variable. A majority of these models do include an affective component, often as a result of or precursor to risk assessments (e.g., Griffin et al. 1999; Kahlor 2010). However, the type of affect represented in these models is almost always anxiety, whereas other emotional motivators for seeking have received little attention (for exceptions, see Afifi and Morse 2009; Brashers, Goldsmith, and Hsieh 2002). Furthermore, there is little known about how emotions that occur in response to a search impact post-search behaviors.

In an effort to explore why and how feelings of fear or anxiety motivate health information seeking, as well as to explore the possible effects of other emotions on health information seeking, it is helpful to look at theories from communication and psychology that deal directly with emotions.

Appraisal Theories of Emotion

Perceptions of uncertainty that are at the heart of many models of health information seeking are also an important component of emotion elicitation. Appraisal theories of emotion, as discussed in chapter 1, postulate that emotions arise from cognitive appraisals of a situation (often automatic in nature), such that each emotion is differentiated from another by its specific pattern of appraisals (Lazarus 1991; Roseman 1984; Scherer 1984; Scherer, Schorr, and Johnstone 2001; C. A. Smith and Ellsworth 1985). Appraisals of goal relevance, goal congruency, ego involvement, agency, coping potential, and future expectancies/certainty distinguish discrete emotions from each other (Lazarus). These discrete emotions are also associated with unique

action tendencies (Frijda, Kuipers, and ter Schure 1989; Lazarus 1991; Roseman, Wiest, and Swartz 1994). For example, the action tendency associated
with fear is to seek protection from the imminent threat, while the action
tendency associated with anger is to attack the agent responsible for the
offense (Lazarus). Emotional appraisals, action tendencies, and emotion-
based goals should influence the initial motivation to search for health information because seeking health information is often a response to an uncertain
situation.

Emotion Regulation and Mood Management

The concept of emotion regulation (i.e., the process of changing emotional
states) is one aspect of the link between emotions and behavior. Emotion
regulation is a broad term for the many ways in which people attempt to
regulate or control their own emotions (Gross and Thompson 2007). This
type of regulation may be automatic or controlled, and it also plays an important role in media processes and effects.

One often-overlooked conceptualization of information seeking is that it
can be thought of as a form of media or message choice. The searcher,
curious about health prevention and/or early detection, sets out to weed
through a plethora of possible health media options in order to find useful or
comforting information. As such, theories of mood management and selective exposure can help explain *why* people seek out certain types of health
messages and skip over others. Additionally, a number of conceptual frameworks specific to health information seeking provide guidance as to the
circumstances that spur health information seeking.

In a mediated health message context, an individual's current emotional
state can motivate that person to selectively attend to some aspects of a
message, or to certain types of messages, instead of others (Zillmann and
Bryant 1985). This happens such that the individual can change or maintain
her current emotional state, depending on if that state is aversive or hedonically pleasing, respectively. Zillmann (1988) posits that "the consumption of
messages . . . is capable of prevailing mood states, and the selection of
specific messages for consumption often serves the regulation of mood
states" (327). For instance, if one were feeling fearful, seeking out positively
toned health information may help alleviate the negative emotional state and
make the individual feel better. Indeed, research indicates that experiencing
positive emotions has been found to down-regulate a previous experience of
negative emotions (Fredrickson and Levenson 1998; Fredrickson, Mancuso,
Branigan, and Tugade 2000).

Furthermore, an individual's current level of arousal or emotional intensity can influence which types of media that person consumes. Research on
mood management indicates that individuals who are stressed tend to choose

calming media, while bored individuals are more likely to choose arousing media (Bryant and Zillmann 1984). For example, someone who is stressed about the potential of catching a particularly severe strain of influenza may be overwhelmed by an informational video animation with fast-paced music and instead prefer a website with a less-arousing, text-based list of information about the influenza strain and nearby locations for receiving the vaccination.

Zillmann (1988) argues that individuals need not be consciously aware of the underlying affective motivations prompting their media choices for those emotions to impact media choice. Mood-influenced media selection, according to principles of mood management, is impacted by content characteristics, such as excitatory potential, hedonic valence, semantic affinity to an individual's current state, and absorption potential (for a review, see Oliver 2003). If a potential source of health information is perceived by a searcher as high or low on any one of those four content characteristics, it could either attract or deter that health information seeker from looking at it, depending on the seeker's mood.

The original conceptualization of mood management prescribed that individuals seek certain types of media in order to distract themselves from aversive affective states or to maintain positive states (Zillmann and Bryant 1985). However, ideas about mood management have evolved to acknowledge that hedonic motivations are not the only emotional goals that influence media selection. Instead, people will sometimes consume content that can induce aversive states in order to engage more deeply with the human experience (Oliver 2008). Therefore, individuals may not always avoid reading negatively valenced health information (e.g., the story of a dying cancer patient) if their emotional goal is to connect with other human beings. This can be extremely helpful for spreading prevention information, such as to the individual without cancer who reads the story of a dying cancer patient for the emotional payoff but inadvertently becomes motivated to take her own cancer risks more seriously.

That example is but one of many ways that the process of emotion regulation and mood management via media use has important implications for understanding how emotional states may motivate and/or sustain searches for health information. The ways in which emotions shape media selection and user responses to media can vary across situations and time (Zillmann 1988). Although the majority of the research on mood management in the communication literature focuses on entertainment media, the ability of emotions to impact media selection across contexts makes the theory applicable to the selection of health-related messages.

Positive Emotions

As discussed above, anxiety and fear are the oft-cited emotional motivators for health information seeking. Besides the fact that focusing only on those emotions is conceptually limiting, health communication scholars would be well served by examining how other emotions impact search motivations, search behaviors, and post-search behaviors, especially as anxiety and fear have potentially negative consequences related to health. As stated by Loewenstein et al. (2001):

> Anxiety induction is not, however, a panacea when it comes to promoting self-protective behavior. Besides the fact that evoking anxiety saddles people with the hedonic burden of the anxiety itself, it can also induce defensive reactions that undermine efforts at risk mitigation. (275)

Although anxiety and fear are borne of appraisals of uncertainty and have been found to motivate health information searches, they are not the only emotions associated with uncertainty. Uncertainty appraisals are also a key component leading to feelings of hope (Lazarus 1991; 1999). If the outcome were certain, one would not need to hope and instead could only acknowledge the facts or wish the situation were somehow different.

As Brashers (2001) stated, the "fundamental challenge of refining theories of communication and uncertainty is to abandon the assumption that uncertainty will produce anxiety" (447). He cited appraisal theory as the basis for his prediction that when appraisals of uncertainty lead to anxiety, fear, or other negative emotions, people might seek information to gain knowledge or improve their understanding of complex issues. However, when appraisals of uncertainty lead people to experience positive emotions, Brashers posited that they might choose to avoid additional information that could be potentially stressful or unwelcome.

Currently, few models of health information seeking include positive emotions as a precursor to information searches or information avoidance. However, based on appraisal theories of emotion and on Brashers's work, Afifi and Morse (2009) expanded the TMIM to include all types of uncertainty-based emotions. Afifi and Morse argue that positive emotions, such as hope, can motivate information seeking in certain situations.

But in one of the very few empirical tests of the effects of positive emotions on information seeking–intentions (although not in the context of health), Yang and Kahlor (2013) found the experience of positive affect encouraged information avoidance while negative affect drove information seeking about climate change. However, the researchers' measures of positive and negative affect combined multiple discrete emotions, each with differing sets of appraisals and action tendencies. The positive emotion items in Yang and Kahlor's measures included excitement, hope, and happiness, while the negative items included concern, worry, anxiety, and general negative feelings. This grouping of emotions can mask different effects of discrete emotions on communication behaviors (Dillard and Seo 2013), such as information seeking. Additional research is needed to test if and how different discrete positive emotions motivate health information seeking or avoidance. Below, two discrete positive emotions, in particular, are discussed in relation to their potential to motivate prevention-oriented health information searches.

Hope

Hope is an emotion characterized by appraisals of uncertainty and future expectancy, and has an action tendency that motivates individuals to make a desired goal happen (Roseman 2011; Roseman et al. 1994) (see chapter 9). Lazarus (1999) defined hope as an emotion that serves as a coping resource for individuals. He stated, "To hope is to believe that something positive, which does not presently apply to one's life, could still materialize, and so we yearn for it" (653). This conceptualization emphasizes the belief that a goal *could* be reached, informing a hypothesis that hope would spur searchers for information that would help one achieve the desired goal. Afifi and Morse (2009) posit that feeling hopeful is an important motivator of health information seeking because it imbues individuals with positive future expectancies and elevated coping potential. These are the types of resources that would help individuals dig through large amounts of health information in order to find the relevant, trustworthy, and/or comforting material.

Interest

Interest is considered a "knowledge emotion" (Silvia 2008, 57) (see chapter 8). It is associated with all the components that make a discrete emotion, such as unique physiological changes, facial and vocal expressions, and appraisal patterns (Silvia 2005; 2008). Feelings of interest come about when an individual appraises the situation as both novel-complex and as comprehensible—that is, the individual has either the skills, knowledge, or resources to deal with the situation (Silvia 2005). The function of interest is to provide people with intrinsic motivation to learn and explore (Silvia 2006).

Kashdan (2004) argued that interest can serve as a counterweight to feelings of uncertainty or anxiety, which can have negative effects on individuals or unnecessarily narrow the focus of a search if not kept in balance. As Silvia (2006) stated,

> Interest motivates learning about something new and complex; once people understand the thing, it is not interesting anymore. The new knowledge, in turn, enables more things to be interesting. For appraisals of novelty-complex-

ity, knowledge about an area enables people to see subtle differences and contrasting perspectives that aren't apparent to novices. (59)

The implications of interest serving as a motivation for prevention-oriented health information seeking are many. Information about health and medical conditions is often complex, and if individuals seek it out of interest then they may be more open to consuming information that may not be simple or straightforward but is perhaps more accurate or helpful.

Additionally, feelings of interest could motivate people to seek information about health topics even if they do not perceive themselves to be at an immediate risk for the condition. The benefit of this type of health information seeking would be improved public knowledge of and possibly empathy for those who are affected by various health issues. The resultant knowledge and feelings could be translated to support and advocacy for important public health policies. Additionally, the information encountered in such an interest-inspired search could then motivate prevention behaviors if any self-relevant information is encountered during that search.

Mixed Emotions

It is also possible to experience more than one emotion at the same time (Larsen, McGraw, and Cacioppo 2001), and therefore, the impact of mixed emotions on motivations to seek health information should be considered. The experience of mixed emotions has been found to motivate people to connect with humanity, explore the human experience, and find meaning in life (Oliver 2008; Oliver and Bartsch 2011). This is a promising area of emotion research in the field of communication, but especially so for those interested in health communication who want to promote a holistic view of health and well-being as part of a meaningful life. Additionally, because mixed emotional appeals contain both positively and negatively valenced components, they may prevent some of the defensive reactions that sometimes accompany negative emotions and would keep individuals from wanting to seek more information about potential health threats.

Feeling tender, moved, inspired, or compassionate are types of affective blends containing both negative and positive affective components (Oliver and Bartsch 2010; Oliver, Hartmann, and Woolley 2012). Mixed emotions can foster greater cognitive reflection of message content after exposure (Bartsch and Kalch 2012; Bartsch and Oliver 2011), and information seeking may be one behavior individuals undertake as part of a quest to reflect on their mixed emotional experience. One can imagine watching a very moving and tender advertisement for the American Cancer Society about a cancer survivor who cares for cancer patients in hospice. The viewer could feel hopeful and happy for the survivor, but also sad about the fate of those in hospice. By end of the ad, the viewer would likely feel touched and moved, and might then feel motivated to search for more information about cancer and or organizations that fund cancer research and survivorship programs. This is but one example of how mixed emotions may facilitate information searchers, particularly searches for social information, or information presented in a social environment such as via social media or an online support group, such that the search would help the user connect with humanity (Oliver 2008; Oliver and Bartsch 2011).

HOW WE SEARCH

The literature on emotions and emotional communication processes point to a number of ways in which emotions motivate people to search for health information. However, emotions can also shape how people search for such information—the actual process of searching. Which search terms are entered into a search engine, or which questions are asked in a health-related chat room? Which links are chosen or personal blogs read? How long do individuals search for health information, and when do they stop searching? These are the questions that have received relatively little scholarly attention as compared to why people search for health information.

Additionally, the massive amount of health information to be found via media makes the process of health information searching a navigational feat. Given the near-infinite amount of health information through which to search, people must make a dizzying number of decisions about what content to consume and how to consume it from among an array of results. Without gatekeepers to instill credibility and relevance to the information, the task of sifting through search engine results, for example, can be onerous (see Kalyanaraman and Sundar 2008). How do people deal with this information overload in a health information context? Many of the same emotion theories discussed above provide some possible insight, as do additional frameworks from the social psychology literature.

Appraisal Theories

Once someone has decided to search for information, appraisals, emotions, and action tendencies can shape the nature of that search. In a three-factor between-subjects experiment about how people search online for information about influenza, it was found that participants induced to feel fearful or to be in a neutral emotional state were significantly more likely to think of search query terms related to death than were those induced to feel hopeful (citation withheld for blind review). This is preliminary evidence that even at the earliest stages of a health information search, emotions can influence the nature of the search.

Emotions will also impact the actual process of searching by shaping preferences for different types of content. The affective component of information seeking helps information seekers regulate the cognitive processing of information by prioritizing certain search goals over others (Nahl 1998; 2004). As Nabi (1999) hypothesized, based on the tenets of appraisal theories and the action tendencies associated with discrete emotions, "if afraid, receivers seek information about protection; if angry, about retribution; if sad, about coping with loss; if disgusted, about avoidance of the noxious element; and if guilt ridden, about proper reparation" (305).

To test a portion of this hypothesis, Nabi (2003) designed an experiment to test if feelings of fear versus anger impacted participant's desire to seek different types of information about drunk driving. Her predictions were confirmed when those participants induced to feel fear were more likely to desire protection-related information while those induced to feel anger were more likely to desire retribution-related information. This study demonstrated how after people have already decided to search for health information, action tendencies can influence what content they chose to consume during their search.

Lerner and Keltner's (2000; 2001) extension of appraisal theories—the Appraisal Tendency Framework (ATF)—outlines the ways in which initial appraisals associated with an emotional reaction can also influence subsequent cognitions and decisions. They found feelings of fear led to pessimistic risk estimates while feelings of anger led to optimistic risk estimates, in line with appraisals of certainty and control. In another instance, Winterich, Han, and Lerner (2010) used the ATF to show that feelings of sadness (anger) can blunt a subsequent experience of anger (sadness), and that these effects are mediated by the different appraisals of agency associated with sadness (situational control) and anger (individual control), respectively.

If one source of health information encountered during a search leads the searcher to feel one way, say anxious, while the next morsel of information encountered in a search would normally induce a different emotion, say anger, then the ATF would predict that the initial emotion will alter that secondary emotional experience in ways that would shape how the searcher judges the latter piece of information. Given the vast number of decision points during an information search (e.g., which search queries to use, which source of information to chose, when to move on to a new source, when to ask a medical professional about information found during an initial search, when to ask for help, when to stop searching, etc.), the ATF suggests an important avenue for future research on health information searches is one that tests who inter-media or inter-message emotions impact the processing of and reactions to subsequent health information.

The Mood-as-Resource Hypothesis

Another way the emotional state of the user may influence preferences for certain types of content during a search can be explained by the mood-as-resource hypothesis (Raghunathan and Trope 2002; Trope and Pomerantz 1998). This framework argues that positive emotional states provide individuals with a buffer, or resource, they can then use to consume potentially self-threatening information. Research bears out this idea that positive affect can promote information consumption that would benefit long-term instead of short-term interests of the individual. Trope and Neter (1994) found that participants in a positive mood were more likely to seek information about their weaknesses than their strengths than were participants in a negative mood. Similarly, Kustubayeva, Matthews, and Panganiban (2011) showed that the affective state of a video game player influences what types of information the player sought from the program during a decision-making task. Players who had been experimentally induced to be in a negative mood were more likely to sample positive information from the game than those who were induced to be in a positive mood, whereas those in a positive mood sampled more negative information about their progress in the game.

It benefits individuals to consume self-threatening information—including information about health threats and risks—so that they may learn and improve in the long term despite the short-term discomfort. While it may be unpleasant for a healthy individual in her twenties to imagine having breast cancer in her fifties, doing so may motivate her to take the necessary preventative actions of exercising and eating a healthier diet. However, because individuals are often motivated to protect their egos and self-identities, they are often inclined to avoid such information so they can maintain short-term positive feelings and self-images.

The mood-as-resource perspective indicates that if health information seekers perceive potential sources of health information as self-relevant, then those individuals already experiencing a positive emotion, such as hope, would be more likely to pay attention to potentially self-threatening health information that could help them prevent a future health threat. On the other hand, searchers experiencing an aversive negative state such as anxiety may unconsciously avoid information that would tell them their true risks of a health threat, and instead favoring more reassuring information. These different types of health searches would likely have important impacts on post-search behavior, but empirical evidence is needed to test this assumption.

Emotion Regulation and Mood Management

Literature in the tradition of emotion regulation and mood management also demonstrates how emotions generated by one event can impact perceptions of subsequent stimuli. And when searching for health information, the searcher is likely to encounter multiple stimuli. Research on inter-media effects demonstrates the connections between emotions resulting from one media stimulus and reactions to another. Holbert and Hansen (2008) showed that when people felt angry after viewing the movie *Fahrenheit 9/11* (which criticized the George W. Bush administration) prior to watching a presidential debate between Bush and his Democratic challenger, John Kerry, that anger from the movie explained partisan preferences and audiences' perceptions of the subsequent debate.

Just as a desire to manage one's affective state may motivate a search for health information, that initial emotion may impact how searchers interpret and react to information they find *during* the search process. Additionally, emotional reactions to information found at the beginning of the search process may then shape how users respond to information found at the end of the search. However, an initial emotional reaction may also impede subsequent emotional responses. In a paper called "Now that I'm sad, it's hard to be mad," Winterich et al. (2010) found that a specific emotion can blunt the experience of a subsequent emotion when the two emotions are defined by contrasting appraisal tendencies. For instance, sadness is defined by appraisals of situational agency (i.e., the situation is to blame, not any one person), whereas anger arises from appraisals of individual agency, making it hard to be mad immediately after feeling sad. When searching for health information, similar influences on subsequent emotions and attitudes could occur, but additional research is needed to test this hypothesis.

The intensity of an emotion state may also impact how people search. Zillmann and colleagues (Tannenbaum and Zillmann 1975; Zillmann 1971) demonstrated that excitation (i.e., an increase in sympathetic activity of the autonomic nervous system) can transfer from one mediated experience to another, and that audiences typically misattribute the transferred arousal from the primary message to the secondary one. Excitation could transfer from the initial event that motivated an information search (e.g., a curious-looking mole) to the content found while searching (e.g., the first website in a Google search results page), leading the searcher to perceive the information as more arousing than it would if she happened upon it in a calmer context. Likewise, a source of information found early in a search, such as a fast-paced public service announcement with graphic images of a health threat, could have carry-over arousal for subsequent information sources found during the source. While arousal levels may not alter the nature of cognitions or behaviors that result from the information-seeking process, it may amplify their intensity or immediacy (Roseman 2011).

Expanding the excitation transfer framework Internet use, Mastro, Eastin, and Tamborini (2002) found that high levels of stress in participants resulted in participants viewing fewer websites than those who were bored. Meanwhile, participants experiencing high levels of boredom searched through higher numbers of websites within the same amount of time. Therefore, online health information searches may result in better health outcomes if the searcher is not overly aroused and spends more time sorting through the vast amount of the health information found online, much of it of dubious quality (Eysenbach, Powell, Kuss, and Sa 2002). Future research could test this proposition in experimental and naturalistic settings.

Researchers have also found that individuals expect events that match the valence of their mood states to be more likely to occur than ones that are different from their current mood (E. J. Johnson and Tversky 1983). That is, people in a sad mood think sad events are more likely to occur in the future than are happy events. DeSteno, Petty, Wegener, and Rucker (2000) demonstrated that this effect held true for discrete emotions as well, with those participants who were sad (angry) being more likely to except future sad (angering) events. The researchers also found that the informational value of discrete emotions mediated the relationship between emotional state and outcome expectancies. Basically, the initial emotion state was provided evidence that events of a similar-emotional tone are likely to happen, and therefore could easily happen again in the future.

Because of this relationship between emotions and outcome expectancies, Afifi and his colleagues (Afifi and Morse 2009; Afifi and Weiner 2004) included a direct link between emotions and outcome expectancies in the TMIM. This literature should encourage researchers to not only measure concurrent affective states during searches but also assess how searchers imagine they will feel after searching in order to help explain mood management outcomes and variance in actual search behaviors (e.g., choosing certain sources over others or terminating a search earlier or later). As in other health domains, both current and anticipated emotional states of searchers would likely shape the search process.

WHAT HAPPENS AFTER A SEARCH

After a search for health information, will users change their health behaviors for the better? Will they contact a medical professional, or talk to friends or family about the health issue at hand? Will they use social media to reach out to others in a similar situation or ask for help finding more information? Will they turn to the Internet again if more questions arise about a health issue? The answers to these questions are likely influenced by the emotions users experience at the end their search. These emotions are temporally more proximate to the behaviors that can occur once a searcher closes the laptop.

Research indicates that the emotions felt at the peak and at the end of an experience dominate individuals' retrospective evaluations of that experience

(Kahneman, Fredrickson, Schreiber, and Redelmeier 1993). This finding implies that the emotions users feel at the end of a search, as well as the most intense emotions felt during the search, could help explain what users do with the information they find after searching. Preliminary experimental evidence indicates that post-search emotions do, indeed, have an impact on what people do after they search for health information. In a study of online searches for information about influenza, Myrick (2014) found that post-search feelings of fear and hope were both positive predictors of intentions to get an influenza vaccine. Additionally, feeling content after a search was directly related to positive attitudes toward a beta version of a search engine created solely to retrieve online health information, while feeling interested in the topic of influenza/the influenza vaccine increased positive outcome expectancies related to future health information searches, indirectly increased self-efficacy for searching for health information, and was indirectly related to positive attitudes toward the search engine. Feelings of fear after searching, however, decreased the positive outcome expectancies related to future searches for health information. Additional work is needed to also test the effects of peak search emotions in juxtaposition to these post-search emotions.

Mixed Emotions

Throughout the health information–seeking process, users are likely to be exposed to a variety of information, presented via a variety of emotional overtones, and eliciting a variety of emotional responses. As has been mentioned previously in this book, health messages can evoke multiple emotions in audiences, from fear and sadness to anger, guilt, hope, and many others (Dillard, Plotnick, Godblod, Freimuth, and Edgar 1996; Nabi 2015; S. W. Smith et al. 2010; Williams-Piehota, Pizarro, Schneider, Mowad, and Salovey 2005). In an online search context, one link on a search results page may scare the user, while the next provides the user with reassurance, but the third link spurs a mix of emotional reactions in the user. To date, little research has examined the impact of mixed emotions following a health information search, be they the result of consuming multiple types of search results or from a single search result that evokes multiple emotions simultaneously.

Experiencing mixed emotions while or after searching could increase the chances that the searcher will share the encountered information with others (Myrick and Oliver 2014), and such sharing could greatly increase the number of people exposed to a preventative health message. Emotional states are often short-lived (Lazarus 1991), making the link between emotions and subsequent behaviors difficult to trace (Baumeister, Vohs, Nathan DeWall, and Zhang 2007). However, in a hyper-connected online environment, users can share information almost instantly while the present emotion is still salient. This technological affordance means that the sharing of information with others could be one of the more common behaviors to result from experiencing emotions while using the Internet for health information seeking, as opposed to behaviors that take longer to implement or that occur after the initial emotion dissipates.

A mixed emotional experience that motivates health information seekers to share what they find can also motivate users to continue to ponder the information found during a search as mixed emotions have been found to stimulate cognitive reflection (see Bartsch and Oliver 2011; Oliver and Woolley 2011). Because a healthy lifestyle cannot be achieved through one search for information alone, it is important that health information–seeking research include the study of emotional responses that foster further reflection on the information found in that search. Search results that evoke mixed emotions are one route through which information seeking may foster such reflection, and future work could continue to test the processes and effects related to mixed emotions information seeking.

A NOTE ON METHODOLOGY

Many tests of health information–seeking models use cross-sectional survey data (e.g., Kahlor 2010; Yang and Kahlor 2012). While this method provides a nice snapshot of how individuals think about health information seeking at one moment in time, the use of experiments should be added to the methodological arsenal to better test causal chains of effects of health information seeking. Experiments using affective measures other than self-reports, such as facial action coding (Ekman and Rosenberg 1998), or psychophysiological measures such as skin conductance and heart rate (Lang, Potter, and Bolls 2009), or even implicit affective evaluations (Payne, Cheng, Govorun, and Stewart 2005), could also help researchers better understand the impact of emotions throughout the health information–seeking processes.

Longitudinal data could also help reveal how improvements over time in a user's searching ability and/or self-efficacy for finding useful health information during a search impact post-search emotions and behaviors. Longitudinal and unobtrusive measurements of search behaviors via search-monitoring software is another promising methodological innovation for those wanting to study health information seeking. This type of data, especially if it is combined with longitudinal data on emotional reactions (be it self-report or more implicitly measured), would provide scholars with valuable insights related to the connection between emotional reactions and actual search behaviors. Longitudinal observations and self-report data would also help scholars tease apart conceptual and empirical differences in scanning (i.e., health information gathered via routine media use) versus purposeful health information seeking (see Kelly et al. 2010; Kelly, Niederdeppe, and Hornik 2009; Shim et al. 2006).

CONCLUSION

Theory and research on discrete emotions provide communication researchers with many avenues for investigating and explaining health information–seeking behaviors, particularly as they pertain to searches that aim to prevent illness and disease. Studying emotional reactions to health information other than fear and anxiety are ripe conceptual areas for investigation. As health communication scholars begin to branch out in their quest to understand what motivates people to seek health information, and to understand what users do with that information once they've found it, expanding theoretical and methodological boundaries is of the utmost importance.

This chapter is not an exhaustive list of the ways in which emotions impact health information seeking. Rather, it is meant to be a springboard for additional theory building and empirical research of health information seeking and post-search preventative health behaviors. Conceptual and methodological innovations in the study of how people search for, find, and make use of quality, relevant, and helpful health information are particularly needed in the digital age in which people can find vast amounts of health information online, anytime, day or night.

REFERENCES

Afifi, W. A., and C. R. Morse. 2009. Expanding the role of emotion in the theory of motivated information management. In T. D. Afifi and W. A. Afifi (Eds.), *Uncertainty, information management, and disclosure decisions: Theories and applications* (pp. 87–105). New York: Routledge.

Afifi, W. A., and J. L. Weiner. 2004. Toward a theory of motivated information management. *Communication Theory* 14(2):167–90. doi: 10.1111/j.1468-2885.2004.tb00310.x.

Bartsch, A., and A. Kalch. 2012. *Moved to think: The role of emotional media experiences in stimulating reflective thoughts.* Paper presented at the annual conference of the International Communication Association, Phoenix, AZ.

Bartsch, A., and M. B. Oliver. 2011. Making sense of entertainment: On the interplay of emotion and cognition in entertainment experience. *Journal of Media Psychology: Theories, Methods, and Applications* 23(1):12–17. doi: 10.1027/1864-1105/a000026.

Baumeister, R. F., K. D. Vohs, C. Nathan DeWall, and L. Zhang. 2007. How emotion shapes behavior: Feedback, anticipation, and reflection, rather than direct causation. *Personality and Social Psychology Review* 11(2):167–203. doi: 10.1177/1088868307301033.

Brashers, D. E. 2001. Communication and uncertainty management. *Journal of Communication* 51(3):477–97. doi: 10.1111/j.1460-2466.2001.tb02892.x.

Brashers, D. E., D. J. Goldsmith, and E. Hsieh. 2002. Information seeking and avoiding in health contexts. *Human Communication Research* 28(2):258–71. doi: 10.1111/j.1468-2958.2002.tb00807.x.

Bryant, J., and D. Zillmann. 1984. Using television to alleviate boredom and stress: Selective exposure as a function of induced excitational states. *Journal of Broadcasting* 28(1):1–20. doi: 10.1080/08838158409386511.

DeSteno, D., R. E. Petty, D. T. Wegener, and D. D. Rucker. 2000. Beyond valence in the perception of likelihood: The role of emotion specificity. *Journal of Personality and Social Psychology* 78(3):397–416. doi: 10.1037/0022-3514.78.3.397.

Dillard, J. P., C. A. Plotnick, L. C. Godblod, V. S. Freimuth, and T. Edgar. 1996. The multiple affective outcomes of AIDS PSAs: Fear appeals do more than scare people. *Communication Research* 23(1):44–72. doi: 10.1177/009365096023001002.

Dillard, J. P., and K. Seo. 2013. Affect and persuasion. In J. P. Dillard and L. Shen (Eds.), *The SAGE handbook of persuasion: Developments in theory and practice* (Second ed., pp. 150–66). Thousand Oaks, CA: SAGE.

Ekman, P., and E. L. Rosenberg. 1998. *What the face reveals: Basic and applied studies of spontaneous expression using the Facial Action Coding System (FACS)*. Oxford University Press, USA.

Eysenbach, G., J. Powell, O. Kuss, and E.-R. Sa. 2002. Empirical studies assessing the quality of health information for consumers on the world wide web: A systematic review. *JAMA: The Journal of the American Medical Association* 287(20):2691–700. doi: 10.1001/jama.287.20.2691.

Fox, S. 2013. Health online 2013. Retrieved March 3, 2013, from http://www.pewinternet.org/Reports/2013/Health-online.aspx.

Fredrickson, B. L., and R. W. Levenson. 1998. Positive emotions speed recovery from the cardiovascular sequelae of negative emotions. *Cognition and Emotion* 12(2):191–220. doi: 10.1080/026999398379718.

Fredrickson, B. L., R. A. Mancuso, C. Branigan, and M. M. Tugade. 2000. The undoing effect of positive emotion. *Motivation and Emotion* 24(4):237–58. doi: 10.1023/A:1010796329158.

Freimuth, V. S., J. A. Stein, and T. J. Kean. 1989. *Searching for health information: The cancer information service model*. Philadelphia: University of Pennsylvania Press.

Frijda, N. H., P. Kuipers, and E. ter Schure. 1989. Relations among emotion, appraisal, and emotional action readiness. *Journal of Personality and Social Psychology* 57(2):212–28. doi: 10.1037/0022-3514.57.2.212.

Galarce, E. M., S. Ramanadhan, and K. Viswanath. 2011. Health information seeking. In T. L. Thompson, R. Parrott, and J. F. Nussbaum (Eds.), *The Routledge handbook of health communication* (Second ed., pp. 167–80). New York: Routledge.

Griffin, R. J., S. Dunwoody, and K. Neuwirth. 1999. Proposed model of the relationship of risk information seeking and processing to the development of preventive behaviors. *Environmental Research* 80(2):S230–S245. doi: 10.1006/enrs.1998.3940.

Gross, J. J., and R. A. Thompson. 2007. Emotion regulation: Conceptual foundations. In J. J. Gross (Ed.), *Handbook of emotion regulation* (pp. 3–24). New York: Guilford Press.

Holbert, R. L., and G. J. Hansen. 2008. Stepping beyond message specificity in the study of emotion as mediator and inter-emotion associations across attitude objects: Fahrenheit 9/11, anger, and debate superiority. *Media Psychology* 11(1):98–118. doi: 10.1080/15213260701832512.

Johnson, E. J., and A. Tversky. 1983. Affect, generalization, and the perception of risk. *Journal of Personality and Social Psychology* 45(1):20–31. doi: 10.1037/0022-3514.45.1.20.

Johnson, J. D., and H. Meischke. 1993. A comprehensive model of cancer-related information seeking applied to magazines. *Human Communication Research* 19(3):343–67. doi: 10.1111/j.1468-2958.1993.tb00305.x.

Kahlor, L. 2010. PRISM: A planned risk information seeking model. *Health Communication* 25:345–56. doi: 10.1080/10410231003775172.

Kahneman, D., B. L. Fredrickson, C. A. Schreiber, and D. A. Redelmeier. 1993. When more pain is preferred to less: Adding a better end. *Psychological Science* 4(6):401–5. doi: 10.1111/j.1467-9280.1993.tb00589.x.

Kalyanaraman, S., and S. S. Sundar. 2008. Portrait of the portal as a metaphor: Explicating web portals for communication research. *Journalism and Mass Communication Quarterly* 85(2):239–56. doi: 10.1177/107769900808500202.

Kashdan, T. B. 2004. Curiosity. In C. Peterson and M. E. P. Seligman (Eds.), *Character strengths and virtues* (pp. 125–41). New York: Oxford University Press.

Kelly, B., R. Hornik, A. Romantan, J. S. Schwartz, K. Armstrong, A. DeMichele, . . . N. Wong. 2010. Cancer information scanning and seeking in the general population. *Journal of Health Communication* 15(7):734–53. doi: 10.1080/10810730.2010.514029.

Kelly, B., J. Niederdeppe, and R. Hornik. 2009. Validating measures of scanned information exposure in the context of cancer prevention and screening behaviors. *Journal of Health Communication* 14(8):721–40. doi: 10.1080/10810730903295559.

Kuhlthau, C. C. 1991. Inside the search process: Information seeking from the user's perspective. *Journal of the American Society for Information Science* 42(5):361–71. doi: 10.1002/(sici)1097-4571(199106)42:5***l361::aid-asi6***r3.0.co;2-#.

Kustubayeva, A., G. Matthews, and A. Panganiban. 2011. Emotion and information search in tactical decision-making: Moderator effects of feedback. *Motivation and Emotion*, 1–15. doi: 10.1007/s11031-011-9270-5.

Lang, A., R. F. Potter, and P. Bolls. 2009. Where psychophysiology meets the media: Taking the effects out of mass media research. In J. Bryant and M. B. Oliver (Eds.), *Media effects: Advances in theory and research* (Third ed., pp. 185–206). New York: Routledge.

Larsen, J. T., A. P. McGraw, and J. T. Cacioppo. 2001. Can people feel happy and sad at the same time? *Journal of Personality and Social Psychology* 81(4):684–96. doi: 10.1037/0022-3514.81.4.684.

Lazarus, R. S. 1991. *Emotion and adaptation.* New York: Oxford University Press.

———. 1999. Hope: An emotion and a vital coping resource against despair. *Social Research* 66(2):653–78.

Lerner, J. S., and D. Keltner. 2000. Beyond valence: Toward a model of emotion-specific influences on judgment and choice. *Cognition and Emotion* 14(4):473–93. doi: 10.1080/026999300402763.

———. 2001. Fear, anger, and risk. *Journal of Personality and Social Psychology* 81(1):146–59. doi: 10.1037/0022-3514.81.1.146.

Loewenstein, G. F., E. U. Weber, C. K. Hsee, and N. Welch. 2001. Risk as feelings. *Psychological Bulletin* 127(2):267–86. doi: 10.1037/0033-2909.127.2.267.

Mastro, D. E., M. S. Eastin, and R. Tamborini. 2002. Internet search behaviors and mood alterations: A selective exposure approach. *Media Psychology* 4(2):157–72. doi: 10.1207/S1532785XMEP0402_03.

Morahan-Martin, J. M. 2004. How Internet users find, evaluate, and use online health information: A cross-cultural review. *Cyberpsychology and Behavior* 7(5):497–510. doi: 10.1089/cpb.2004.7.497.

Myrick, J. G. 2014. *The role of emotions and social cognitive variables in health information seeking: A tailored approach.* Paper presented at the Kentucky Conference on Health Communication, Lexington, KY.

Myrick, J. G., and M. B. Oliver. 2014. Laughing and crying: Mixed emotions, compassion, and the effectiveness of a YouTube PSA about skin cancer. *Health Communication*, 1–10. doi: 10.1080/10410236.2013.845729.

Nabi, R. L. 1999. A cognitive-functional model for the effects of discrete negative emotions on information processing, attitude change, and recall. *Communication Theory* 9(3):292–320. doi: 10.1111/j.1468-2885.1999.tb00172.x.

———. 2003. Exploring the framing effects of emotion. *Communication Research* 30(2):224–47. doi: 10.1177/0093650202250881.

———. 2015. Emotional flow in persuasive health messages. *Health Communication* 30(2):114–24. doi: 10.1080/10410236.2014.974129.

Nahl, D. 1998. Ethnography of novices' first use of web search engines. *Internet Reference Services Quarterly* 3(2):51–72. doi: 10.1300/J136v03n02_09.

———. 2004. Measuring the affective information environment of web searchers. *Proceedings of the American Society for Information Science and Technology* 41(1):191–97. doi: 10.1002/meet.1450410122.

Oliver, M. B. 2003. Mood management and selective exposure. In J. Bryant, D. Roskos-Ewoldsen, and J. Cantor (Eds.), *Communication and emotion* (pp. 85–106). Mahway, NJ: Lawrence Erlbaum Associates.

———. 2008. Tender affective states as predictors of entertainment preference. *Journal of Communication* 58(1):40–61. doi: 10.1111/j.1460-2466.2007.00373.x.

Oliver, M. B., and A. Bartsch. 2010. Appreciation as audience response: Exploring entertainment gratifications beyond hedonism. *Human Communication Research* 36(1):53–81. doi: 10.1111/j.1468-2958.2009.01368.x.

———. 2011. Appreciation of entertainment: The importance of meaningfulness via virtue and wisdom. *Journal of Media Psychology: Theories, Methods, and Applications* 23(1):29–33. doi: 10.1027/1864-1105/a000029.

Oliver, M. B., T. Hartmann, and J. K. Woolley. 2012. Elevation in response to entertainment portrayals of moral virtue. *Human Communication Research* 38(3):360–78. doi: 10.1111/j.1468-2958.2012.01427.x.

Oliver, M. B., and J. K. Woolley. 2011. Tragic and poignant entertainment: The gratifications of meaningfulness as emotional response. In K. Döveling, C. von Scheve, and E. A. Konijn (Eds.), *The Routledge handbook of emotions and mass media* (pp. 134–47). New York: Routledge.

Panksepp, J. 2007. Neurologizing the psychology of affects: How appraisal-based constructivism and basic emotion theory can coexist. *Perspectives on Psychological Science* 2(3):281–96.

Payne, B. K., C. M. Cheng, O. Govorun, and B. D. Stewart. 2005. An inkblot for attitudes: Affect misattribution as implicit measurement. *Journal of Personality and Social Psychology* 89(3):227–93. doi: 10.1037/0022-3514.89.3.277.

Pirolli, P., and S. Card. 1999. Information foraging. *Psychological Review* 106(4):643–75.

Raghunathan, R., and Y. Trope. 2002. Walking the tightrope between feeling good and being accurate: Mood as a resource in processing persuasive messages. *Journal of Personality and Social Psychology* 83(3):510–25. doi: 10.1037/0022-3514.83.3.510.

Rimal, R. N., and K. Real. 2003. Perceived risk and efficacy beliefs as motivators of change: Use of the risk perception attitude (RPA) framework to understand health behaviors. *Human Communication Research* 29(3):370–99. doi: 10.1111/j.1468-2958.2003.tb00844.x.

Roseman, I. J. 1984. Cognitive determinants of emotion: A structural theory. *Review of Personality and Social Psychology* 5:11–36.

———. 2011. Emotional behaviors, emotivational goals, emotion strategies: Multiple levels of organization integrate variable and consistent responses. *Emotion Review* 3(4):434–43. doi: 10.1177/1754073911410744.

Roseman, I. J., C. Wiest, and T. S. Swartz. 1994. Phenomenology, behaviors, and goals differentiate discrete emotions. *Journal of Personality and Social Psychology* 67(2):206–21. doi: 10.1037/0022-3514.67.2.206.

Rutten, L. J. F., L. Squiers, and B. Hesse. 2006. Cancer-related information seeking: Hints from the 2003 health information national trends survey (HINTS). *Journal of Health Communication* 11(s1):147–56. doi: 10.1080/10810730600637574.

Scherer, K. R. 1984. On the nature and function of emotion: A component process approach. In K. R. Scherer and P. Ekman (Eds.), *Approaches to emotions* (pp. 293–318). Hillsdale, NJ: Lawrence Erlbaum.

Scherer, K. R., A. Schorr, and T. Johnstone. 2001. *Appraisal processes in emotion: Theory, methods, research.* Oxford: Oxford University Press.

Shim, M., B. Kelly, and R. Hornik. 2006. Cancer information scanning and seeking behavior is associated with knowledge, lifestyle choices, and screening. *Journal of Health Communication* 11(S1):157–72. doi: 10.1080/10810730600637475.

Silvia, P. J. 2005. What is interesting? Exploring the appraisal structure of interest. *Emotion* 5(1):89–102. doi: 10.1037/1528-3542.5.1.89.

———. 2006. *Exploring the psychology of interest.* New York: Oxford University Press.

———. 2008. Interest—The curious emotion. *Current Directions in Psychological Science* 17(1):57–60. doi: 10.1111/j.1467-8721.2008.00548.x.

Smith, C. A., and P. C. Ellsworth. 1985. Patterns of cognitive appraisal in emotion. *Journal of Personality and Social Psychology* 48(4):813–38. doi: 10.1037/0022-3514.48.4.813.

Smith, S. W., L. M. Hamel, M. R. Kotowski, S. Nazione, C. LaPlante, and C. K. Atkin. 2010. Action tendency emotions evoked by memorable breast cancer messages and their association with prevention and detection behaviors. *Health Communication* 25:737–46.

Tannenbaum, P. H., and D. Zillmann. 1975. Emotional arousal in the facilitation of aggression through communication. In B. Leonard (Ed.), *Advances in Experimental Social Psychology* (Vol. 8, pp. 149–92): Academic Press.

Tian, Y., and J. D. Robinson. 2008. Media use and health information seeking: An empirical test of complementarity theory. *Health Communication* 23(2):184–90. doi: 10.1080/10410230801968260.

Trope, Y., and E. Neter. 1994. Reconciling competing motives in self-evaluation: The role of self-control in feedback seeking. *Journal of Personality and Social Psychology* 66(4):646–57. doi: 10.1037/0022-3514.66.4.646.

Trope, Y., and E. M. Pomerantz. 1998. Resolving conflicts among self-evaluative motives: Positive experiences as a resource for overcoming defensiveness. *Motivation and Emotion* 22(1):53–72. doi: 10.1023/a:1023044625309.

Williams-Piehota, P., J. Pizarro, T. R. Schneider, L. Mowad, and P. Salovey. 2005. Matching health messages to monitor-blunter coping styles to motivate screening mammography. *Health Psychology* 24(1):58–67. doi: 10.1037/0278-6133.24.1.58.

Winterich, K. P., S. Han, and J. S. Lerner. 2010. Now that I'm sad, it's hard to be mad: The role of cognitive appraisals in emotional blunting. *Personality and Social Psychology Bulletin* 36(11):1467–83. doi: 10.1177/0146167210384710.

Yang, Z. J., and L. Kahlor. 2013. What, me worry? The role of affect in information seeking and avoidance. *Science Communication* 35(2):189–212. doi: 10.1177/1075547012441873.

Zillmann, D. 1971. Excitation transfer in communication-mediated aggressive behavior. *Journal of Experimental Social Psychology* 7(4):419–34. doi: 10.1016/0022-1031(71)90075-8.

———. 1988. Mood management through communication choices. *American Behavioral Scientist* 31(3):327–40. doi: 10.1177/000276488031003005.

Zillmann, D., and J. Bryant. 1985. *Selective exposure to communication*. Hillsdale, NJ: Erlbaum Associates.

Chapter Fourteen

eHealth

In response to the seeming omnipresence of interactive communication technologies (ICTs), a growing number of health communication researchers are studying and using modern technology as a tool for fostering health behavior change (Sundar, Rice, Kim, and Sciamanna 2011). This work is generally referred to as "eHealth," which is "the use of emerging information and communication technology, especially the Internet, to improve or enable health and health care" (Eng 2001, 1). Simply put, eHealth is the use of digital communication tools to improve health. A growing body of research examines eHealth applications and their implications for public health (Noar and Harrington 2012). This includes the use of the Internet, computers, and/or mobile devices to disseminate health information and social support to individuals who may need it. Examples of eHealth include text messages to assist smokers in their quest to quit, online health information websites, computer-tailored exercise routines with tracking and feedback features, and even video games that require physical activity that aim to prevent obesity and type 2 diabetes.

This study of eHealth is part of a larger research paradigm investigating the effects of communication technology on users. Communication technology scholars have long recognized the important role of emotions in shaping attitudes and behaviors related to information transferred via technology (Picard 1997). Affective computing, a term coined by Picard, embodies the view that computers can be programed to recognize emotions and respond to users in an appropriate manner based on their emotional states. Because computers store and utilize large amounts of information, computer programs can take advantage of affective information provided by users in deciding how to respond to various user inputs (Clore and Palmer 2009). The ability of computers to capture, analyze, and respond to digital health information has allowed researchers to monitor influenza outbreaks (Cook, Conrad, Fowlkes, and Mohebbi 2011) and gain valuable insight into public reactions to health campaigns (Emery, Szczypka, Abril, Kim, and Vera 2014).

Despite the cold, hard, physical features of mechanical devices, users tend to respond to computers rather naturally, as if they were interacting with another human (Nass and Yen 2010; Reeves and Nass 1996). The media equation (Reeves and Nass) states that human users perceive computers to be social actors and, therefore, user interactions with computers (and other ICTs) are quite similar to interactions users might have with another human. According to the media equation, people will identify what they believe to be good or bad behavior, react differently to positive and negative stimuli, and experience various levels of emotional arousal when interacting with ICTs, just as they would when interacting with another person or event in a non-technological environment.

Besides being a factor in how users interact with ICTs, emotion is an essential component of interface design in a digital environment (Ji 2013). From emoji (computer symbols that display cartoon images of emotional facial expressions) to the choice of color of various widgets or the type of audio used, emotion-evoking structural features and content abounds in electronic media. For example, in a study of audience reactions to audio news stories, Nass, Foehr, Brave, and Somoza (2001) had participants listen to the same stories presented via either a happy-toned or sad-toned computerized voice. The researchers found that the emotional tone of the computer's voice impacted users' perception of the news content's valence, likability, and trustworthiness.

Furthermore, embodied computing agents can display empathy toward human users. Research indicates that when a computer displays empathy, users report liking and trusting the computer agent more than if it did not portray compassion toward the user (Brave, Nass, and Hutchinson 2005). Brave et al. found that people who interact with such empathic computerized agents report greater perceived caring and felt as though they had received social support. Given the beneficial health outcomes associated with social support (Sherbourne and Stewart 1991; Shumaker and Brownell 1984; Uchino, Cacioppo, and Kiecolt-Glaser 1996), computing agents that can recognize user emotion and respond with empathy for individuals struggling to implement challenging preventative behaviors (like healthy diet and exercise regimens) are promising prospects for eHealth applications.

Given the ability of computing agents and electronic interfaces to represent emotion and empathy, which in turn influences users' affective, cognitive, and behavioral responses to technology, it would be a smart move for those studying user responses to eHealth applications to analyze and understand the role of emotion in various digital-based prevention contexts. This chapter first discusses conceptual considerations for understanding eHealth processes and effects before discussing the role of emotions in four specific eHealth domains: tailored information, mobile health, virtual reality and serious games, and social media. Finally, this chapter suggests many future avenues for integrating the study of emotion and affect in research on and applications of eHealth to promote health prevention behaviors.

CONCEPTUAL CONSIDERATIONS: INTERACTIVITY AND TAILORING

Interaction between two people, or two agents, is the backbone of an interactive experience (Sundar 2007). Conceptually, interactivity is rooted in the idea of contingency. That is, new messages are contingent upon previous messages in an interactive environment, and each response builds upon the prior one (Sundar, Kalyanaraman, and Brown 2003). The contingency view of interactivity results in a loop of interdependent messages. These contingent messages are fairly easy for users to generate in face-to-face and computer-mediated communications (CMC), but more challenging to foster in a human-computer interaction (HCI) context where an electronic agent or device must use algorithms in order to respond to the user (Sundar, Bellur, Oh, Jia, and Kim 2014).

Research demonstrates that perceptions of interactivity can shape the attitudes and behavioral intentions of ICT users. For example, users' perceptions of interactivity of a website can increase perceptions of source credibility, with more interactive websites associated with more credibility (Sundar 2007; Sundar et al. 2003; Tao and Bucy 2007). Perceptions of website interactivity can also foster increased user engagement and, subsequently, positive attitudes toward the a site (Sundar et al. 2014). Multiple structural features of websites can increase perceptions of interactivity, from live chat conversations and presenting messages based on interaction history to features that offer users a choice (e.g., drop-down menus) or the opportunity to interact with other users. In short, though, it is the perception of interactivity and not necessarily objective measures of objectivity, such as the number of certain features on a website, that shapes user attitudes and behavior.

Understanding and analyzing interactivity in eHealth programs can help health communication researchers understand which digital features will foster user engagement and positive attitudes—both outcomes with implications for emotion arousal. For instance, inclusion of high levels of interactivity in an eHealth program that allows users to get answers to specific questions for improving their diets could evoke positive emotional reactions, such as hope that one will be able eventually to achieve a healthier body. Moreover, computer-mediated interaction with other people via an eHealth interface could foster perceptions of social and emotional support, which in turn contributes to improved psychological and physical health (Reblin and Uchino 2008; Uchino 2006; Uchino et al. 1996).

In addition to understanding interactivity, knowledge about tailoring is helpful for comprehending and advancing eHealth research. Kreuter, Farrell, Olevitch, and Brennan (2000) define tailoring as the process of providing each individual unique content based on feedback as well as personal needs. An example of tailored health information is a pamphlet about mammography created based on individual's answers to a survey assessing risk for breast cancer, past screening behavior, time since last screening, and perceptions about susceptibility of breast cancer as well as benefits and barriers to mammography (Jensen, King, Carcioppolo, and Davis 2012). Tailoring is different from targeting in that tailoring is predicated on the provision of unique information to each individual, while targeting is the act of presenting information based on a group identity. By tailoring messages via ICTs, health information that was once relegated to mass media channels can instead be made to appear like interpersonal communication between individuals in a shared community (Beniger 1987).

ICTs can employ algorithms, tracking of past behaviors, and user input to efficiently tailor information to individual users. In their list of basic tenets of effective health communication in the eHealth era, Neuhauser and Kreps (2003) asserted that "tailored communication is more effective than generic messages" (11). Indeed, matching messages to user characteristics or preferences has proven to be an effective way to improve user attitudes toward digital content and interfaces (Kalyanaraman and Sundar 2006). The literature on tailoring of health information, specifically, reveals that tailoring generally produces positive effects on user attitudes and also on compliance with target health behaviors (Noar, Benac, and Harris 2007; Noar, Grant Harrington, Van Stee, and Shemanski Aldrich 2011). These meta-analytic reviews have shown that when health messages correspond with some aspect of the self related to demographics, individual differences, or psychological concepts, they are more effective in changing behaviors than are generic messages (Noar et al. 2007; 2011).

Although many tailored health interventions have resulted in attitude and behavior change, less is known about exactly *why* they were effective (Noar et al. 2011). How personally relevant message recipients perceive the message to be is one likely driver behind tailoring effects (Rimal and Adkins 2003). Tailored health messages are, indeed, perceived by users as more relevant to them than are non-tailored, generic health messages (Resnicow et al. 2009; Strecher, Shiffman, and West 2006). In a study of tailored breast cancer materials, Jensen, King, Carcioppolo, and Davis (2012) found participants who viewed illustrated pamphlets tailored to their self-reported personal risk factors and preferences for visual information responded to the tailored pamphlets with stronger intentions to get a mammogram than did participants who saw non-tailored information. Mediation analyses revealed that the positive effect of tailored illustrations on intentions to perform mammography was fully mediated by perceived relevance of the material in the pamphlet. However, perceived relevance did not mediate the relationship when participants saw charts or graphs instead of illustrations. While this study provided initial evidence of relevance as a mediator of tailoring effects, it left the door open to the existence of many potential other mediators of these effects.

Perceived relevance is also a primary appraisal required for the evocation of emotions (Lazarus 1991). Once an emotion is activated by an appraisal's self-relevance, the attendant action tendencies of their emotional states motivates people to try to adapt to their situation and make progress toward emotion-induced goals (Zeelenberg, Nelissen, Breugelmans, and Pieters 2008). Therefore, the evocation of emotions occurs in an inherently self-relevant manner, and tailored messages presenting audience members with self-relevant information are likely to evoke emotion in users. This connection between appraisal theory and the effects of tailored information requires empirical analysis, but presents a promising route for future research aiming to understand additional mechanisms of tailoring effects.

Health communication researchers might also consider using emotional content tailored to users' emotional states. The literature on emotion is sprinkled with clues that matching messages to some aspect of one's present emotional state may promote message acceptance and, eventually, behavioral compliance. For instance, scholars who matched the content of messages with the same discrete emotional states of participants found that emotion-matched messages were more persuasive than messages matched to other emotions (DeSteno, Petty, Rucker, Wegener, and Braverman 2004; DeSteno, Petty, Wegener, and Rucker 2000).

Tailoring health messages to the action tendencies of ICT users' current emotional states may also be an avenue for promoting message acceptance (Lerner and Keltner 2000; 2001). For example, Nabi (2003a) found that individuals primed to feel either angry or afraid with regard to a public health issue were more likely to seek out information that suggested policy changes that matched the action tendencies of their respective present emotional states (Nabi 2003a). If ICTs provide users with prevention-oriented health information that embodies their underlying emotional motivations, then perhaps the users will be more likely to embark on preventative health-related actions than if they receive information that does not conform to their emotion-related motivations (Myrick 2014). Future work could test the impact of emotional tailoring in any number of health contexts, from online information seeking to virtual reality simulations that can adapt instantly to users' emotional states.

To supplement the discussion of conceptual variables (i.e., interactivity and tailoring) central to understanding the role of emotions in eHealth research, this chapter will now review four specific eHealth domains: mobile health (mHealth), video games, virtual reality, and social media. For each of these eHealth contexts, the discussion centers on connections between the domains and emotional arousal as well as opportunities for future research.

MOBILE HEALTH (MHEALTH)

Mobile health, or mHealth, is the use of mobile electronic technology to improve health care, monitor health, promote self-management, and/or encourage healthy behaviors (Kumar et al. 2013). Specific to prevention, mobile devices have been used for interventions aimed at smoking cessation, body weight loss, reducing alcohol consumption, preventing sexually transmitted infections and their spread (see Cole-Lewis and Kershaw 2010), among other behaviors. Often, mHealth involves sending text messages (i.e., short message service, or SMS) to target populations. Other mHealth programs operate via applications on smartphones. mHealth has been an especially promising strategy for persuasive health communication and interventions in developing countries or in low-income populations where cell phones are low in cost but commonly used (Mechael 2009).

Mobile devices can be effective platforms for health communication and fostering healthy behaviors because these devices are almost always on individuals, can be personalized, can respond intelligently, and can help connect users to other people who are then able to provide information and/or social support (Fogg and Adler 2009). These capabilities, the spread of mobile technology to all corners of the globe (thanks to satellite technology), and the relatively low price of cell phones as compared to other electronics has encouraged health communication researchers to investigate why and how mHealth can help prevent disease.

In fact, researchers are beginning to find patterns that can predict which mHealth programs will be effective and which will not. Abroms, Padmanabhan, and Evans (2012) delineate six common approaches taken by effective mHealth text messaging programs: 1) providing health information/advice in a tailored format; 2) asking users to set goals; 3) providing reinforcement for goals that are met; 4) offering reminders; 5) providing opportunities for tracking progress; and, 6) offering social support. Many of these tactics involve psychological processes related to emotions. For instance, goals can be shaped by emotional action tendencies (Roseman 2011; Zeelenberg and Pieters 2006), while receiving reinforcement for progress and/or receiving social support can elicit positive emotional responses from users (Sarason, Sarason, and Pierce 1990; Uchino 2006). Furthermore, emotional support is an important component of social support (Sherbourne and Stewart 1991), and one commonly found in online social support programs related to health conditions (Klemm and Wheeler 2005; Yoo et al. 2014) that could also possibly be applied to interactive text messaging programs.

Below, two successful prevention-focused mHealth programs are briefly outlined as case studies of how mobile platforms can be used for preventative health purposes as well as how mHealth applications may shape users' emotional reactions to health information and potential threats.

Text4baby

Text4baby is a SMS-based program that delivers messages to traditionally underserved pregnant women and new mothers (text4baby 2014). The program sends the same set of messages to anyone who signs up for the service. The particular messages differ based on the stage of the user's pregnancy and eventually on their infant's ages. Sample messages include "Free t4b msg: Morning sickness may be caused by a change in your hormones. Try eating crackers or dry cereal. Eat small meals often. Don't go without eating"; and "Free msg: Not sure if your car seat is installed right? Get it inspected. Department of Transportation can help. Call 888-327-4236 for locations near you." (text4baby).

Text4baby was the first free national mobile health service in the United States (Remick and Kendrick 2013). The goal of the program, which came about via a public-private partnership, is to use timely text messages to help improve the health of mothers *and* babies from underserved populations. Message creators designed the text messages with the goals of increasing self-efficacy, outcome expectations for successful post-pregnancy outcomes, and health literacy among users (Evans, Wallace, and Snider 2012). Initial evaluations of text4baby found that underserved pregnant women and their infants did benefit from using the program (Evans et al. 2014; Evans et al. 2012).

The early evaluations of text4baby are promising for mHealth advocates. Nonetheless, these studies did not analyze any emotional motivations for using the service or emotional reactions to receiving the text messages. Researching both selective exposure to the service and affective reactions to it could help unveil reasons for its preliminary success as well as ways to improve the program to be even more efficacious. For instance, some women may have decided to sign up for the program due to anxiety or fears that they did not know enough about staying healthy during pregnancy or taking care of a baby. Those anxious women may respond better to texts with differently framed messages that match the action tendencies of anxiety than would those women who came to the service feeling hopeful about providing a better future for their child. Moreover, receiving the texts might evoke feelings of relief and even hope in users, while the information in the texts might make others realize how little they know and instead spark feelings of anxiety. Those users who become anxious after receiving the messages may do better if they received supplemental social support texts or other forms of pregnancy information.

Health communication researchers have also pointed to the need to tailor information provided by mHealth applications targeting female users, in particular, to women's information-gathering practices (Xue et al. 2013). According to Xue et al., these practices include a desire for information to provide flexiblity, responsiveness, and empathy. Gender differences have also been found in other emotion, health, and communication contexts (e.g., Andsager, Austin, and Pinkleton 2002; Biswas, Riffe, and Zillmann 1994; Guadagno, Blascovich, Bailenson, and McCall 2007; Wirth and Bodenhausen 2009). The findings from this body of research could be applied to improve programs such as text4baby based on differences in gender-based communication preferences or habits. Emotions and related concepts like empathy should be considered at the beginning of a user-centered design process and not just during evaluation of mHealth programs in order to improve their efficacy.

text2quit

As the name implies, text2quit is a mHealth program that helps its users quit smoking. Unlike text4baby, which provided one-way communication in the form of uniform messages being sent to all users based on pregnancy stage, text2quit is an interactive and personalized text-messaging system (Abroms, Ahuja, et al. 2012). Using a cell phone, any text2quit user can track quitting progress, ask for tips to control cravings, and find information on why others quit.

Preliminary evaluations of the program found that text2quit is relatively well received by its users (Abroms, Ahuja, et al. 2012). Additionally, a randomized trial revealed that 11 percent of smokers who used text2quit had actually quit after six months, compared to only 5 percent in the control group (Abroms, Boal, Simmens, Mendel, and Windsor 2014). Although the margin of success is relatively small (89 percent of those who received text messages from the program did not quit), the program appears to be more effective than no program at all. Given the severe negative impact smoking has on individual and public health, even small gains in cessation are noteworthy. However, less is know about *why* programs like text2quit are somewhat effective at promoting cessation. Investigating the processes behind mHealth effects, such as emotional reactions to the information and support provided by these text messages, can help researchers improve the programs to make them more effective, too.

Understanding emotional reactions as possible mechanisms of mHealth effects would likely explain additional variance in outcomes related to attitudes and behavior change, particularly in the realm of smoking cessation, which previous research has linked to affective motivations and the nonrational process of addiction (Kourosh, Harrington, and Adinoff 2010; Thompson, Barnett, and Pearce 2009). For instance, a review of the literature on text messaging–based smoking cessation interventions found that these programs are typically grounded in principles of social cognitive theory that guide message designers as they create messages for smokers (Kong, Ells, Camenga, and Krishnan-Sarin 2014). However, application-based mobile smoking cessation programs have also been found to have rather low levels of adherence (Abroms, Lee Westmaas, Bontemps-Jones, Ramani, and Mellerson 2013). Perhaps the attempts to foster social cognitive outcomes, such as increased self-efficacy and positive outcome expectations, are falling short because emotional factors, such as feelings of shame or anxiety from not quitting as soon as users had hoped, are not also considered.

Additionally, generating positive emotions via positively toned text messages may be an effective way to improve increase self-efficacy and positive outcome expectations related to smoking cessation. As Cappella and colleagues (2002; 2006) have demonstrated, anticipated feelings of pride and hope are positive predictors of smoking cessation intentions. Crafting text messages in smoking cessation mHealth messages that embody the corerelational themes of pride and hope may help foster similar feelings in users, and therefore improve adherence and eventually cessation.

VIDEO GAMES

As video games have gained popularity, they have also evolved to the point where researchers and companies have started using games to help improve health education and behavior. The term "serious games" is used to describe games designed for the purposes of education and positive behavior change, versus games made solely for entertainment (McCallum 2012). Researchers have shown that these serious games can be an effective way to promote many types of health-related behaviors (Baranowski, Buday, Thompson, and Baranowski 2008; Lieberman 2012).

Health games are commonly used specifically to promote prevention behaviors. For example, many serious games are designed to promote exercise (Lieberman et al. 2011), called exergames (McCallum 2012). A review of studies testing the effects of exergames that target childhood obesity revealed that most games were commercially available to the public (Lu, Kharrazi, Gharghabi, and Thompson 2013). This review also found that about 40 percent of the studies on exergames targeting childhood obesity prevention reported positive outcomes associated with game use. Serious games have also been applied in other prevention contexts, from pregnancy prevention (Paperny and Starn 1989) to smoking prevention (Lieberman 1997).

How, exactly, do these health games relate to emotions? There are multiple potential connections that beg for further inquiry. For instance, mastering health-related skills, such as exercising, while using an exergame could result in feelings of pride in users, one that could motivate continued physical activity (see chapter 7 about pride, this volume). Additionally, video games may result in greater feelings of interest toward the target behavior, such as exercise—a mundane activity when performed alone in a gym turns into an enjoyable leisure pursuit when using a Wii (see chapter 8 about interest, this volume).

Doing well in a prevention-focused video game may also provide users with hope that they will be able to improve or maintain their well-being outside of the game environment. Conversely, if a health-related serious game is too difficult for a user or the user has a negative in-game experience, then anxiety and frustration may result and carry over into post-game health-related outcomes. Future research would greatly advance our understanding of the processes behind health game effects by measuring emotional reactions to game play, as well as changes in emotions throughout game play, and how those affective reactions help shape post-game behaviors.

Furthermore, serious games, similar to entertainment games, often use narratives to help communicate health information to players, and emotional arousal is an inevitable component and result of narrative engagement (Green 2006; Green and Brock 2000). Narratives presented in health-related games may also evoke a variety of emotions in players, from elevation and hope to fear and anger, depending on the outcome of the game. These emotional reactions to the game could change as the game progresses. Research indicates that the most intense emotions as well as the final emotions experienced during an event can have the strongest lasting impressions of that event, with feelings at the end being particularly impactful (Kahneman, Fredrickson, Schreiber, and Redelmeier 1993). Therefore, health game designers could pay particular attention to the emotional ramifications at the end of levels and the end of the entire game in order to ensure users come away from the experience with an overall positive impression, one that they may share with others.

Narratives also contribute to story immersion, or the process of totally immersing oneself into the narrative world, which in turn can facilitate positive outcomes in health-focused games. For instance, Lu, Thompson, Baranowski, Buday, and Baranowski (2012) found that children who thought themselves to be very similar to the protagonist in a health video game were more likely to be immersed in the story. This story immersion correlated with increases in preferences for fruits and vegetables, intrinsic motivation to drink water, and self-efficacy for eating vegetables and for partaking in physical activity—all valuable activities for promoting health and preventing illness.

Researchers may also turn to the literature on emotions to understand why people would chose to play health games on their own, outside of interventions or controlled laboratory experiments. Mood management research in the entertainment literature has addressed why individuals play video games and how game play can alter and regulate emotional states (Vorderer and Bryant 2006). Given that extant research points to health games effectively communicating health information, improving health outcomes, and having great appeal for many traditionally hard-to-reach audiences (Lieberman 2012), more work testing selective exposure and mood management via health games would help increase their diffusion to target populations.

Moreover, investigating health-related actions or plots in non-serious games may also be a promising route for research on the impact of video games on health. For instance, avatars in a war game could benefit from virtual exercise and healthy diets in order to gain strength and be better fighters. Additionally, research on serious games could be advanced by studying how interpersonal relationships and corresponding emotional attachment to game characters, or other players in multiplayer games, impact health-related outcomes. In short, there are many avenues of research for investigating how serious games related to health may attract users, may evoke emotions in users, and how those emotional reactions combine with increased self-efficacy and/or health knowledge from playing that may influence health behaviors and well-being.

Another concept related to video games is gamification. Gamification is the application of game elements to non-game contexts in order to improve user experience and engagement (Deterding, Dixon, Khaled, and Nacke 2011). Game elements include (but are not limited to) avatars, three-dimensional environments, narratives, feedback/interactivity, levels, status/rank, competition, rules, time pressure, and teams (Reeves and Read 2009). The success of the location-based service Foursquare, where users can check in at any location and the user with the most check-ins becomes the Foursquare mayor of that location, as well as other popular gamified marketing experiences, has sparked interest from the business world in applying game principles to any number of messages or audience-engagement activities (Deterding et al. 2011). Health communicators could likewise adopt gamification techniques to spark interest in preventative health information and behaviors (McCallum 2012).

VIRTUAL REALITY

Virtual reality technology, often employed in games, digital simulations, and other types of virtual worlds, provides users with a personalized mediated experience, one where an avatar can be created based on a user's actual image (Bailenson 2012; Bailenson, Blascovich, and Guadagno 2008; J. Fox and Bailenson 2009). Virtual reality also gives users the ability to vicariously experience an imagined-yet-possible iteration of their own self-concepts. Possible selves, as conceptualized by Markus and Nurius (1986), are the parts of an individual's self-concept concerned with what one thinks of herself, her potential, and her future. Possible selves can be both feared and desired. For example, a young gymnast might experience hope when envisioning herself as a future Olympic champion-turned-national-hero, a desired possible self. But she might fear the possible self that is a chronically injured adult in constant pain after years of physically demanding training.

Research suggests that possible selves are influential in promoting behavior change, likely because imagining a possible self makes an abstract notion (e.g., living a healthy life) more concrete (e.g., I will start a walking routine tomorrow morning) (Comello 2009; Markus and Nurius 1986). Because possible selves are linked to anticipated emotions, they have many ramifications for understanding how virtual representations of the self taking part in preventative health behaviors may evoke such emotions in users. In order to regulate those anticipated emotions, users may decide to change their real-world behavior after their virtual experience.

Moreover, acting as one's possible self via an avatar could either lessen or deepen the impact of discrepancies between actual and desired versions of the self. The magnitude of this incongruity between selves can motivate behavior, as predicted by self-discrepancy theory (Higgins 1987). A related benefit of using virtual reality to communicate health information is that it can improve self-efficacy for performing health behaviors (J. Fox 2012). Feelings of fear and hope can decrease or increase self-efficacy, respectively (see chapters 2 about fear and 9 about hope, this volume). Therefore, feeling hopeful and/or feeling less anxious while acting out prevention behaviors via an avatar may be the mechanisms behind increased self-efficacy and positive outcome expectations resulting from virtual reality–based health activities.

In the future, virtual reality is likely to be more commonplace and a oft-turned-to source of health information, and may even be a common channel for interacting with health care providers (J. Fox 2012). Virtual reality technology can easily tailor messages and experiences to individual users. And virtual reality can be highly interactive as well, making it an eHealth medium that can easily engage users. Given the vividness and intimacy of virtual reality, emotional reactions to encountering other avatars, or to experiencing emotionally arousing events with one's own avatar, are likely common experiences in this realm. Yet little research has propped the ways in which this ICT may foster discrete emotional reactions in users.

Many researchers have already taken advantage of highly engaging virtual worlds as platforms for promoting health education and behavior change. A virtual interactive intervention is an intervention delivered via digital media that includes social interaction with either real or perceived others (Miller et al. 2012; 2011). Designers program these virtual interactive interventions with the goal of improving users' health choices. Miller and colleagues (2012; 2011) point out, though, that most virtual interactive interventions tend to neglect the affective concepts that facilitate health behavior changes, and therefore could be improved.

To begin to overcome this shortfall, the researchers developed SOLVE (Socially Optimized Learning in Virtual Environments) as a way to model safer sex behaviors for men having sex with men (Miller et al., 2012; 2011). They made sure the virtual interactive intervention contained scenarios that created sexual arousal so that the intervention would better simulate real-world, emotionally charged sexual encounters where users would have to make difficult decisions about their behavior. Additionally, the SOLVE virtual intervention included a unit that helped users deal with the shame associated with stigmatized sexual behavior. SOLVE could serve as a model for how to more fully integrate emotional considerations into the design and evaluation of virtual reality applications meant to prevent illness.

SOCIAL MEDIA

Social media are digital spaces where users can communicate with other members of their online social networks. Popular platforms for social media include such websites as Facebook, Twitter, Google Plus, YouTube, and less popular sites dedicated to specific topics. PatientsLikeMe.com, for example, is a social media website dedicated to connecting patients with various conditions to each other and providing tools for interaction and health tracking. Social media is a space where anyone with Internet access can participate, speak their minds, and interact with others, but it also allows traditional mass media outlets a way to share content with users, who in turn can reshare and/or comment on that content.

These online platforms can also be a space where users express and share emotions as well as find content that can evoke, change, or dissipate their feelings. Early research in computer-mediated communication established that the use of ICTs to communicate with other people does not preclude or even diminish the emotional nature of communication between individuals. Rice and Love (1987) found that nearly a third of all messages in the most popular computer network of the time were socioemotional in nature (i.e., the messages touched on topics such as unity, tension, agreement, or conflict). Since the 1980s, the dissemination and popularization of the Internet has put digital social networks, and therefore large quantities of socioemotional content, at the fingertips of billions of users.

The amount of information shared and spread across the Internet is enormous, and health information is an important component of the online information ecosystem (Eysenbach 2008; Eysenbach, Powell, Englesakis, Rizo, and Stern 2004; Eysenbach, Powell, Kuss, and Sa 2002). Much of this online health information is social in nature, too. In a given year, more than a quarter of Internet users read about or watch someone else's health-related experiences, while 16 percent of Internet users go online to look for other people who might share similar health concerns (S. Fox 2013). The growing reliance on social media for health information has both benefits and drawbacks for users. Social media is a low cost and quick way to disseminate health information to multiple audiences and to promote interaction and conversation. However, social media also allows anyone, including non-experts, to disseminate health information, resulting in a plethora of health-related misinformation floating around the Internet (Vance, Howe, and Dellavalle 2009).

Nonetheless, health information from a variety of sources can evoke emotions in social media users or reflect the spread of emotions across social networks. A moving video PSA telling the stories of skin cancer patients and their family members made YouTube users feel sad, happy, fearful, and compassionate (Myrick and Oliver 2014). And tweets about a national anti-smoking campaign reflected Twitter users' fear of negative health outcomes related to tobacco use (Emery et al. 2014).

Emotion-evoking health social media content can also spread quickly as users share and comment on social media posts. For example, Kramer, Guillory, and Hancock (2014) used a large-scale study ($N = 689,003$) to show how emotional content portrayed on Facebook can transfer to other users. When the researchers experimentally decreased the amount of positive content in some users' Facebook feeds, those users included more negative words and fewer positive words in their own Facebook statuses. Likewise, when negative content was decreased, the opposite effects occurred. Users were not aware of the manipulation or of the change in their own behavior. Even without direct interaction between individuals and in the complete absence of nonverbal cues, Kramer et al. established that emotional contagion across online social networks is a real phenomenon. Additional work is needed to test if emotions related to health information or health narratives moves differently across social media than does other types of content.

Besides evoking emotional reactions in users, emotional content found online is more likely to be shared and go viral than is non-emotional content (Berger 2013; Berger and Milkman 2012). A diary study of consumers' information sharing via mobile phones found that more than 40 percent of all shared information contained expressions of emotions, with positive emotions dominating (Goh, Ang, Chua, and Lee 2009). In a health context, Myrick and Oliver (2014) found that emotional versions of a YouTube skin cancer public service announcement were more effective at motivating viewers to share the video than was a low-emotion, highly logical, and even-keeled video of a doctor discussing skin cancer. Clearly, emotional reactions are involved in individual's decisions as to what makes information worth sharing online, including health information. If that health content is shared via social media alongside emotional expressions, it could likewise traverse quickly through social networks.

It is important to recognize that many social media messages are short and constrained by the properties of the interface. That is, complex health topics may not be well explained in a single social media post. However, health communicators who want to infuse emotion into their social media messages in order to encourage users to share them could easily use or add visuals to their messages to give them additional explanatory power. Visuals are very efficient at evoking emotions in viewers (e.g, Lang, Greenwald, Bradley, and Hamm 1993; Nabi 2003b), can be very persuasive (e.g., Huddy and Gunnthorsdottir 2000; Joffe 2008), and can even improve message recall (e.g., Graber 1990). Although not studied as thoroughly as text-based messages, visuals are important components of health communication, too (Osborne 2006) and could be applied to improving the use of social media as a conduit of health information.

The sharing of preventative health messages through free social media accounts would seem, on the surface, quite beneficial for promoting prevention behaviors, especially given the small budgets of many public health organizations that cannot afford prominent paid media placements. However, there are also pitfalls to consider when using social media for health communication. Southwell (2013) points out that various segments of the population are not equally connected to the Internet and social media, meaning that existing health disparities can be exaggerated when organizations rely too heavily on social media for spreading health messages. Moreover, social media users tend to be younger than non-social media users, making the platform ill suited for directly reaching older populations (Chou, Hunt, Beckjord, Moser, and Hesse 2009).

Personal blogs are another social form of Internet-based media that have attracted the attention of health communication scholars. Despite their anecdotal nature, they can be relatable and quite convincing for those seeking information or a connection with someone else concerned about the same health topics. Neubaum and Krämer (2014) found in an experiment that the personal blogs of people living with HIV were more effective at promoting the use of condoms in readers (who were HIV negative) than was an institutional HIV website. The stronger relationship between reading the personal blogs and intentions to prevent HIV occurred despite the fact that participants rated the institutional website as more credible than the personal blogs.

The implication of this study is that credibility, while an important consideration for many Internet users seeking health information (Eastin 2001), needs to be considered within a broader context that takes into account socioemotional predictors of behavior. As Zillmann (2006) has shown, exemplars are often more powerful than statistics in shaping risk perceptions and even behavior because individuals react emotionally to exemplars in a way that they do not react to statistics.

Future work could explore how and when emotional responses to online personal blogs about health interact with user evaluations of information credibility, as well as other cognitive factors and information processing variables, to influence subsequent prevention behaviors. The specific health context is likely of great importance in how Internet users react to online health information (Hu and Shyam Sundar 2010) as personal blogs may be deemed more appropriate sources for engaging with certain types of health information (e.g., information about sexual or mental health where it is difficult to talk about with a strange doctor due to stigma and embarrassment) than for others (e.g., a serious condition where the value of expert medical advice outweighs the emotional attachment to a blogger).

CONCLUSION

Since the emergence of ICTs, health communication researchers have been investing considerable effort into the impact of eHealth messages on health behavior. Interactivity and tailoring are particularly important conceptual variables for understanding these potential effects in realms from mobile health interventions to video games to social media messages. Each of these eHealth domains differs in the degree to which they are interactive or can be tailored, and each differs with respect to its typical users and as appropriate avenues for prevention-oriented health messages on different health topics. As ICTs continue to diffuse across populations and gain in popularity, eHealth will likewise continue to garner attention as a promising approach for disease prevention and the promotion of well-being.

As discussed above, the intersections of eHealth, prevention, and emotions are many. However, little existing work directly explores or has empirically tested the connections between eHealth applications and discrete emotional reactions. This means that many opportunities exist to increase the efficacy of eHealth interventions by analyzing the emotional tones of these messages and users' discrete emotional reactions to them. The ability of digital interfaces to recognize user emotions via video readings of facial expressions, sensor tracking of heart rate or galvanic skin response, or via self-reports provides researchers with many opportunities for collecting data relating eHealth programs and applications to emotional arousal and effects. As affective computing advances, so too will the potential for eHealth messages to foster prevention behaviors.

REFERENCES

Abroms, L. C., M. Ahuja, Y. Kodl, L. Thaweethai, J. Sims, J. P. Winickoff, and R. A. Windsor. 2012. Text2quit: Results from a pilot test of a personalized, interactive mobile health smoking cessation program. *Journal of Health Communication* 17(sup1):44–53. doi: 10.1080/10810730.2011.649159.

Abroms, L. C., A. L. Boal, S. J. Simmens, J. A. Mendel, and R. A. Windsor. 2014. A randomized trial of text2quit: A text messaging program for smoking cessation. *American Journal of Preventive Medicine*(0). doi: http://dx.doi.org/10.1016/j.amepre.2014.04.010.

Abroms, L. C., J. Lee Westmaas, J. Bontemps-Jones, R. Ramani, and J. Mellerson. 2013. A content analysis of popular smartphone apps for smoking cessation. *American Journal of Preventive Medicine* 45(6):732–36. doi: 10.1016/j.amepre.2013.07.008.

Abroms, L. C., N. Padmanabhan, and W. D. Evans. 2012. Mobile phones for health communication to promote behavior change. In S. M. Noar and N. G. Harrington (Eds.), *eHealth applications: Promising strategies for behavior change* (pp. 147–66). New York: Routledge.

Andsager, J. L., E. W. Austin, and B. E. Pinkleton. 2002. Gender as a variable in interpretation of alcohol-related messages. *Communication Research* 29(3):246–69. doi: 10.1177/0093650202029003002.

Bailenson, J. N. 2012. Doppelgängers—a new form of self? *Psychologist* 25(1):36–38.

Bailenson, J. N., J. Blascovich, and R. E. Guadagno. 2008. Self-representations in immersive virtual environments. *Journal of Applied Social Psychology* 38(11):2673–90. doi: 10.1111/j.1559-1816.2008.00409.x.

Baranowski, T., R. Buday, D. I. Thompson, and J. Baranowski. 2008. Playing for real. *American Journal of Preventive Medicine* 34(1):74–82.e10. doi: 10.1016/j.amepre.2007.09.027.

Beniger, J. R. 1987. Personalization of mass media and the growth of pseudo-community. *Communication Research* 14:352–71.

Berger, J. 2013. *Contagious: Why things catch on.* New York: Simon and Schuster.

Berger, J., and K. L. Milkman. 2012. What makes online content viral? *Journal of Marketing Research* 49(2):192–205. doi: 10.1509/jmr.10.0353.

Biswas, R., D. Riffe, and D. Zillmann. 1994. Mood influence on the appeal of bad news. *Journalism and Mass Communication Quarterly* 71(3):689–96. doi: 10.1177/107769909407100319.

Brave, S., C. Nass, and K. Hutchinson. 2005. Computers that care: Investigating the effects of orientation of emotion exhibited by an embodied computer agent. *International Journal of Human-Computer Studies* 62(2):161–78. doi: 10.1016/j.ijhcs.2004.11.002.

Cappella, J. N., A. Romantan, and C. Lerman. 2002. *Emotional bases for quitting smoking: Extending the integrated theory of behavior change.* Annenberg Public Policy Center, University of Pennsylvania. Philadelphia, PA.

Cappella, J. N., A. Romantan, F. Patterson, and C. Lerman. 2006. *The emotional basis for quitting smoking: Anticipated emotions as predictors of intention and behavior.* [Unpublished manuscript]. Philadelphia.

Chou, W. Y., Y. M. Hunt, E. B. Beckjord, R. P. Moser, and B. W. Hesse. 2009. Social media use in the United States: Implications for health communication. *Journal of Medical Internet Research* 11(4):e48. doi: 10.2196/jmir.1249.

Clore, G. L., and J. Palmer. 2009. Affective guidance of intelligent agents: How emotion controls cognition. *Cognitive Systems Research* 10:21–30.

Cole-Lewis, H., and T. Kershaw. 2010. Text messaging as a tool for behavior change in disease prevention and management. *Epidemiology Review* 32(1):56–69. doi: 10.1093/epirev/mxq004.

Comello, M. L. G. 2009. William James on "possible selves": Implications for studying identity in communication contexts. *Communication Theory* 19(3):337–50. doi: 10.1111/j.1468-2885.2009.01346.x.

Cook, S., C. Conrad, A. L. Fowlkes, and M. H. Mohebbi. 2011. Assessing Google flu trends performance in the United States during the 2009 influenza virus A (H1N1) pandemic. *PLoS ONE* 6(8):1–8. doi: 10.1371/journal.pone.0023610.

DeSteno, D., R. E. Petty, D. D. Rucker, D. T. Wegener, and J. Braverman. 2004. Discrete emotions and persuasion: The role of emotion-induced expectancies. *Journal of Personality and Social Psychology* 86(1):43–56. doi: 10.1037/0022-3514.86.1.43.

DeSteno, D., R. E. Petty, D. T. Wegener, and D. D. Rucker. 2000. Beyond valence in the perception of likelihood: The role of emotion specificity. *Journal of Personality and Social Psychology* 78(3):397–416. doi: 10.1037/0022-3514.78.3.397.

Deterding, S., D. Dixon, R. Khaled, and L. Nacke. 2011. *From game design elements to gamefulness: Defining gamification.* Paper presented at the Proceedings of the 15th International Academic MindTrek Conference: Envisioning Future Media Environments.

Eastin, M. S. 2001. Credibility assessments of online health information: The effects of source expertise and knowledge of content. *Journal of Computer-Mediated Communication* 6(4). doi: 10.1111/j.1083-6101.2001.tb00126.x.

Emery, S. L., G. Szczypka, E. P. Abril, Y. Kim, and L. Vera. 2014. Are you scared yet? Evaluating fear appeal messages in tweets about the tips campaign. *Journal of Communication* 64(2):278–95. doi: 10.1111/jcom.12083.

Eng, T. R. 2001. *The eHealth landscape: A terrain map of emerging information and communication technologies in health and health care.* Princeton, NJ: Roert Wood Johnson Foundation.

Evans, W. D., J. Wallace Bihm, D. Szekely, P. Nielsen, E. Murray, L. Abroms, and J. Snider. 2014. Initial outcomes from a 4-week follow-up study of the text4baby program in the military women's population: Randomized controlled trial. *Journal of Medical Internet Research* 16(5):e131.

Evans, W. D., J. L. Wallace, and J. Snider. 2012. Pilot evaluation of the text4baby mobile health program. *BMC Public Health* 12:1031. doi: 10.1186/1471-2458-12-1031.

Eysenbach, G. 2008. Medicine 2.0: social networking, collaboration, participation, apomediation, and openness. *Journal of Medical Internet Research* 10(3):e22. doi: 10.2196/jmir.1030.

Eysenbach, G., J. Powell, M. Englesakis, C. Rizo, and A. Stern. 2004. Health related virtual communities and electronic support groups: Systematic review of the effects of online peer to peer interactions. *BMJ* 328(7449):1166. doi: 10.1136/bmj.328.7449.1166.

Eysenbach, G., J. Powell, O. Kuss, and E.-R. Sa. 2002. Empirical studies assessing the quality of health information for consumers on the world wide web: A systematic review. *JAMA: The Journal of the American Medical Association* 287(20):2691–700. doi: 10.1001/jama.287.20.2691.

Fogg, B. J., and R. Adler (Eds.). 2009. *Texting 4 health: A simple, powerful way to change lives.* Stanford University: Captology Media.

Fox, J. 2012. Avatars for health behavior change. In S. M. Noar and N. G. Harrington (Eds.), *eHealth applications: Promising strategies for behavior change* (pp. 96–109). New York: Routledge.

Fox, J., and J. N. Bailenson. 2009. Virtual self-modeling: The effects of vicarious reinforcement and identification on exercise behaviors. *Media Psychology* 12(1):1–25. doi: 10.1080/15213260802669474.

Fox, S. 2013. Health online 2013. Retrieved June 17, 2014, from http://www.pewinternet.org/2013/01/15/health-online-2013/.

Goh, D., R. Ang, A. Chua, and C. Lee. 2009. Why we share: A study of motivations for mobile media sharing. In J. Liu, J. Wu, Y. Yao, and T. Nishida (Eds.), *Active Media Technology* (Vol. 5820, pp. 195–206): Springer Berlin / Heidelberg.

Graber, D. A. 1990. Seeing is remembering: How visuals contribute to learning from television news. *Journal of Communication* 40(3):134–56. doi: 10.1111/j.1460-2466.1990.tb02275.x.

Green, M. C. 2006. Narratives and cancer communication. *Journal of Communication* 56:S163–S183. doi: 10.1111/j.1460-2466.2006.00288.x.

Green, M. C., and T. C. Brock. 2000. The role of transportation in the persuasiveness of public narratives. *Journal of Personality and Social Psychology* 79(5):701–21.

Guadagno, R. E., J. Blascovich, J. N. Bailenson, and C. McCall. 2007. Virtual humans and persuasion: The effects of agency and behavioral realism. *Media Psychology* 10(1):1–22. doi: 10.1080/15213260701300865.

Higgins, E. T. 1987. Self-discrepancy: A theory relating self and affect. *Psychological Review* 94(3):319–40. doi: 10.1037/0033-295X.94.3.319.

Hu, Y., and S. Shyam Sundar. 2010. Effects of online health sources on credibility and behavioral intentions. *Communication Research* 37(1):105–32. doi: 10.1177/0093650209351512.

Huddy, L., and A. H. Gunnthorsdottir. 2000. The persuasive effects of emotive visual imagery: Superficial manipulation or the product of passionate reason? *Political Psychology* 21(4):745–78. doi: 10.1111/0162-895X.00215.

Jensen, J. D., A. J. King, N. Carcioppolo, and L. Davis. 2012. Why are tailored messages more effective? A multiple mediation analysis of a breast cancer screening intervention. *Journal of Communication* 62(5):851–68. doi: 10.1111/j.1460-2466.2012.01668.x.

Ji, Y. G. 2013. *Advances in affective and pleasurable design.* Boca Raton, FL: CRC Press/ Taylor and Francis.

Joffe, H. 2008. The power of visual material: Persuasion, emotion and identification. *Diogenes* 55(1):84–93. doi: 10.1177/0392192107087919.

Kahneman, D., B. L. Fredrickson, C. A. Schreiber, and D. A. Redelmeier. 1993. When more pain is preferred to less: Adding a better end. *Psychological Science* 4(6):401–5. doi: 10.1111/j.1467-9280.1993.tb00589.x.

Kalyanaraman, S., and S. S. Sundar. 2006. The psychological appeal of personalized content in web portals: Does customization affect attitudes and behavior? *Journal of Communication* 56:110–32. doi: 10.1111/j.1460-2466.2006.00006.x.

Klemm, P., and E. Wheeler. 2005. Cancer caregivers online: Hope, emotional roller coaster, and physical/emotional/psychological responses. *Computers, Informatics, Nursing* 23(1):38–45. doi: http://journals.lww.com/cinjournal/Fulltext/2005/01000/Cancer_Caregivers_Online__Hope,_Emotional_Roller.8.aspx.

Kong, G., D. M. Ells, D. R. Camenga, and S. Krishnan-Sarin. 2014. Text messaging-based smoking cessation intervention: A narrative review. *Addictive Behaviors* 39(5):907–17. doi: 10.1016/j.addbeh.2013.11.024.

Kourosh, A. S., C. R. Harrington, and B. Adinoff. 2010. Tanning as behavioral addiction. *The American Journal of Drug and Alcohol Abuse* 36:284–90.

Kramer, A. D. I., J. E. Guillory, and J. T. Hancock. 2014. Experimental evidence of massive-scale emotional contagion through social networks. *Proceedings of the National Academy of Sciences.* doi: 10.1073/pnas.1320040111.

Kreuter, M. W., D. Farrell, L. Olevitch, and L. Brennan. 2000. *Tailoring health messages: Customizing communication with computer technology.* Mahwah, NJ: Lawrence Erlbaum Associates.

Kumar, S., W. J. Nilsen, A. Abernethy, A. Atienza, K. Patrick, M. Pavel, . . . D. Swendeman. 2013. Mobile health technology evaluation. *American Journal of Preventive Medicine* 45(2):228–36. doi: 10.1016/j.amepre.2013.03.017.

Lang, P. J., M. K. Greenwald, M. M. Bradley, and A. O. Hamm. 1993. Looking at pictures: Affective, facial, visceral, and behavioral reactions. *Psychophysiology* 30(3):261–73. doi: 10.1111/j.1469-8986.1993.tb03352.x.

Lazarus, R. S. 1991. *Emotion and adaptation.* New York: Oxford University Press.

Lerner, J. S., and D. Keltner. 2000. Beyond valence: Toward a model of emotion-specific influences on judgment and choice. *Cognition and Emotion* 14(4):473–93. doi: 10.1080/026999300402763.

———. 2001. Fear, anger, and risk. *Journal of Personality and Social Psychology* 81(1):146–59. doi: 10.1037/0022-3514.81.1.146.

Lieberman, D. A. 1997. Interactive video games for health promotion: Effects on knowledge, self-efficacy, social support, and health. In R. L. Street, W. R. Gold, and T. R. Manning (Eds.), *Health promotion and interactive technology: Theoretical applications and future directions* (pp. 103–20). Mahwah, NJ, US: Lawrence Erlbaum Associates.

———. 2012. Digital games for health behavior change: Research, design, and future directions. In S. M. Noar and N. G. Harrington (Eds.), *eHealth applications: Promising strategies for behavior change* (pp. 110–27). New York: Routledge.

Lieberman, D. A., B. Chamberlin, E. Medina, B. A. Franklin, B. M. Sanner, and D. K. Vafiadis. 2011. The power of play: Innovations in getting active summit 2011: A science panel proceedings report from the American Heart Association. *Circulation* 123(21):2507–16. doi: 10.1161/CIR.0b013e318219661d.

Lu, A. S., H. Kharrazi, F. Gharghabi, and D. I. Thompson. 2013. A systematic review of health videogames on childhood obesity prevention and intervention. *Games for Health Journal* 2(3):131–41. doi: 10.1089/g4h.2013.0025.

Lu, A. S., D. I. Thompson, J. Baranowski, R. Buday, and T. Baranowski. 2012. Story immersion in a health videogame for childhood obesity prevention. *Games for Health Journal* 1(1):37–44. doi: 10.1089/g4h.2011.0011.

Markus, H., and P. Nurius. 1986. Possible selves. *American Psychologist* 41(9):954–69. doi: 10.1037/0003-066X.41.9.954.

McCallum, S. 2012. Gamification and serious games for personalized health. *Studies in Health Technology and Informatics* 177:85–96. doi: 10.3233/978-1-61499-069-7-85.

Mechael, P. N. 2009. The case for mHealth in developing countries. *Innovations: Technology, Governance, Globalization* 4(1):103–18. doi: 10.1162/itgg.2009.4.1.103.

Miller, L. C., P. R. Appleby, J. L. Christensen, C. Godoy, M. Si, C. Corsbie-Massay, . . . J. Klatt. 2012. Virtual interactive interventions for reducing risky sex: Adaptations, integrations, and innovations. In S. M. Noar and N. G. Harrington (Eds.), *eHealth applications: Promising strategies for behavior change* (pp. 79–95). New York: Routledge.

Miller, L. C., S. Marsella, T. Dey, P. R. Appleby, J. L. Christensen, J. Klatt, and S. J. Read. 2011. Socially Optimized Learning in Virtual Environments (SOLVE). In M. Si, D. Thue, E. André, J. Lester, J. Tanenbaum, and V. Zammitto (Eds.), *Interactive Storytelling* (Vol. 7069, pp. 182–92): Springer Berlin Heidelberg.

Myrick, J. G. 2014. *The role of emotions and social cognitive variables in health information seeking: A tailored approach.* Paper presented at the Kentucky Conference on Health Communication, Lexington, KY.

Myrick, J. G., and M. B. Oliver. 2014. Laughing and crying: Mixed emotions, compassion, and the effectiveness of a YouTube PSA about skin cancer. *Health Communication*, 1–10. doi: 10.1080/10410236.2013.845729.

Nabi, R. L. 2003a. Exploring the framing effects of emotion. *Communication Research* 30(2):224–47. doi: 10.1177/0093650202250881.

———. 2003b. "Feeling" resistance: Exploring the role of emotionally evocative visuals in inducing inoculation. *Media Psychology* 5(2):199–223. doi: 10.1207/S1532785XMEP0502_4.

Nass, C., U. Foehr, S. Brave, and M. Somoza. 2001. *The effects of emotion of voice in synthesized and recorded speech.* Paper presented at the Proceedings of the AAAI Symposium: Emotional and Intelligent II: The Tangled Knot of Social Cognition, North Falmouth, MA.

Nass, C., and C. Yen. 2010. *The man who lied to his laptop: What machines teach us about human relationships.* New York: Current.

Neubaum, G., and N. C. Krämer. 2014. Let's blog about health! Exploring the persuasiveness of a personal HIV blog compared to an institutional HIV website. *Health Communication*, 1–12. doi: 10.1080/10410236.2013.856742.

Neuhauser, L., and G. L. Kreps. 2003. Rethinking communication in the ehealth era. *Journal of Health Psychology* 8(1):7–23. doi: 10.1177/1359105303008001426.

Noar, S. M., C. N. Benac, and M. S. Harris. 2007. Does tailoring matter? Meta-analytic review of tailored print health behavior change interventions. *Psychological Bulletin* 133(4):673–93. doi: 10.1037/0033-2909.133.4.673.

Noar, S. M., and N. G. Harrington (Eds.). 2012. *eHealth applications: Promising strategies for behavior change*. New York: Routledge.

Noar, S. M., N. G. Harrington, S. K. Van Stee, and R. Shemanski Aldrich. 2011. Tailored health communication to change lifestyle behaviors. *American Journal of Lifestyle Medicine* 5(2):112–22. doi: 10.1177/1559827610387255.

Osborne, H. 2006. Health literacy: How visuals can help tell the healthcare story. *Journal of Visual Communication in Medicine* 29(1):28–32. doi: doi:10.1080/01405110600772830.

Paperny, D. M., and J. R. Starn. 1989. Adolescent pregnancy prevention by health education computer games: Computer-assisted instruction of knowledge and attitudes. *Pediatrics* 83(5):742–52.

Picard, R. W. 1997. *Affective computing*. Cambridge, MA: MIT Press.

Reblin, M., and B. N. Uchino. 2008. Social and emotional support and its implication for health. *Curr Opin Psychiatry* 21(2):201–5. doi: 10.1097/YCO.0b013e3282f3ad89.

Reeves, B., and C. Nass. 1996. *The media equation: How people treat computers, television, and new media like real people and places*. Stanford, CA: CSLI Publications.

Reeves, B., and J. L. Read. 2009. *Total engagement: Using games and virtual worlds to change the way people work and businesses compete*. Boston, MA: Harvard Business School Press.

Remick, A. P., and J. S. Kendrick. 2013. Breaking new ground: The text4baby program. *American Journal of Health Promotion* 27(sp3):S4–S6. doi: 10.4278/ajhp.27.3.c2.

Resnicow, K., R. Davis, N. Zhang, V. Strecher, D. Tolsma, J. Calvi, . . . W. E. Cross. 2009. Tailoring a fruit and vegetable intervention on ethnic identity: Results of a randomized study. *Health Psychology* 28(4):394–403.

Rice, R. E., and G. Love. 1987. Electronic emotion: Socioemotional content in a computer-mediated communication network. *Communication Research* 14(1):85–108. doi: 10.1177/009365087014001005.

Rimal, R. N., and A. D. Adkins. 2003. Using computers to narrowcast health messages: The role of audience segmentation, targeting, and tailoring in health promotion. In T. L. Thompson, A. M. Dorsey, K. I. Miller, and R. Parrott (Eds.), *Handbook of health communication* (pp. 497–513). Mahwah, NJ: Lawrence Erlbaum Associates Publishers.

Roseman, I. J. 2011. Emotional behaviors, emotivational goals, emotion strategies: Multiple levels of organization integrate variable and consistent responses. *Emotion Review* 3(4):434–43. doi: 10.1177/1754073911410744.

Sarason, B. R., I. G. Sarason, and G. R. Pierce. 1990. *Social support: An interactional view*. New York: Wiley.

Sherbourne, C. D., and A. L. Stewart. 1991. The MOS social support survey. *Social Science and Medicine* 32(6):705–14. doi: http://dx.doi.org/10.1016/0277-9536(91)90150-B.

Shumaker, S. A., and A. Brownell. 1984. Toward a theory of social support: Closing conceptual gaps. *Journal of Social Issues* 40(4):11–36. doi: 10.1111/j.1540-4560.1984.tb01105.x.

Southwell, B. G. 2013. *Social networks and popular understanding of science and health: Sharing disparities*. Baltimore, MD/Research Triangle Park, NC: Johns Hopkins University Press/RTI Press.

Strecher, V. J., S. Shiffman, and R. West. 2006. Moderators and mediators of a web-based computer-tailored smoking cessation program among nicotine patch users. *Nicotine and Tobacco Research* 8(Suppl 1):S95–S101. doi: 10.1080/14622200601039444.

Sundar, S. S. 2007. The MAIN Model: A heuristic approach to understanding technology effects on credibility. In M. J. Metzger and A. J. Flanagin (Eds.), *The John D. and Catherine T. MacArthur Foundation Series on Digital Media and Learning* (pp. 73–100). Cambridge, MA: MIT Press.

Sundar, S. S., S. Bellur, J. Oh, H. Jia, and H.-S. Kim. 2014. Theoretical importance of contingency in human-computer interaction: Effects of message interactivity on user engagement. *Communication Research*. doi: 10.1177/0093650214534962.

Sundar, S. S., S. Kalyanaraman, and J. Brown. 2003. Explicating web site interactivity. *Communication Research* 30(1):30–59. doi: 10.1177/0093650202239025.

Sundar, S. S., R. E. Rice, H.-S. Kim, and C. N. Sciamanna. 2011. Online health information: Conceptual challenges and theoretical opportunities. In T. L. Thompson, R. Parrott, and J. F. Nussbaum (Eds.), *The Routledge handbook of health communication* (pp. 181–202). New York: Routledge.

Tao, C.-C., and E. P. Bucy. 2007. Conceptualizing media stimuli in experimental research: Psychological versus attribute-based definitions. *Human Communication Research* 33(4):397–426. doi: 10.1111/j.1468-2958.2007.00305.x.

text4baby. 2014. text4baby. Retrieved June 15, 2014, from https://http://www.text4baby.org/.

Thompson, L. E., J. R. Barnett, and J. R. Pearce. 2009. Scared straight? Fear-appeal anti-smoking campaigns, risk, self-efficacy and addiction. *Health, Risk and Society* 11(2):181–96. doi: 10.1080/13698570902784281.

Uchino, B. N. 2006. Social support and health: A review of physiological processes potentially underlying links to disease outcomes. *Journal of Behavioral Medicine* 29(4):377–87. doi: 10.1007/s10865-006-9056-5.

Uchino, B. N., J. T. Cacioppo, and J. K. Kiecolt-Glaser. 1996. The relationship between social support and physiological processes: A review with emphasis on underlying mechanisms and implications for health. *Psychological Bulletin* 119(3):488–531. doi: 10.1037/0033-2909.119.3.488.

Vance, K., W. Howe, and R. P. Dellavalle. 2009. Social Internet sites as a source of public health information. *Dermatology Clinics* 27(2):133–36. doi: 10.1016/j.det.2008.11.010.

Vorderer, P., and J. Bryant (Eds.). 2006. *Playing video games: Motives, responses, and consequences.* Mawhaw, NJ: Lawrence Erlbaum Associates.

Wirth, J. H., and G. V. Bodenhausen. 2009. The role of gender in mental-illness stigma: A national experiment. *Psychological Science* 20(2):169–73. doi: 10.1111/j.1467-9280.2009.02282.x.

Xue, L., C. C. Yen, L. Chang, B. C. Tai, H. C. Chan, H. B.-L. Duh, and M. Choolani. 2013. Journeying toward female-focused m-Health applications. *Advances in Affective and Pleasurable Design* (pp. 295–305). Boca Raton, FL: CRC Press/Taylor and Francis.

Yoo, W., K. Namkoong, M. Choi, D. V. Shah, S. Tsang, Y. Hong, . . . D. H. Gustafson. 2014. Giving and receiving emotional support online: Communication competence as a moderator of psychosocial benefits for women with breast cancer. *Computers in Human Behavior* 30:13–22. doi: http://dx.doi.org/10.1016/j.chb.2013.07.024.

Zeelenberg, M., R. M. A. Nelissen, S. M. Breugelmans, and R. Pieters. 2008. On emotion specificity in decision making: Why feeling is for doing. *Judgment and Decision Making* 3(1):18–27.

Zeelenberg, M., and R. Pieters. 2006. Feeling is for doing: A pragmatic approach to the study of emotions in economic behavior. In M. DeCremer, M. Zeelenberg, and J. K. Murnighan (Eds.), *Social psychology and economics* (pp. 117–37). Mahway, NJ: Erlbaum.

Zillmann, D. 2006. Exemplification effects in the promotion of safety and health. *Journal of Communication* 56:S221–S237. doi: 10.1111/j.1460-2466.2006.00291.x.

Conclusion

Future Directions for Research on Emotions and Prevention-Focused Health Messages

This book undertook a formidable task: to review, analyze, and expand upon the role of discrete emotions as they may impact the public's reactions to prevention-focused health messages. By breaking this task into smaller parts, from theoretical foundations to a discussion of specific emotions and then finally an overview of different health communication contexts, the process of understanding how audience emotions can impact message outcomes became more manageable. After those incremental steps were taken, it is also helpful to take a step back and examine the content in the book as a whole. This opportunity to look at the big picture provides a chance to identify common themes and additional points of interest related to the study of emotions and preventative health message effects.

THEMES

As certain statements found themselves reappearing in chapter after chapter, it became clear that some ideas crossed all boundaries of this area of research. One important theme mentioned throughout this book is that the audiences' emotional reactions to health media are multifaceted and nuanced. These reactions differ by valence (positive or negative) and level of arousal (intense or calm), but they also differ based on their unique appraisal patterns and action tendencies. Furthermore, emotions can take place in the present, but the ability of humans to project into the future also allows for anticipated emotional reactions to likewise influence the audiences' thoughts and behaviors. While the parsimony of looking at emotional reactions as positive or negative or as arousing or calming can be appealing and does provide important insights as to the role of emotions in media effects, researchers should acknowledge the loss of the additional explanatory power involved. The discrete approach, with its nuances and relationship to action tendencies, can help advance the field's understanding of when and why prevention messages can motivate health behavior changes.

Another theme of this book is that emotion and cognition work in conjunction to impact individuals' reactions to prevention-focused health messages, including the reaction of ultimate interest to public health advocates: behavior. Researchers must not forget that affect and cognition work in tandem and influence each other (Frijda, Manstead, and Bem 2000). In fact, appraisal theory relies on the premise that automatic cognitions about one's situation (i.e., appraisals) are the basis of emotional experience. Emotions can also shape subsequent cognitive appraisals of risk and outcome expectations, for example. As the comedian Ellen DeGeneres (2011) advises her audiences, "Emote. It's okay. It shows you are thinking and feeling" (240). Work that aims to advance knowledge of the connection between the two psychological processes can result in analyses that explain a greater portion of the variance in health-related media effects.

One more important theme of note is the link between emotions evoked by health messages and ensuing behavior. The founding premise of this book is that it is challenging to get seemingly healthy individuals to undertake often difficult or annoying prevention behaviors (e.g., exercising, eating healthy foods, quitting smoking, etc.). This is because their present healthy (or at least non-ill) state leaves them demotivated to spend energy on an activity that may or not prevent disease. However, because the functional, adaptive purpose of emotions is to motivate people to take situation-appropriate actions, using health messages that make audiences feel *something* with regard to a health issue is one way to promote behavior change. The message-relevant emotion-to-behavior link is not always direct (e.g., "A PSA about skin cancer frightened me about my own risk for the disease, therefore I will go to the store, buy sunscreen, and apply it before I go to the beach again."). Instead, emotional reactions to health messages may often take indirect routes to fostering behavior change. Discrete emotional states may alter the way audiences seek health information, or they may promote further reflection on message content, which then eventually leads to behavior change. Regardless of the nature of the path (i.e., direct or indirect), the strong relationship between emotion and behavior is what makes this area of research so important for advancing health communication theory and its practical applications.

METHODOLOGICAL ISSUES

The empirical study of communication is a relatively young area of research compared to its forbearers: psychology, biology, and sociology, among others (Rogers 1994). As the field advances, so too do methodological approaches to analyzing communication phenomenon like emotional reactions. However, much room remains for improvement in the methodology used to test and assess emotional reactions to media. Below, three potential areas for improving methodological approaches to this area are outlined.

Design

As with other subfields of communication based in the social scientific paradigm, cross-sectional surveys and one-shot experiments dominated the health communication literature cited in this book. And many of these studies, due to constraints on time and resources, only assess intentions to act and not actual health behavior changes. However, employing longitudinal designs that incorporate measures of actual post-message behavior would be immensely helpful for determining the long-term effects of emotionally evocative health messages on a variety of audiences. Be it a longitudinal survey or an experiment with multiple collection points, longitudinal work will help determine if and how short-lived emotional reactions to media messages shape actual behaviors. Applying additional methodologies, such as diary studies that have participants record their emotional reactions throughout the day or the collection of heart rate data via mobile tracking devices that also track media consumption, could also provide interesting longitudinal data to researchers in this field.

Furthermore, in order for theories that integrate emotion into explanations of health message effects to gain steam, the field needs more studies that compare theories against each other in order to see which work best and which need revisions. This type of comparative design is rarely used in health communication or health behavior work (for an exception, see Gerend and Shepherd 2012). However, more and more health communication scholars are calling for an increase in the use of comparative design (Jensen 2014; Noar and Zimmerman 2005; Slater and Gleason 2012). Comparative design may be particularly useful for researchers utilizing emotion-based theories in their work because it can help demonstrate the efficacy of including emotion and emotion-related variables in theoretical models of health message effects (as compared to models that do not analyze discrete emotions). Practically, comparing theories and finding the ones that best apply themselves to real-world media contexts would also be very valuable for cash-strapped public health organizations. These groups may not have the resources to design intricate messages based on numerous theoretical components, but they likely could manage to incorporate one specific theoretical perspective into their messages.

Dissecting messages into more specific components and directly assessing the relationships between message features and psychological states would also help alleviate some methodological concerns regarding audience reactions to emotion-evoking messages (O'Keefe 2003). However, as noted by Dillard and Seo (2013), messages vary on many dimensions, making it difficult to decipher which features are evoking emotions and which are not. For example, exemplification theory posits that showing individuals directly affected by a health issue influences health news consumers' perceptions more than do statistics because exemplars are more emotionally evocative than numbers (Zillmann 2006). But to truly test this hypothesis, it would be necessary to see if non-emotion-evoking exemplars had different effects on audience members than did emotionally evocative exemplars. Yet because people often relate to and empathize with the stories of exemplars who are facing health issues, and because stories that mention health threats and depict them in concrete terms are likely to evoke at least some anxiety/fear in regard to the threat, it would be extremely difficult to find a health-related exemplar who evoked no emotion in news audiences.

Another difficulty in separating out the message features that evoke emotions in audiences from other features of messages is that chopping up a message into its component parts can make it seem fake or unrealistic. That is, even if researchers have theoretical reasons to suspect one particular component of a message is evoking a particular emotion, it can be difficult to remove or manipulate the content feature without harming ecological validity. For example, many PSAs or web videos have some type of background music or sound effects, and audio is one feature that can spur emotional reactions in audiences (e.g., Bolls, Lang, and Potter 2001; Dillman, Carpentier, and Potter 2007). For example, an experimenter may want to test how different types of background music impact emotional reactions to anti-drug PSAs. If the experimenter edited one version of a video PSA about the dangers of taking illegal drugs to have uplifting music in the background, that might seem very odd to the participants used to hearing frightening music in anti-drug PSAs. That could leave the participants overly focused on the peculiarity of the music and skew the results related to emotional reactions and behavioral intentions related to the health message itself.

Nonetheless, just because separating message features into components that represent important research concepts may be difficult does not mean researchers should avoid it entirely. Rather, caution and creativity will be needed to ensure such studies maintain adequate ecological validity. The translation of a finding from the psychology literature into a reliable finding in the study of media effects is not always a straight line, and the challenge of matching message components to these psychological concepts is likely one reason why (O'Keefe 2012).

Media effects researchers should also be aware of the relativity of emotional reactions when designing studies that analyze audiences' emotional reactions (Cacioppo and Gardner 1999). That is, emotions are relative to each individual's appraisal of his or her own person-environment relationship. A PSA about the dangers of tobacco may frighten one viewer who perceives lung cancer as a serious threat while the very same PSA angers another viewer who feels manipulated by the message sender. One option for dealing with emotional relativity is to thoroughly pretest stimuli and discard any that evoke extremely varied emotional responses in the target audience. Other options include using multiple stimuli to represent a particular media phenomenon, employing mixed (between- and within-subjects) designs, and replicating findings in multiple populations to ensure that no one particular message or one participant sample is responsible for study outcomes.

Additionally, research designs in this would be wise to take into consideration the realities of health disparities, particularly for experiments that manipulate content in order to evoke discrete emotions in participants. While many communication studies rely on white, eighteen- to twenty-two-year-old undergraduate students as participants, the demographics of the people most impacted by health issues are vastly different than those at most American research-intensive universities. The federal government has documented noticeable differences in insurance coverage, mortality, morbidity, and risky behaviors based on race, ethnicity, and socioeconomic status (Centers for Disease Control and Prevention 2011).

The populations negatively impacted by health disparities may be desensitized to the supposedly frightening health threats pictured in fear appeals because they see them more frequently than others. Moreover, they may also be skeptical of promises of good health portrayed in media messages with positive emotional overtones because their life experiences have included worse health and watching many loved ones suffer from illness and disease. Additional research is needed to confirm how these different life experiences relate to the ease with which prevention messages can evoke emotions in populations that have long dealt with poor health and other social justice issues.

Because these traditionally underserved populations are also the ones who could be most helped by prevention behaviors and changes in policies advocated for in preventive health messages, keeping in mind differences in the content and structure of messages that will evoke emotions in these populations should be an important study and message design consideration for health communication scholars. Likewise, actively recruiting members of these underserved populations to be subjects in health-related media effects research will also improve the generalizability of such studies. This is not necessarily an easy task given resource and time constraints for research, but it would be a worthwhile one that could potentially be supported by seeking grants and external funding.

Measurement

As discussed in the introduction and theoretical foundations chapters of this book, there are many ways to conceptualize and operationalize emotions, providing researchers with multiple options for measuring the concept. A majority of research on emotions in the realm of health communication has relied on self-reports of post-message exposure emotion. While this type of measurement is informative and has been validated, it only captures one part of the multifaceted impact of emotions on communication processes and effects. Additionally, reliable and validated multi-item emotion scales exist that could improve the measurement of self-reports of discrete emotions across the field (e.g., Dillard and Shen 2007).

Using continuous or multipoint measurements of emotions before, during, and after media exposure would also provide insights as to how changes in emotional reactions to various parts of a message can influence post-message effects on audiences (Nabi 2015). Furthermore, finding ways to employ implicit measures, such as the affect misattribution procedure (Payne, Cheng, Govorun, and Stewart 2005) or linguistic analysis (Pennebaker, Mehl, and Niederhoffer 2003), as well as psychophysiological measures of bodily and neural responses alongside self-report measures, could greatly advance our understanding of the role of emotions in health message effects.

Additionally, including measures of trait levels of emotions and affect-related concepts (e.g., trait anxiety, trait optimism, trait empathy, need for affect, etc.) as control variables may help statistically isolate the impact of health messages on behavior in the midst of individual differences in reactivity. Although adding such measures may result in lengthy questionnaires, the additional knowledge gained about what audiences bring with them to health messaging situations would be very valuable. This type of information could help message designers tailor health messages to these individual traits that impact emotional reactions to messages, and it could also aid targeting messages for specific sub-populations.

Analysis

Emotional responses to media often serve as mediators, or mechanisms, of the effects of media messages on audiences. For example, media effects research using meditational analyses reveals that reading a narrative news account about the challenges facing a stigmatized group (e.g., people with a mental illness) can increase feelings of compassion for members of those groups, and these feelings of compassion then lead participants to report greater intentions to aid members of the stigmatized groups (Oliver, Dillard, Bae, and Tamul 2012). Testing indirect effects typically involves using path analyses or structural equation modeling, statistical techniques that have grown in popularity during the last few decades (Kline 2011).

Given their increasing usage in the field, health communication scholars are more frequently turning to these types of process-based statistical analyses to help explain why exactly effects happen, and not just that they happen. The creation of user-friendly macros for existing statistical packages (Hayes 2013) makes this type of analysis even more accessible to health communication researchers than ever before. Multilevel modeling that takes into account group characteristics that might also help improve the analysis of health communication data in ways that better explain the complex processes at play. Researchers wanting to study emotion in the context of health messages would be well served to embrace the wide variety of statistical tools available to them in order to better capture the nuanced role that message-relevant emotions may have on audience behavior.

Another analysis issue involves grouping items that measure emotional reactions by valence alone. Even when researchers do measure multiple discrete emotional reactions in their studies, they often run an exploratory factor analysis (EFA) and decide to group these different emotions into one of two categories: positive or negative (e.g., Murphy, Frank, Moran, and Patnoe-Woodley 2011). As Dillard and Seo (2013) note, EFAs are usually meant for analyzing groups of items where there is not existing theoretical guidance for how best to group them. However, appraisal theory *does* provide researchers with guidance on which emotion items belong together. Important distinctions in appraisals and action tendencies exist between emotions of the same valence. Although both fear and anger, for instance, are negative, fear is an avoidance emotion, and anger is an approach emotion.

By reducing emotional measures to a couple of valence-based categories, researchers may be unintentionally masking the separate effects of discrete emotions. While factor reduction is a useful and important tool in quantitative research, the theoretical importance of testing the effects of discrete emotion may override the need to reduce emotion down its valence. If the individual discrete emotion indices display adequate reliability and are not multicolinear, it would be worthwhile to analyze them both as discrete entities and as general valence groups in order to see if there are any differences in effects.

FUTURE DIRECTIONS

One of the most repeated phrases in this book goes something like this: "While there is little research in this area, related work and theory indicate that [insert emotion name] could be influential in shaping the effects of preventative health messages on audiences." This absence of literature is particularly evident if we look at work on emotions and health communication that is not dedicated to studying fear appeals. The lack of research on emotions other than fear in the context of preventative health communication is a huge barrier in making accurate predictions about what types of messages will be most effective in motivating positive health changes. However, this gap in the literature also provides exciting new avenues of work for researchers who are ready to embrace the notion that human behavior is dependent on both affect and cognition.

The nuance of the discrete emotional perspective is compounded by the fact that prevention messages can easily evoke multiple emotions in audiences. Work on multiple-emotional reactions and mixed-valence emotions (e.g., elevation, which is generally positive but also negative in valence) is only beginning to permeate the communication literature. As health communication researchers strive to study ecologically valid media effects, a deeper understanding of the effects of simultaneously experiencing multiple emotions and/or experiencing mixed emotions will help advance the literature on media effects and health communication.

Along those lines, emotional reactions that transfer across mediated experiences (i.e., inter-media emotional reactions) is another area ripe for study in the health communication context. The emotions generated by one mediated experience (e.g., watching a news report of the Ebola virus spreading across countries) can influence subsequent mediated and interpersonal experiences (e.g., using the Internet to look up more information on the virus and the current situation and then sharing some of that information via a social media network). In a media-saturated environment, multiple-media studies are just as important as studying multiple emotions related to preventative health communication. Furthermore, additional work on the role of modality, be it text, audio, video, virtual reality, or combinations of these, could advance our understanding of how discrete emotions and emotional arousal effects differ depending on the delivery mechanism of the preventative health message.

The development of conceptual models or theories that integrate emotion and cognition would help researchers better predict the effects of emotions on health message consumers. While theories exist to explain the role of some negative emotions, like fear (e.g., Nabi 1999; Witte 1992), on communication outcomes, communication and media theories have yet to regularly integrate discrete positive or mixed emotions into theoretical frameworks. In the realm of interpersonal health information seeking, Afifi and Morse

(2009) began a conversation about the ways in which positive emotions can motivate behavior based on the premises of the theory of motivated information management. However, continued work in this domain and in that of numerous other health communication contexts is needed to fill the void left by the lack of emotional components in many communication and health behavior theories.

Beyond the nine discrete emotions examined in this book, many other emotions and emotion blends can influence the effects of health messages on audiences. For instance, anticipated regret has been shown to be a mechanism that can promote healthy eating behaviors post-health message exposure (van Koningsbruggen et al. 2014), while another study found that anticipated regret was a better predictor of influenza vaccination than was perceived risk (Chapman and Coups 2006). Other work demonstrates the emotion of disgust is an important predictor of how audiences will react to health messages that utilize graphic images (Jónsdóttir, Holm, Poltavski, and Vogeltanz-Holm 2014; Leshner, Vultee, Bolls, and Moore 2010; Morales, Wu, and Fitzsimons 2012).

Other emotions that could potentially provide insights into health message effects are jealousy/envy (e.g., wanting the level of health that others have may motivate people to take action) or gratitude (e.g., feeling thankful for good health may promote behaviors to maintain that gift). Beyond these, there are many more options for studying the role of discrete emotions in health communication processes. Although research on discrete emotions and health message effects, particularly from a prevention perspective, remains in its infancy, the upward trend in the number of health communication scholars studying emotions is encouraging.

CLOSING THOUGHTS

Prevention has not always been the focus of the health and medical communities (Rose 1992). However, the tide is changing. The United States no longer has the Centers for Disease Control. Instead, it has the Centers for Disease Control and Prevention. Sobering statistics have dictated such changes. In America, chronic illnesses (e.g., heart disease, cancer, and diabetes) cause seven out of every ten deaths and account for 75 percent of the nation's health spending (Centers for Disease Control and Prevention 2013). The CDC (2013) also reports that Americans use preventive health services at about half the recommended rate, further demonstrating the public's current lack of commitment to prevention behaviors.

As this turn toward prevention continues to wash over government, nonprofit, and commercial entities, more messages will need to be created to inform the public about and encourage them to adopt prevention behaviors or use preventive health services. And these organizations recognize the need for research that studies the effects of health-related media as well as application of that research in order to improve health communication practices. The CDC website even has a "Gateway to Health Communication and Social Marketing Practice" sub-site aimed at informing researchers and public health advocates about effective messaging strategies and tactics (Centers for Disease Control and Prevention 2014). Further research on the role of discrete emotions in motivating audiences to take action to prevent illness in themselves and those around them is a crucial step for improving the ability of these messaging strategies and tactics to change behavior.

In sum, prevention-oriented health behaviors and policies are vitally important for improving individual and public health. Yet gaining the attention of healthy audiences and then changing their behavior is no easy task. One psychological force is particularly adept at capturing attention and motivating action. Combining the study of emotion with the study of preventative health message effects is a productive and worthwhile venture for health communication and media researchers hoping to stop illnesses before they start.

REFERENCES

Afifi, W. A., and C. R. Morse. 2009. Expanding the role of emotion in the theory of motivated information management. In T. D. Afifi and W. A. Afifi (Eds.), *Uncertainty, information management, and disclosure decisions: Theories and applications* (pp. 87–105). New York: Routledge.

Baumeister, R. F., K. D. Vohs, C. Nathan DeWall, and L. Zhang. 2007. How emotion shapes behavior: Feedback, anticipation, and reflection, rather than direct causation. *Personality and Social Psychology Review* 11(2):167–203. doi: 10.1177/1088868307301033.

Bolls, P. D., A. Lang, and R. F. Potter. 2001. The effects of message valence and listener arousal on attention, memory, and facial muscular responses to radio advertisements. *Communication Research* 28(5):627–51. doi: 10.1177/009365001028005003.

Cacioppo, J. T., and W. L. Gardner. 1999. Emotion. *Annual Review of Psychology* 50(1):191–214. doi: 10.1146/annurev.psych.50.1.191.

Centers for Disease Control and Prevention. 2011. CDC health disparities and inequalities report—United States 2011. *MMWR Morbidity and Mortality Weekly Report*.

———. 2013. Gateway to health communication and social marketing practice: Preventive health care. Retrieved January 26, 2015, from http://www.cdc.gov/healthcommunication/toolstemplates/entertainmented/tips/preventivehealth.html.

———. 2014. Gateway to health communication and social marketing practice. Retrieved January 26, 2015, from http://www.cdc.gov/healthcommunication/index.html.

Chapman, G. B., and E. J. Coups. 2006. Emotions and preventive health behavior: Worry, regret, and influenza vaccination. *Health Psychology* 25(1):82–90. doi: 10.1037/0278-6133.25.1.82.

DeGeneres, E. 2011. *Seriously . . . I'm kidding*. New York: Grand Central Publishing.

Dillard, J. P., and K. Seo. 2013. Affect and persuasion. In J. P. Dillard and L. Shen (Eds.), *The SAGE handbook of persuasion: Developments in theory and practice* (Second ed., pp. 150–66). Thousand Oaks, CA: SAGE.

Dillard, J. P., and L. Shen. 2007. Self-report measures of discrete emotions. In R. A. Reynolds, R. Woods, and J. D. Baker (Eds.), *Handbook of research on electronic surveys and measurements* (pp. 330–33). Hershey, PA: Idea Group Reference.

Dillman Carpentier, F. R., and R. F. Potter. 2007. Effects of music on physiological arousal: Explorations into tempo and genre. *Media Psychology* 10(3):339–63. doi: 10.1080/15213260701533045.

Frijda, N. H., A. S. R. Manstead, and S. Bem. 2000. *Emotions and beliefs: How feelings influence thoughts.* Cambridge: Cambridge University Press.

Gerend, M., and J. Shepherd. 2012. Predicting human papillomavirus vaccine uptake in young adult women: Comparing the health belief model and theory of planned behavior. *Annals of Behavioral Medicine* 44(2):171–80. doi: 10.1007/s12160-012-9366-5.

Hayes, A. F. 2013. *Introduction to mediation, moderation, and conditional process analysis: A regression-based approach.* New York: Guilford.

Jensen, J. D. 2014. Comparison as a basic component of communication research: A call to action. *Green Papers in Communication* 1(1):1–2. http://www.ncahealthcom.org/green/1_1.pdf.

Jónsdóttir, H. L., J. E. Holm, D. Poltavski, and N. Vogeltanz-Holm. 2014. The role of fear and disgust in predicting the effectiveness of television advertisements that graphically depict the health harms of smoking. *Preventing Chronic Disease* 11:E218. doi: 10.5888/pcd11.140326.

Kline, R. B. 2011. *Principles and practice of structural equation modeling* (Third ed.). New York: Guilford Press.

Leshner, G., F. Vultee, P. D. Bolls, and J. Moore. 2010. When a fear appeal isn't just a fear appeal: The effects of graphic anti-tobacco messages. *Journal of Broadcasting and Electronic Media* 54(3):485–507. doi: 10.1080/08838151.2010.498850.

Morales, A. C., E. C. Wu, and G. J. Fitzsimons. 2012. How disgust enhances the effectiveness of fear appeals. *Journal of Marketing Research* 49(3):383–93. doi: 10.1509/jmr.07.0364.

Murphy, S. T., L. B. Frank, M. B. Moran, and P. Patnoe-Woodley. 2011. Involved, transported, or emotional? Exploring the determinants of change in knowledge, attitudes, and behavior in entertainment-education. *Journal of Communication* 61(3):407–31. doi: 10.1111/j.1460-2466.2011.01554.x.

Nabi, R. L. 1999. A cognitive-functional model for the effects of discrete negative emotions on information processing, attitude change, and recall. *Communication Theory* 9(3):292–320. doi: 10.1111/j.1468-2885.1999.tb00172.x.

———. 2015. Emotional flow in persuasive health messages. *Health Communication* 30(2):114–24. doi: 10.1080/10410236.2014.974129.

Noar, S. M., and R. S. Zimmerman. 2005. Health behavior theory and cumulative knowledge regarding health behaviors: Are we moving in the right direction? *Health Education Research* 20(3):275–90. doi: 10.1093/her/cyg113.

O'Keefe, D. J. 2003. Message properties, mediating states, and manipulation checks: Claims, evidence, and data analysis in experimental persuasive message effects research. *Communication Theory* 13(3):251–74. doi: 10.1111/j.1468-2885.2003.tb00292.x.

———. 2012. From psychological theory to message design: Lessons from the story of gain-framed and loss-framed persuasive messages. In H. Cho (Ed.), *Health communication message design: Theory and practice* (pp. 3–20). Los Angeles: SAGE.

Oliver, M. B., J. P. Dillard, K. Bae, and D. J. Tamul. 2012. The effect of narrative news format on empathy for stigmatized groups. *Journalism and Mass Communication Quarterly* 89(2):205–24. doi: 10.1177/1077699012439020.

Payne, B. K., C. M. Cheng, O. Govorun, and B. D. Stewart. 2005. An inkblot for attitudes: Affect misattribution as implicit measurement. *Journal of Personality and Social Psychology* 89(3):227–93. doi: 10.1037/0022-3514.89.3.277.

Pennebaker, J. W., M. R. Mehl, and K. G. Niederhoffer. 2003. Psychological aspects of natural language use: Our words, our selves. *Annual Review of Psychology* 54(1):547.

Rogers, E. M. 1994. *A history of communication study: A biographical approach.* New York: The Free Press.

Rose, G. 1992. *The strategy of preventive medicine.* New York, NY: Oxford University Press.

Slater, M. D., and L. S. Gleason. 2012. Contributing to theory and knowledge in quantitative communication science. *Communication Methods and Measures* 6(4):215–36. doi: 10.1080/19312458.2012.732626.

van Koningsbruggen, G. M., P. R. Harris, A. J. Smits, B. Schüz, U. Scholz, and R. Cooke. 2014. Self-affirmation before exposure to health communications promotes intentions and health behavior change by increasing anticipated regret. *Communication Research*. doi: 10.1177/0093650214555180.

Witte, K. 1992. Putting the fear back into fear appeals: The extended parallel process model. *Communication Monographs* 12(4):329–49. doi: 10.1080/03637759209376276.

Zillmann, D. 2006. Exemplification effects in the promotion of safety and health. *Journal of Communication* 56:S221–S237. doi: 10.1111/j.1460-2466.2006.00291.x.

Appendix

Additional Theoretical Perspectives on Emotions,
Social Psychology, and Media

AFFECT-AS-INFORMATION: EMOTION AS A CUE

Schwarz and Clore (1983; 1988; 2003) developed the affect-as-information framework while studying the ways in which incidental mood states can influence judgments. In a series of experiments they found that participants were more likely to report greater happiness and life satisfaction when they were in a good mood than when they were in a bad mood. One study in this line of research employed the weather as a mood manipulation to test this hypotheses. That is, participants surveyed on a rainy day were relegated to the bad mood condition, and participants surveyed on a sunny day were in the good mood condition (1983).

However, when participants were made aware of *why* they were in a particular mood (i.e., they were told about an experimental manipulation or reminded of the weather), those who had been in the bad mood no longer reported more negative judgments of well-being. But the participants in a positive mood maintained that they had higher levels of happiness and life-satisfaction even after being told about the external influences on their mood. These findings indicate that affective states can serve as cues, or as a source of information, about perceptions and judgments. Affect provides individuals with guidance they can use to make judgments about their situations, be it about their personal well-being or evaluations of objects, people, or behaviors. The logic goes that if people feel good, they will use that information as evidence they are making a correct judgment, whereas bad feelings indicate something should change.

As demonstrated by Schwarz and Clore (1983; 1988; 2003), the valence of affect is an important part of this informational process. By signaling that something is impeding one's goals, the affect-as-information paradigm posits that negative moods prod individuals to become more attentive to their surroundings in order to better grasp the context behind their negative state, and then possibly alleviate it (e.g., Bless, Bohner, Schwarz, and Strack 1990; Bless et al. 1996; Bodenhausen 1993). That is, individuals experiencing negative affect are more likely to seek out external information above and beyond the information provided by their emotional state, likely due to their desire to dissipate negative feelings. Raghunathan and Corfman (2004) were able to extend the affect-as-information framework to discrete negative emotions in the context of consumer behavior, finding that sadness leads individuals to seek pleasurable stimuli whereas anxiety leads them to be more attentive than sad or happy individuals.

Affect-as-information is not the only framework where pre-existing emotional states influence subsequent evaluations of messages. Zillmann's (1971) work on excitation transfer demonstrates that if the emotional arousal from a previous experience has not fully dissipated before individuals encounter another message, their arousal will transfer over to the present context. This transfer of arousal is non-conscious, and individuals typically misattribute their highly aroused state to the latter experience, one that when experienced on its own without the prior arousal would not be judged to be as exciting.

Excitation transfer shows that arousal can also serve an informative function for individuals. Likewise is Damasio's (2006) somatic marker hypothesis, which is the idea that we associate past decisions with their affective consequences and automatically rely on these learned associates when making current decisions. The somatic marker hypothesis underscores the intertwining of biology and emotion, similar to how the physiological arousal discussed in excitation transfer impacts evaluations of subsequent situations.

Similar to affect-as-information, the affect heuristic plays an important function in explaining the role of emotions with regard to risk perceptions. The affect heuristic is an ingrained reliance on affect to make judgments about risk (Slovic, Finucane, Peters, and MacGregor 2004; Slovic and Peters 2006; Slovic, Peters, Finucane, and Macgregor 2005). One's feelings, particularly if one is experiencing dread, serve as a cognitive shortcut to evaluating the risk of a potential behavior—the greater the feelings of dread, the greater the perceived risk. Although previous work on risk perception relied heavily on cognitive approaches, research on the affect heuristic demonstrates that affect has a very powerful role to play in determining risk. When affective and cognitive reactions to a risk differ, it is the affective response that guides risk perceptions in most cases (Loewenstein, Weber, Hsee, and Welch 2001).

From a motivational perspective, affective reactions can also provide information about progress toward one's pursuit of an important goal. Carver and Scheier's (1998) model of self-regulation distinguishes between approach goals, where individuals want to move toward a desired end, and avoidance goals, where individuals want to stay away from an undesired outcome. For approach goals, individuals appraise their progress toward the desired state. If they are making good progress, they will likely experience feelings of elation or joy, whereas a lack of progress can evoke feelings of depression. Avoidance goals, on the other hand, are associated with feelings of relief when individuals make adequate progress and feelings of anxiety when they are not progressing toward the goal.

Another conceptual perspective akin to affect-as-information and the ability of emotion to serve as a mental shortcut providing guidance on how to respond to a particular situation is the emotions-as-frames paradigm (Nabi 2003). Nabi argues that emotions can serve as frames for issues because they privilege certain information in terms of accessibility. The appraisals of a particular emotion make information similar to those appraisals more assessable, and this connection between the emotional state of the individual and the content of the message guides subsequent decision-making.

In a test of the emotion-as-frames perspective examining participants' reactions to social problems, Nabi (2003) found that feelings of fear were connected with the attribution of responsibility to societal causes, whereas anger was linked to blaming individuals, matching the respective appraisals of each emotion (uncertainty for fear and blame for anger). Furthermore, participants primed to feel fear were more likely to suggest solutions that would provide for protection from harm, whereas angry participants suggested retributive solutions to the social problems. Fearful participants also expressed a desire to seek information about susceptibility to a danger and efficacy for threat-reduction, whereas angry participants intended to seek information about the source of the offense and how others could be held accountable. The findings suggest that solutions and information seeking differing by emotion prime matched the action tendency properties of each emotion—the action tendency to seek safety for fear and to seek retribution for anger.

However, she also found these differences were moderated by schema development. The emotional states of participants framed, or shaped, their perceptions of a social issue with which they were highly familiar (i.e., drunk driving). Yet there were not significant differences between the emotional prime groups for an issue for which the participants did not have high levels of schema development (i.e., gun violence). Additional work has supported the predictive power of the emotions-as-frames perspective (Kim and Cameron 2011; Kühne and Schemer 2013), and points the way to additional work applying this framework to the realm of health communication.

In sum, a variety of conceptual frameworks describe the ways in which emotions and moods can cue or inform particular judgments or behaviors. Emotions provide individuals information about the nature of their relationship with their environments, make certain information more accessible than other information, and provide guidance and mental shortcuts for making judgments and decisions about behavior.

EMOTION REGULATION AND MOOD MANAGEMENT

Because emotions are dynamic and not static, the concept of emotion regulation must be considered when studying the effects of media on audience members' emotions and other reactions. Emotion regulation is a broad term for the many ways people attempt to regulate, or control, their own emotions (Gross and Thompson 2007). Emotion regulation is often automatic and takes place without conscious awareness; however, individuals may also try to purposefully change their emotional state. In a media context, pre-existing affective states can lead audiences to chose certain types of media with the goal (often a subconscious one) of changing or maintaining their affective states (Zillmann and Bryant 1985). Zillmann (1988) posited that "the consumption of messages . . . is capable of prevailing mood states, and the selection of specific messages for consumption often serves the regulation of mood states" (327). Goals related to emotion regulation, frequently referred to as mood management in the context of media consumption, can motivate audiences to choose certain genres of media over others in the hope that they will be able to manage their moods or to cultivate desired emotional states (for a review, see Oliver 2003).

The original conceptualization of mood management in communication research prescribed that people seek certain types of media in order to distract themselves from aversive affective states or to maintain positive affective states (Zillmann and Bryant 1985). However, mood management theory has since expanded to acknowledge motivations to seek certain types of media not only to distract from negative states but also to repair or cope with negative moods (Knobloch-Westerwick 2006). Mastro, Eastin, and Tamborini (2002) also extended mood-management principles to Internet-based media use by showing how high levels of stress resulted in participants viewing fewer websites while high levels of boredom resulted in higher numbers of websites visited within the same amount of time. Preventative health messages do not exist in isolation, and the mood-management paradigm could help researchers understand how pre-existing affective states influence audience reactions to health message.

LIMITED CAPACITY MODEL OF MOTIVATED
MEDIATED MESSAGE PROCESSING (LC4MP)

A. Lang's (2000) Limited Capacity Model of Motivated Mediated Message Processing is a framework that focuses on the motivational mechanisms behind information processing and memory-related outcomes of media use. The model has five main assumptions. The first is that individuals can only process so much information at any one time. That is, the human capacity to process information is limited. Furthermore, there are multiple information processing sub-tasks for which this capacity is needed: perception, encoding, storage, and retrieval. The second assumption of the LC4MP is that there are two automatically engaged motivational systems guiding how individuals spend their limited cognitive resources. The appetitive system controls approach motivation while the aversive system directs avoidance motivation. Emotions can activate both of these motivational systems (Bolls, Lang, and Potter 2001; Lang and Yegiyan 2008), as can changes in emotional states (Lang, Sanders-Jackson, Wang, and Rubenking 2012). Furthermore, individuals vary in their trait levels of motivational reactivity (Lang, Bradley, Sparks, and Lee 2007).

The third assumption of the LC4MP is that there are many sources and types of information portrayed via media. Individuals use their senses of sight, sounds, and touch to consume information of various formats, from text to still images to video. Fourth, the LC4MP recognizes that behavior, cognition, and affect are all dynamic processes that vary over time. The fifth statement of the model is that communication is an interactive process that takes place over time between the motivated information-processing system and the communication message itself.

The five assumptions of the model can help researchers predict how individuals will react to mediated messages, including prevention-oriented health messages. The existence of limits on cognitive resources suggests that individuals cannot always allocate sufficient information to each sub-process (encoding, storage, and retrieval). Therefore, the LC4MP predicts that motivational activation (aversive, appetitive, or simultaneous activation of both systems), message structure, content, and viewer goals will all interact to determine resource allocation when consuming a message (Lang 2000). Appetitive activation can result from positive stimuli, and it increases allocation to encoding and storage, thereby promoting information intake. Aversive activation, on the other hand, results from negative stimuli and motivates individuals to seek protection. At low levels of aversive activation, an individual allocates information to encoding, but at higher levels an individual is quickly aware of the threat and instead allocates more resources to retrieval in order to decide, based on past experience, how best to avoid the present threat.

By analyzing the interrelationships between message stimuli, audience motivations, and allocation of resources to various sub-processes, health message creators can design media based on their strategic goals (Lang 2006). For instance, if a local health department wants citizens to learn more about a new free exercise program in the community, using positive messages to activate the appetitive system could foster information intake. However, if the same health department wants to promote influenza vaccination, they may need to avoid using overly negative messages so that citizens will not stop encoding the threat-relevant information and rely too much on their past behavior, which for two-thirds of the American public would be avoiding the vaccine (Williams, Lu, Lindley, Kennedy, and Singleton 2012).

Furthermore, the LC4MP provides guidance about which media channels would be most appropriate to use for specific types of messages (Lang, Bolls, Potter, and Kawahara 1999). For instance, video is very good at gaining attention (i.e., eliciting an orienting response) and is emotionally evocative, which in turn activates motivational systems. However, video also presents audiences with much more information than do audio or text messages, making information overload likely and allocation of sufficient resources to all of the sub-processes unlikely. Therefore, if a health message is presented via video, then message designers need to be sure to use certain structural features (e.g., speed of cuts, image framing, pans, zooms, colors, overlay of audio, etc.) that help viewers dedicate sufficient resources to encoding the most important information in the video.

As Lang (2006) warns, the use of graphic, negatively valenced images can gain attention and activate the aversive motivation system, but this type of content often leads to poor memory for the information presented within it. She explains in more detail how the LC4MP can direct message design that prevents information overload by using combinations of message features, depending on the goal of the message: "The keys to attention are eliciting orienting responses and using motivationally relevant elements in your message. The keys to good memory are controlled resource allocation (e.g., cognitive effort), the automatic allocation of resources to encoding, and the creation of arousal in viewers through the use of either arousing content or fast-paced structure" (S74).

There have been multiple applications of the LC4MP to the context of health communication, from studying the effects of emotions and visual complexity on processing of prescription drug advertisements (Norris, Bailey, Bolls, and Wise 2011) to differences in how children respond to images of taboo products that can hurt health, such as beer, liquor, and cigarettes (Lang and Lee 2014). For another example, Lang and Yegiyan (2008) found that the intense emotional appeals used in many anti-drug PSAs are ineffective when the verbal claims in these PSAs are not also strong. Furthermore, the researchers found that stronger verbal claims were better remembered for negatively valenced than for positively valenced PSAs, demonstrating an interaction between emotional valence and memory. Future work expanding the LC4MP's assumptions to work on preventative health communication and discrete emotions could provide researchers with many valuable insights regarding message processes and effects.

THE BROADEN-AND-BUILD THEORY

While the majority of the theoretical developments and empirical tests of emotional influences on audiences have focused on negative emotions, positive emotions also have an important role to play in shaping how individuals react to messages, including preventative health messages. In fact, some scholars posit that an overuse of negative emotions in prevention messages is hampering efforts to effectively communicate health information to the public: "[We] end up telling people that if the cigarettes don't get them, a drunk driver, sexually transmitted disease or an over-abundance of butter surely will. The net effect is to turn health promotion from a tremendous opportunity for people to enhance their enjoyment of life, into a clutch of disparate and capricious threats" (Hastings and MacFadyen 2002, 74).

The burgeoning field of positive psychology provides media effects and health communication researchers with guidance as to the functions and effects of positive emotions. In particular, Fredrickson's (1998; 2001) broaden-and-build theory is useful for researchers wanting to apply positive psychology to prevention-oriented health communication. Fredrickson argues that, unlike negative emotions, positive emotions exist in order to broaden an individual's scope of attention, cognition, and action, while also helping the individual build skills for the future. Both of these outcomes (broadening and building) prove useful for individuals attempting to overcome obstacles and flourish in the long run.

Empirical research validates the propositions made by the broaden-and-build theory. For instance, in support of the "broaden" portion of the hypothesis, Fredrickson and Branigan (2005) found that the experience of positive emotions (versus negative emotions) led participants to exhibit a global (versus local) bias in a visual-processing task and to produce a longer and broader array of responses to an open-ended question. As for the "build" portion of the hypothesis, research indicates that positive emotions help individuals come back from negative experiences by building resilience and the necessary skills to flourish (Tugade and Fredrickson 2004). Furthermore, building health-related skills and building personal relationships with others who may later provide social support would also help those seeking to improve their health. For example, social support related to health issues is an oft-cited contributor to better health and well-being (Klemm and Wheeler 2005; White and Dorman 2001). Additionally, experiencing positive emotions has been found to down-regulate a previous experience of negative emotions (Fredrickson and Levenson 1998; Fredrickson, Mancuso, Branigan, and Tugade 2000).

There are many potential advantages to using positive emotions in preventative health messages. For one, health messages laced with positive affect can gain the audience's attention, lead to greater receptiveness, prompt reconsideration of an issue, facilitate recall, and lead to more positive attitudes toward the message (Monahan 1995). In general, individuals have an inclination to avoid threatening information about themselves in order to maintain a positive self-image (Baumeister 2010). However, positive emotions have been shown to motivate people to attend to self-relevant threats—information that will help them improve and benefit later in life (Das and Fennis 2008; Raghunathan and Trope 2002; Trope and Neter 1994; Trope and Pomerantz 1998). The broaden-and-build framework provides health communication researchers with a conceptual basis for determining which situations may favor the use of positive emotional appeals or positively toned information in order to help individuals achieve better health.

OTHER THEORETICAL PERSPECTIVES TO CONSIDER

While a complete overview of all the theories, models, and conceptual frameworks that are relevant to the study of emotion in the context of preventative health messages is beyond the scope of this chapter or this book, these five frameworks provide a decent start. Additional frameworks of relevance for health communication scholars include theories such as the Elaboration Likelihood Model and the Heuristic/Systematic Model, Social Cognitive Theory, Self-Determination Theory, and terror management perspectives, to name only a few. Many of these theories are briefly outlined in individual chapters throughout the book.

RELATED CONCEPTS

Emotion stands alone as a complete psychological concept. However, numerous related concepts include aspects of affect or emotional involvement that are important for understanding the role of emotion—broadly defined—in preventation-focused health communication. This appendix describes five such concepts: empathy, identification, parasocial interaction, transportation, and meta-emotions. Furthermore, many of these concepts involve the intertwined effects of narratives, or stories, on audiences. As such, health-related narratives are also discussed below. In reviewing these five concepts and the use of the narrative format, the aim is to demonstrate the many ways in which emotion can impact preventative health communication beyond the direct arousal of discrete emotions.

EMPATHY

Empathy is the process by which people come to understand each other and form deeper connections (Campbell and Babrow 2004; Lazarus 1991). Batson et al. (1997) define empathy as "an other-oriented emotional response congruent with another's perceived welfare" (105). In addition to its strong affective roots, empathy includes the cognitive component of perspective taking. When an individual experiences empathy, that person imagines the circumstances of another (Ickes 1993). To underscore the dual affective-cognitive nature of empathy, neuroimaging research has found that experiencing empathy for another simultaneously activates portions of the brain dedicated to affective and cognitive processing (Panksepp 2011). Indeed, the affective and cognitive components of empathy are closely related as they both entail a vicarious experience of another person's experiences—feelings and thoughts, respectively (Batson 2011; Shamay-Tsoory, Aharon-Peretz, and Perry 2009).

Empathy is closely related to the concept of emotional contagion, which is the phenomenon in which witnessing the emotions of another leads the observer to experience similar emotional responses (Hatfield, Cacioppo, and Rapson 1993). The witnessing of another individual's emotional expressions can take place face-to-face or via media. Researchers have found that when an observer views the actions and emotional reactions of another, mirror neurons fire in the observer's brain as if she were actually behaving in the same manner as the other person (Jabbi, Swart, and Keysers 2007; Rizzolatti 2008). Even observing other individuals' emotions via social media posts can change the valence of one's own social media status updates to more closely match the emotional tone of the user's social network (Kramer, Guillory, and Hancock 2014).

While empathy is often thought of as a negatively valenced response to the distress of another individual, it can also be positively valenced (e.g., feeling happy for another person's good fortune). Empathy may be defined as either a context-specific reaction or a more stable individual difference variable (Stiff, Dillard, Somera, Kim, and Sleight 1988). Moreover, those individuals exhibiting higher levels of trait empathy are more likely to exhibit higher levels of state empathy.

Campbell and Babrow (2004) propose a theoretical take on the role of empathy in persuasive health communication. The researchers contend that empathy has multiple components, including the abilities to identify with another, understand the path that led a person to that situation, experience similar emotions as the other person, feel concern for the other, and believe that the context is either true or realistic. As for the mechanics of empathy in a health communication context, Campbell and Brabow argue that feelings of empathy with a model portraying elements of health risk and efficacy should evoke empathy, which in turn deepens the audience member's cognitive and emotional understanding of the health risk. They found support for their model connecting empathy for a model, understanding of risk, and persuasion in the context of HIV/AIDS prevention PSAs.

Many health communication studies have found that empathy can facilitate message acceptance and behavior change. For instance, Pechmann and Reibling (2006) showed that adolescents who viewed anti-tobacco advertisements portraying individuals who were suffering from tobacco-related illnesses experienced more empathy than did those adolescents who did *not* view disease-related suffering. Consequently, the adolescents who experienced empathy in response to the anti-tobacco advertisements reported a decrease in their intentions to smoke, demonstrating the ability of empathy for others to impact individual health behaviors.

Work on health messages has also established the value of researching empathic responses in conjunction with emotional reactions. For instance, Shen (2011) used an experiment to compare the effectiveness of empathy-versus fear-arousing anti-smoking PSAs. He found that both types of PSAs could be effective when compared to a control advertisement. However, the empathy-arousing PSAs were more persuasive than the fear-arousing ones. This lower level of effectiveness for the fear appeal advertisements was due to the emotion's negative indirect effect on persuasion: fear induced higher levels of reactance, which in turn decreased persuasion. Other research confirms that creating health messages that produce empathy in audience members is an effective way to mitigate reactance against such messages (Shen 2010). Given these findings, empathy is clearly an important concept for health communication scholars and message designers to keep in mind.

Identification

The process of identification occurs when one assumes the identity of another (Cohen 2001). In taking on another person's identity, the thoughts and feelings of the other start to merge with the observer's and become one. According to Cohen, the intensity of identification with a mediated other depends on how fully one assumes the other's perspective and is able to momentarily leave behind her own thoughts and feelings. Although the literature on empathy and identification often cross paths, with some scholars even including identification as a sub-component of empathy (Campbell and Babrow 2004; Stiff et al. 1988), identification is sufficiently different conceptually to merit individual examination. Individuals can experience empathy for another without merging identities, making it important to study empathy and identification as separate, although related, concepts.

Identification has been a particularly fruitful concept for researchers aiming to understand when and how news of celebrity illnesses can influence individuals to change their own health behaviors. For example, Brown and Basil (1995) and Basil (1996) investigated reactions to basketball star Earvin "Magic" Johnson's HIV diagnosis and found that the impact of Johnson's announcement on the individual's personal concern, perceived risk of HIV, and sexual behaviors was shaped by their sense of identification with Johnson. Those who identified more with Johnson were more likely to adopt preventative behaviors. Many studies of other celebrities, from athletes to politicians to royalty, have found a similar relationship between identification with the celebrity and health-related outcomes (Brown and Basil 2010).

Recent work has found that the process of identification with celebrities experiencing health problems also involves emotional reactions to news of the celebrity's illness or death. One study examined young adults' reactions to the death of Apple co-founder and CEO Steve Jobs from pancreatic cancer. The researchers found that feelings of sadness related to his death partially mediated the impact of identification on both interpersonal conversation and on information seeking related to Jobs's cancer (Myrick, Willoughby, Noar, and Brown 2013). However, a similar study using a sample of older and more diverse participants found that cancer worry, and not sadness, partially mediated the relationship between identification with Jobs and both conversation and information seeking about cancer (Myrick, Noar, Willoughby, and Brown 2014). The different emotional reactions to identifying with Jobs may be due to the fact that older news audiences are more susceptible to cancer. Therefore, it makes sense that seeing a similar other fall to the disease would cause worry, whereas young people who witness someone they felt a connection with succumb to this disease would, instead, feel sad about it. Together, these findings indicate that identification with celebrities featured in the media during their struggles with a health issue can have both direct and indirect (via emotional reactions to the news) on health behaviors, and those individual differences like age may change the nature of the relationship between identification, emotional responses, and behavioral responses.

In sum, identification with a media persona fosters audience perceptions and emotions similar to that of the persona. Early research in this paradigm found that identification with media characters or public figures was directly related to health behaviors, whereas more recent work points to the ability of assuming another's identity to elicit emotional reactions that likewise contribute to health and communication outcomes. However, most of the research examining these links has utilized cross-sectional survey designs, leaving up for debate the causal direction between identification and behavior. Future research could utilize experimental and time-series designs to help establish causality in this relationship.

Parasocial Interaction

While the concept of identification focuses on the situation where a media consumer assumes the identity of a media character or persona, parasocial interaction focuses on the building of kinship with a mediated persona. Horton and Wohl (1956) first defined a parasocial relationship as the bond that develops between a media character and the viewer. Over time, parasocial interactions can result in a pseudo-friendship or sense of intimacy with a mediated other (Brown, Basil, and Bocarnea 2003). The parasocial relationship assumes many of the qualities of a real, face-to-face relationship, despite the fact that an actual relationship with the mediated character is (typically) only an illusion (Horton and Wohl 1956).

These parasocial relationships can develop between audiences and fictional characters as well as with actual public figures, from celebrities to politicians to athletes (Bocarnea and Brown 2007). Just as real relationships have many emotional components, so do parasocial ones. When a mediated "friend" acts in ways that please an audience member, that audience member may feel pride or joy, whereas bad behavior on the part of the mediated character may result in negative emotions like shame or disgust. Likewise, when this mediated friend is facing danger or is actually in pain (mental or physical), then audience members who are experiencing parasocial interaction may experience feelings of fear or sadness, respectively.

In the realm of health communication, celebrity announcements of illness can also impact the public via parasocial interaction with the famous individual. Similar to the way identification mediated the effects of exposure to news of Magic Johnson's HIV diagnosis on behavioral intentions, Brown and Basil (1995) found that those who were emotionally involved with Johnson via the process of parasocial interaction were more likely to show greater personal concern about AIDS and greater perceptions of the risk of AIDS for heterosexuals. Those who experienced parasocial interaction with Johnson were also more likely to report intentions to reduce high-risk sexual behaviors. Importantly, Brown and Basil found that those who knew about Johnson's diagnosis but did *not* report feeling emotionally involved with him did not display significant reactions to his disclosure.

Identification and parasocial interaction seem to have very similar roles in shaping how the public responds to celebrity announcements of illness. However, as mentioned above, both are distinct concepts with unique contributions to explaining variance in communication and health outcomes. Brown, Basil, and Bocarnea (2003) outline two important differences: "First, a parasocial relationship is conceived of as a psychological state of involvement with a media personality through an imagined or perceived friendship. The relationship is an entity in itself and not a facet of persuasive influence. Second, parasocial interaction does not require adopting another person's attitudes, values or behaviors although this often occurs" (47).

Likewise, both identification and parasocial interaction can influence reactions to health media. Tian and Yoo (2014) found that individuals who watched the reality television show *The Biggest Loser* experienced both parasocial interaction and identification with contestants. The show involves obese contestants competing with each other to see who can lose the most weight, with "the biggest loser" winning a large cash prize at the end of the season. The researchers showed that parasocial interaction with *Biggest Loser* contestants was positively related to exercise self-efficacy, whereas identification was negatively associated with exercise self-efficacy. The researchers posit that this pattern of effects occurred because identifying with contestants may have made viewers feel as though they were less capable of exercising, given the contestants visible struggles with the activity. On the other hand, parasocial interaction with the contestants, or feeling like contestants were their friends, may have led audience members to want to encourage the participants (just like the show's coaches do) and therefore they felt better about their own ability to exercise. Tian and Yoo also found that exercise self-efficacy was positively associated with exercise behavior, meaning that both processes—identification and parasocial interaction—can have important indirect effects on health behavior.

This study is but one of many finding links between these audience involvement variables and health outcomes. Beyond impacting personal behaviors, parasocial interaction with media persona can also influence how individuals react to others dealing with health conditions (Hoffner and Cohen 2012). While they may have different effects in different contexts, identification and parasocial interaction can each evoke emotional reactions to health-related messages. Therefore, they are important considerations for research tackling the role of emotion in preventative health messages, particularly if the message is a narrative that involves mediated characters or if the message includes public figures with whom audiences have pre-existing emotional involvement.

Transportation

Another concept vital for understanding emotional, cognitive, and behavioral reactions to health narratives is that of transportation. Green and Brock (2000) define transportation as immersion into a story. Being transported is the process of getting lost or entirely absorbed in the narrative. Because the experience of transportation involves an intense focus on the storyline, audiences who are transported leave behind the so-called real world in order to embrace the narrative world. According to Green and Brock, transportation can increase persuasion because individuals are so consumed by the plot and its characters that they fail to counter-argue or contradict claims—be they implicit or explicit—made within the narrative.

Emotional involvement with a storyline is an important facilitator of transportation into a narrative world. Green and Brock (2000) state that "transported readers may experience strong emotions and motivations, even when they know the events in the story are not real" (702). In fact, in a thought-listing task the authors used to assess participants' reactions to a narrative, the majority of responses were global or emotional rather than cognitive in nature. Research indicates that emotional involvement with health-related storylines is can foster health-related behavior change, too. For example, in a study of four organ donation storylines in popular U.S. television shows, Morgan, Movius, and Cody (2009) found in their survey research that viewers of these shows were more likely to become an organ donor if they were emotionally involved in the narrative than if they did not experience a strong enough emotional connection with the plot and characters.

Green (2006) makes a convincing case for embracing highly transporting narratives as a tactic for persuasive cancer communication, in particular. Given that cancer is inextricably tied to emotional reactions like fear, anxiety, and hope (Mukherjee 2010), transportation into a narrative world may help individuals cope with those emotions in a safe space. As Green argues, transportation can foster persuasion because it helps reduce counter-arguing and fosters mental simulations of difficult or frightening health situations (e.g., testing or screening). Narratives with high transportation potential also provide audiences with role models for behavior change. Moreover, transportation elicits both cognitive and emotional reactions that aid in attitude and behavior change. These points about the efficacy of transportation for fostering positive health outcomes can apply to other health contexts beyond cancer, making transportation another important emotion-related concept to study in the realm of preventative health communication.

Meta-Emotions

Emotions can be experienced on multiple levels. The first level is emotion as a direct experience caused by a stimulus (the focus of this book). The second level of emotional experience is more reflective and constitutes an individual's impressions of her own emotional state (Mayer and Gaschke 1988). Meta-emotions are appraisals of one's own feelings (Oliver 1993), akin to how individuals evaluate their own thoughts. Bartsch, Vorderer, Mangold, and Viehoff (2008) describe the concept as such: "Emotions are accompanied by meta-level mental processes that color the experience of emotions and influence how people express and regulate them" (8). Simply stated, meta-emotions are emotions *about* emotions.

Being able to evaluate one's feelings can be a beneficial skill for mastering social situations and achieving personal success, as research in the area of emotional intelligence continues to demonstrate (Mayer and Salovey 1993; Salovey and Mayer 1988). One's environment can also foster differences in meta-emotions (Bartsch et al. 2008). Furthermore, individuals differ in their general preferences for appraising their own emotional states (Maio and Esses 2001). Some individuals are more inclined to reflect on why they are feeling the way they do, while others prefer not to evaluate their own emotional reactions.

To date, the bulk of the research on meta-emotions in the communication field has focused on the entertainment context. A program of research initiated by Oliver (1993) sought to explain why many people enjoy entertainment with strong negative emotional overtones, such as tear jerkers or horror movies. Audience members' voluntary exposure to these genres of media goes against the predictions of the hedonic-based propositions of mood management theory (Zillmann 1988). Oliver's research found that meta-emotions could help explain this paradox. In her study, participants, especially females, who felt sad after watching sad films also experienced greater enjoyment of those films.

Actively reflecting on emotional media content even has benefits for physical health and mental well-being. Research indicates that reflecting on dramatic entertainment is associated with decreases in depression and improvement in affective self-regulatory abilities (Khoo and Graham-Engeland 2014; Khoo and Oliver 2013). While research on meta-emotions and media has focused on the entertainment context, there are important implications for health communication, too. Understanding which features of media content promote meta-emotions would help health communication researchers understand how to foster continued reflection upon health messages long after a PSA has aired or an online news story moves to the bottom of one's social media feed. And continued reflection may spur further information seeking, knowledge gain, and finally health-related behavior change. Bartsch (2008) outlines three such features of media that can spark meta-emotions in audiences: (1) aesthetics; (2) the narrative context (i.e., the plot); and (3) symbolic elements representing cultural norms or values related to emotions.

Research is needed to test how these features may apply to health contexts. But based on those three message features, health messages that are professionally produced (i.e., of very high aesthetic quality) will likely be more aesthetically complex and could better provoke reflection upon the emotional content of the message than amateur content (all other factors held equal). As for the second message feature, a health narrative could include a character who, within the plot, explores her anxiety related to trying to get down to a healthy weight, which in turn might spur similar meta-emotions in viewers who are familiar with that type of anxiety.

The third message feature related to norms coincides with the importance of norms in prominent health behavior theories (Ajzen 1991; Ajzen and Fishbein 1980). Furthermore, violations of social norms result in emotions such as guilt, shame, and embarrassment, while compliance with norms can elicit pride, even hope for future success in fitting into the social scene. Therefore, preventative health messages that project health-related norms and values (e.g., smoking hurts other people and is not socially acceptable in many places anymore) may spur audiences to further reflect on the importance of changing their health behaviors for the better.

Narratives

A unifying theme connecting the aforementioned concepts is that they are all forms of audience involvement with narratives. Audience involvement with a narrative can be generally defined as "the degree to which we invest emotional and mental efforts in decoding the text and making sense of the story" (Tal-Or and Cohen 2010, 402). Humans are story-telling animals, and narratives serve many functions for society. As one reporter put it, "We tell ourselves stories not only for profound reasons but for mundane ones as well: to process the ambiguous and complex events that unfold every day around us" (Greenhouse 2014). Emotions are also key to audience involvement with narratives (Oatley 2002). Without an affective connection to the story and its characters, there is no link between the audience and the characters or plot and little motivation to ruminate about the lessons embedded in the narrative.

In the context of health communication, narratives are often employed in the context of entertainment education. The goal of entertainment education is to incorporate health-related or other prosocial storylines into popular entertainment media fare in order to (1) increase awareness and (2) positively influence audience knowledge levels, attitudes, and behaviors (Kaiser Family Foundation 2004). Entertainment education narratives can evoke multiple forms of audience involvement at once, with identification, parasocial interaction, and transportation having different influences on various mechanisms and outcomes (Moyer-Gusé and Nabi 2010).

The big advantage of using entertainment-based narratives to promote health behaviors is that these stories engage the readers and dissipate counter-arguing such that the format is fairly effective at overcoming audience resistance to health messages (Moyer-Gusé 2008; Slater and Rouner 2002). Moreover, entertainment representations of health behaviors can provide models for audiences, showing them how to deal with similar health-related concerns in their own lives. This modeling of effective health behavior can vicariously increase audience members' self-efficacy for performing the behavior themselves, as predicted by tenets of social cognitive theory (Bandura 2004).

Individuals who immerse themselves in a storyline are more likely to be impacted by a narrative than are those who do not embrace the plot. Busselle and Bilandzic (2009) argue that narrative effects depend on how audiences construct a mental model of the story via various processes related to narrative engagement. The researchers argue that narrative engagement consists of four distinct dimensions: narrative understanding, attentional focus, emotional engagement, and narrative presence. Narrative engagement is important, Busselle and Bilandzic posit, because it facilitates enjoyment and story-consistent attitudes. Attitude consistency is a particularly beneficial outcome for health narratives that aim to persuade audiences to adopt specific behaviors.

As mentioned above, emotional arousal is a central tenant of a narrative, and that holds true for health-related narratives as well. McQueen, Kreuter, Kalesan, and Alcaraz (2011) investigated the effects of narrative versus non-narrative mammography-related videos shown to low-income African American women in St. Louis. They found that the narrative version of the video evoked more positive *and* more negative feelings in participants. In short, it evoked more emotions than the non-narrative version. The increase in negative emotion from watching the narrative version was linked to an increase in participants' perceptions of both breast cancer risk and cancer fear. Meanwhile, the increase in positive affect from the narrative version led to a decrease in perceived barriers to mammography. The narrative version also resulted in greater engagement, which promoted interpersonal conversations that helped improve message recall. The narrative version also increased identification with the message source, which reduced counter-arguing against the message. In sum, both affective reactions (negative and positive) and engagement resulting from exposure to a health narrative had beneficial outcomes in this particular study.

Many other studies have found narratives to be an effective way to promote health behaviors. Murphy, Frank, Chatterjee, and Baezconde-Garbanati (2013) examined the impacts of a fictional narrative versus a traditional nonfiction message about cervical cancer screening. Their experiment revealed that the fictional narrative was more effective than the traditional nonfiction message in increasing knowledge and positive attitudes about cervical cancer screening in audience members. Additionally, data analysis found that transportation, identification with characters, and emotional responses linked with viewing of the fictional narrative contributed to positive changes in knowledge, attitudes, and behavioral intentions. This particular study is particularly important because it compared multiple conceptual explanations for narrative effects (involvement, transportation, and emotions) and found them all to be important variables to consider in conjunction with each other as narrative mechanisms.

Additional research on an entertainment-education storyline in a popular U.S. television drama found that transportation was the best predictor of change in relevant knowledge, attitudes, and behavior, while involvement with a specific character (e.g., identification) was more important for its ability to increase transportation and emotional reactions that subsequently changed in viewers' knowledge, attitudes, and behavior (Murphy, Frank, Moran, and Patnoe-Woodley 2011). In certain contexts, particular variables may take precedence over others as far as having the most impact on audience perceptions and behaviors. Future research could investigate which content and structural features (e.g., multicharacter plotlines versus one focal character, message modality, etc.) as well as which audiences characters (e.g., need for affect, need for cognition, etc.) determine whether character involvement, transportation, or emotional reactions are the best predictors of important health-related outcomes related to narrative exposure.

Non-fictional narratives can also influence health behaviors, as multiple studies have demonstrated. Comparing the effects of news media narratives that involve the stories of individual exemplars to non-narrative news formats that rely on statistics is at the heart of exemplification theory (Gibson and Zillmann 1994; Zillmann 2006; Zillmann and Brosius 2000; Zillmann, Perkins, and Sundar 1992). Zillmann and colleagues have shown that audiences connect on an emotional level with the tales of exemplars and often give greater weight to the exemplars' stories than to base-rate statistics when making judgments about social phenomenon. In the case of health issues, the use of exemplars in news stories can influence audience members' perceived susceptibility for a condition (Aust and Zillmann 1996) or for a certain segment of the population (Gibson and Zillmann 2000). The use of exemplars in health news provides a narrative element and fosters emotional engagement with the content such that these types of news stories have different effects on audiences than do those based primarily on statistics. However, because of the power of the emotional connection with exemplars formed in the course of a news story, the misuse of exemplars in health news can lead to misinformation or misperceptions about disease (see chapter 12 about health journalism, this volume).

Be it a fictional or news narrative, the connection between a strong plot and emotional evocation in audiences is strong. However, most research on narratives focuses on audience and character involvement. If any specific emotional reactions are measured in the studies at all, it is usually only post-exposure emotions. Nabi and Green (2014) make a convincing case that research on narrative effects could be advanced by studying the ways in which emotions shift throughout a story, as well as how these emotional shifts attract potential audiences to narratives in the first place. Shifts in emotional reactions may promote and sustain engagement with a narrative, thereby enhancing the story's ability to persuade audiences. Furthermore,

Nabi and Green state that emotional flow in a narrative likely promotes both short- and long-term attitude change via emotion-driven topic involvement and social sharing. Integrating a more nuanced perspective on the multiple emotions generated throughout a health narrative would significantly advance researchers' understanding of the precise impact of both emotional arousal and changes in emotional arousal on important health-related outcomes. Moreover, Murphy et al. (2013) note that much of the work testing the impact of emotions generated by narratives on audiences has only examined affect from a bivalent (i.e., positive versus negative) orientation, therefore failing to analyze how discrete emotions with different core relational themes and action tendencies may result in distinct responses to a story.

REFERENCES

Ajzen, I. 1991. The theory of planned behavior. *Organizational Behavior and Human Decision Processes* 50(2):179–211. doi: 10.1016/0749-5978(91)90020-t.

Ajzen, I., and M. Fishbein. 1980. *Understanding attitudes and predicting social behavior.* Englewood Cliffs, NJ: Prentice-Hall.

Aust, C. F., and D. Zillmann. 1996. Effects of victim exemplification in television news on viewer perception of social issues. *Journalism and Mass Communication Quarterly* 73(4):787–803. doi: 10.1177/107769909607300403.

Bandura, A. 2004. Social cognitive theory for personal and social change by enabling media. In A. Singhal, M. J. Cody, E. M. Rogers and M. Sabido (Eds.), *Entertainment-education and social change: History, research, and practice* (pp. 75–96). Mahwah, NJ: Lawrence Erlbaum Associates.

Bartsch, A. 2008. Meta-emotion: How films and music videos communicate emotions about emotions. *Projections* 2(1):45–59. doi: 10.3167/proj.2008.020104.

Bartsch, A., P. Vorderer, R. Mangold, and R. Viehoff. 2008. Appraisal of emotions in media use: Toward a process model of meta-emotion and emotion regulation. *Media Psychology* 11(1):7–27.

Basil, M. D. 1996. Identification as a mediator of celebrity effects. *Journal of Broadcasting and Electronic Media* 40(4):478–95. doi: 10.1080/08838159609364370.

Batson, C. D. 2011. *Altruism in humans.* New York: Oxford University Press.

Batson, C. D., M. P. Polycarpou, E. Harmon-Jones, H. J. Imhoff, E. C. Mitchener, L. L. Bednar, . . . L. Highberger. 1997. Empathy and attitudes: Can feeling for a member of a stigmatized group improve feelings toward the group? *Journal of Personality and Social Psychology* 72(1):105–18. doi: 10.1037/0022-3514.72.1.105.

Baumeister, R. F. 2010. The self. In R. F. Baumeister and E. J. Finkel (Eds.), *Advanced social psychology: The state of the science* (pp. 139–75). Oxford: Oxford University Press.

Bless, H., G. Bohner, N. Schwarz, and F. Strack. 1990. Mood and persuasion: A cognitive response analysis. *Personality and Social Psychology Bulletin* 16(2):331–45. doi: 10.1177/0146167290162013.

Bless, H., G. L. Clore, N. Schwarz, V. Golisano, C. Rabe, and M. Wölk. 1996. Mood and the use of scripts: Dose a happy mood really lead to mindlessness? *Journal of Personality and Social Psychology* 71(4):665–79.

Bocarnea, M. C., and W. J. Brown. 2007. Celebrity-persona parasocial interaction scale. In R. A. Reynolds, R. Woods and J. D. Baker (Eds.), *Handbook of research on electronic surveys and measurements* (pp. 309–12). Hershey, PA: Idea Group Reference.

Bodenhausen, G. V. 1993. Emotion, arousal, and stereotypic judgment: A heuristic model of affect and stereotyping. In D. Mackie and D. Hamilton (Eds.), *Affect, cognition, and stereo-*

typing: Interactive processes in intergroup perception (pp. 13–27). San Diego, CA: Academic Press.

Bolls, P. D., A. Lang, and R. F. Potter. 2001. The effects of message valence and listener arousal on attention, memory, and facial muscular responses to radio advertisements. *Communication Research* 28(5):627–51. doi: 10.1177/009365001028005003.

Brown, W. J., and M. D. Basil. 1995. Media celebrities and public health: Responses to "Magic" Johnson's HIV disclosure and its impact on AIDS risk and high-risk behaviors. *Health Communication* 7(4):345–70. doi: 10.1207/s15327027hc0704_4.

———. 2010. Parasocial interaction and identification: Social change processes for effective health interventions. *Health Communication* 25(6/7):601–2. doi: 10.1080/10410236.2010.496830.

Brown, W. J., M. D. Basil, and M. C. Bocarnea. 2003. The influence of famous athletes on health beliefs and practices: Mark McGwire, child abuse prevention, and androstenedione. *Journal of Health Communication* 8(1):41–57. doi: 10.1080/10810730305733.

Busselle, R., and H. Bilandzic. 2009. Measuring narrative engagement. *Media Psychology* 12(4):321–47. doi: 10.1080/15213260903287259.

Campbell, R. G., and A. S. Babrow. 2004. The role of empathy in responses to persuasive risk communication: Overcoming resistance to HIV prevention messages. *Health Communication* 16(2):159–82.

Carver, C. S., and M. F. Scheier. 1998. *On the self-regulation of behavior*. New York: Cambridge University Press.

Cohen, J. 2001. Defining identification: A theoretical look at the identification of audiences with media characters. *Mass Communication and Society* 4(3):245–64. doi: 10.1207/S15327825MCS0403_01.

Damasio, A. R. 2006. *Descartes' error: Emotion, reason, and the human brain*. London: Vintage.

Das, E., and B. M. Fennis. 2008. In the mood to face the facts: When a positive mood promotes systematic processing of self-threatening information. *Motivation and Emotion* 32(3):221–30.

Dillard, J. P., and L. Shen. 2007. Self-report measures of discrete emotions. In R. A. Reynolds, R. Woods and J. D. Baker (Eds.), *Handbook of research on electronic surveys and measurements* (pp. 330–33). Hershey, PA: Idea Group Reference.

Fredrickson, B. L. 1998. What good are positive emotions? *Review of General Psychology* 2(3):300–319. doi: 10.1037/1089-2680.2.3.300.

———. 2001. The role of positive emotions in positive psychology: The broaden-and-build theory of positive emotions. *American Psychologist* 56(3):218–26. doi: 10.1037/0003-066X.56.3.218.

Fredrickson, B. L., and C. Branigan. 2005. Positive emotions broaden the scope of attention and thought-action repertoires. *Cognition and Emotion* 19(3):313–32.

Fredrickson, B. L., and R. W. Levenson. 1998. Positive emotions speed recovery from the cardiovascular sequelae of negative emotions. *Cognition and Emotion* 12(2):191–220. doi: 10.1080/026999398379718.

Fredrickson, B. L., R. A. Mancuso, C. Branigan, and M. M. Tugade. 2000. The undoing effect of positive emotion. *Motivation and Emotion* 24(4):237–58. doi: 10.1023/A:1010796329158.

Gibson, R., and D. Zillmann. 1994. Exaggerated versus representative exemplification in news reports perception of issues and personal consequences. *Communication Research* 21(5):603–24. doi: 10.1177/009365094021005003.

———. 2000. Reading between the photographs: The influence of incidental pictorial information on issue perception. *Journalism and Mass Communication Quarterly* 77(2):355–66.

Green, M. C. 2006. Narratives and cancer communication. *Journal of Communication* 56:S163–S183. doi: 10.1111/j.1460-2466.2006.00288.x.

Green, M. C., and T. C. Brock. 2000. The role of transportation in the persuasiveness of public narratives. *Journal of Personality and Social Psychology* 79(5):701–21.

Greenhouse, L. 2014. The stories we tell. *The New York Times*. http://www.nytimes.com/2014/02/06/opinion/greenhouse-the-stories-we-tell.html?src=rechpand_r=2.

Gross, J. J., and R. A. Thompson. 2007. Emotion regulation: Conceptual foundations. In J. J. Gross (Ed.), *Handbook of emotion regulation* (pp. 3–24). New York: Guilford Press.

Hastings, G., and L. MacFadyen. 2002. The limitations of fear messages. *Tobacco Control* 11(1):73–75. doi: 10.1136/tc.11.1.73.

Hatfield, E., J. T. Cacioppo, and R. L. Rapson. 1993. Emotional contagion. *Current Directions in Psychological Science* 2(3):96–99. doi: 10.2307/20182211.

Hoffner, C. A., and E. L. Cohen. 2012. Responses to obsessive compulsive disorder on *Monk* among series fans: Parasocial relations, presumed media influence, and behavioral outcomes. *Journal of Broadcasting and Electronic Media* 56(4):650–68. doi: 10.1080/08838151.2012.732136.

Horton, D., and R. R. Wohl. 1956. Mass communication and para-social interaction. *Psychiatry: Journal for the Study of Interpersonal Processes* 19:215–29.

Ickes, W. 1993. Empathic accuracy. *Journal of Personality* 61(4):587–610. doi: 10.1111/j.1467-6494.1993.tb00783.x.

Jabbi, M., M. Swart, and C. Keysers. 2007. Empathy for positive and negative emotions in the gustatory cortex. *NeuroImage* 34(4):1744–53. doi: http://dx.doi.org/10.1016/j.neuroimage.2006.10.032.

Kaiser Family Foundation. 2004. Entertainment education and health in the United States: A report to the Kaiser Family Foundation. Menlo Park, CA: Henry J. Kaiser Family Foundation.

Khoo, G. S., and J. E. Graham-Engeland. 2014. The benefits of contemplating tragic drama on self-regulation and health. *Health Promotion International*. doi: 10.1093/heapro/dau056.

Khoo, G. S., and M. B. Oliver. 2013. The therapeutic effects of narrative cinema through clarification: Reexamining catharsis. *Scientific Study of Literature* 3(2):266–93. doi: 10.1075/ssol.3.2.06kho.

Kim, H. J., and G. T. Cameron. 2011. Emotions matter in crisis: The role of anger and sadness in the publics' response to crisis news framing and corporate crisis response. *Communication Research* 38(6):826–55. doi: 10.1177/0093650210385813.

Klemm, P., and E. Wheeler. 2005. Cancer caregivers online: Hope, emotional roller coaster, and physical/emotional/psychological responses. *Computers, Informatics, Nursing* 23(1):38–45. doi: http://journals.lww.com/cinjournal/Fulltext/2005/01000/Cancer_Caregivers_Online__Hope,_Emotional_Roller.8.aspx.

Knobloch-Westerwick, S. 2006. Mood management: Theory, evidence, and advancements. In J. Bryant and P. Vorderer (Eds.), *Psychology of entertainment* (pp. 239–54). Mahwah, NJ: Lawrence Erlbaum Associates.

Kramer, A. D. I., J. E. Guillory, and J. T. Hancock. 2014. Experimental evidence of massive-scale emotional contagion through social networks. *Proceedings of the National Academy of Sciences*. doi: 10.1073/pnas.1320040111.

Kühne, R., and C. Schemer. 2013. The emotional effects of news frames on information processing and opinion formation. *Communication Research*. doi: 10.1177/0093650213514599.

Lang, A. 2000. The limited capacity model of mediated message processing. *Journal of Communication* 50(1):46–70. doi: 10.1111/j.1460-2466.2000.tb02833.x.

———. 2006. Using the Limited Capacity Model of Motivated Mediated Message Processing to design effective cancer communication messages. *Journal of Communication* 56:S57–S80. doi: 10.1111/j.1460-2466.2006.00283.x.

Lang, A., P. Bolls, R. F. Potter, and K. Kawahara. 1999. The effects of production pacing and arousing content on the information processing of television messages. *Journal of Broadcasting and Electronic Media* 43(4):451–75. doi: 10.1080/08838159909364504.

Lang, A., S. D. Bradley, J. V. Sparks, and S. Lee. 2007. The Motivation Activation Measure (MAM): How well does MAM predict individual differences in physiological indicators of appetitive and aversive activation? *Communication Methods and Measures* 1(2):113–36. doi: 10.1080/19312450701399370.

Lang, A., and S. Lee. 2014. Individual differences in trait motivational reactivity influence children and adolescents' responses to pictures of taboo products. *Journal of Health Communication*, 1–17. doi: 10.1080/10810730.2013.864733.

Lang, A., A. Sanders-Jackson, Z. Wang, and B. Rubenking. 2012. Motivated message processing: How motivational activation influences resource allocation, encoding, and storage of TV messages. *Motivation and Emotion*, 1–10. doi: 10.1007/s11031-012-9329-y.

Lang, A., and N. S. Yegiyan. 2008. Understanding the interactive effects of emotional appeal and claim strength in health messages. *Journal of Broadcasting and Electronic Media* 52(3):432–47. doi: 10.1080/08838150802205629.

Lazarus, R. S. 1991. *Emotion and adaptation*. New York: Oxford University Press.

Loewenstein, G. F., E. U. Weber, C. K. Hsee, and N. Welch. 2001. Risk as feelings. *Psychological Bulletin* 127(2):267–86. doi: 10.1037/0033-2909.127.2.267.

Maio, G. R., and V. M. Esses. 2001. The need for affect: Individual differences in the motivation to approach or avoid emotions. *Journal of Personality* 69(4):583–614. doi: 10.1111/1467-6494.694156.

Mastro, D. E., M. S. Eastin, and R. Tamborini. 2002. Internet search behaviors and mood alterations: A selective exposure approach. *Media Psychology* 4(2):157–72. doi: 10.1207/S1532785XMEP0402_03.

Mayer, J. D., and Y. N. Gaschke. 1988. The experience and meta-experience of mood. *Journal of Personality and Social Psychology* 55(1):102–11. doi: 10.1037/0022-3514.55.1.102.

Mayer, J. D., and P. Salovey. 1993. The intelligence of emotional intelligence. *Intelligence* 17(4):433–42. doi: 10.1016/0160-2896(93)90010-3.

McQueen, A., M. W. Kreuter, B. Kalesan, and K. I. Alcaraz. 2011. Understanding narrative effects: The impact of breast cancer survivor stories on message processing, attitudes, and beliefs among African American women. *Health Psychology* 30(6):674–82. doi: 10.1037/a0025395.

Monahan, J. L. 1995. Thinking positively: Using positive affect when designing health messags. In E. W. Maibach and R. Parrott (Eds.), *Designing health messages: Approaches from communication theory and public health practice* (pp. 81–98). Thousand Oaks, CA: SAGE.

Morgan, S. E., L. Movius, and M. J. Cody. 2009. The power of narratives: The effect of entertainment television organ donation storylines on the attitudes, knowledge, and behaviors of donors and nondonors. *Journal of Communication* 59(1):135–51. doi: 10.1111/j.1460-2466.2008.01408.x.

Moyer-Gusé, E. 2008. Toward a theory of entertainment persuasion: Explaining the persuasive effects of entertainment-education messages. *Communication Theory* 18(3):407–25. doi: 10.1111/j.1468-2885.2008.00328.x.

Moyer-Gusé, E., and R. L. Nabi. 2010. Explaining the effects of narrative in an entertainment television program: Overcoming resistance to persuasion. *Human Communication Research* 36(1):26–52. doi: 10.1111/j.1468-2958.2009.01367.x.

Mukherjee, S. 2010. *The emperor of all maladies: A biography of cancer*. New York: Scribner.

Murphy, S. T., L. B. Frank, J. S. Chatterjee, and L. Baezconde-Garbanati. 2013. Narrative versus nonnarrative: The role of identification, transportation, and emotion in reducing health disparities. *Journal of Communication* 63(1):116–37. doi: 10.1111/jcom.12007.

Murphy, S. T., L. B. Frank, M. B. Moran, and P. Patnoe-Woodley. 2011. Involved, transported, or emotional? Exploring the determinants of change in knowledge, attitudes, and behavior in entertainment-education. *Journal of Communication* 61(3):407–31. doi: 10.1111/j.1460-2466.2011.01554.x.

Myrick, J. G., S. M. Noar, J. F. Willoughby, and J. Brown. 2014. Public reaction to the death of Steve Jobs: Implications for cancer communication. *Journal of Health Communication*, 1–18. doi: 10.1080/10810730.2013.872729.

Myrick, J. G., J. F. Willoughby, S. M. Noar, and J. Brown. 2013. Reactions of young adults to the death of Apple CEO Steve Jobs: Implications for cancer communication. *Communication Research Reports* 30(2):115–26. doi: 10.1080/08824096.2012.762906.

Nabi, R. L. 2003. Exploring the framing effects of emotion. *Communication Research* 30(2):224–47. doi: 10.1177/0093650202250881.

Nabi, R. L., and M. C. Green. 2014. The role of a narrative's emotional flow in promoting persuasive outcomes. *Media Psychology*, 1–26. doi: 10.1080/15213269.2014.912585.

Norris, R. L., R. L. Bailey, P. D. Bolls, and K. R. Wise. 2011. Effects of emotional tone and visual complexity on processing health information in prescription drug advertising. *Health Communication* 27(1):42–48. doi: 10.1080/10410236.2011.567450.

Oatley, K. 2002. Emotions and the story worlds of fiction. In M. C. Green, J. J. Strange, and T. C. Brock (Eds.), *Narrative impact: Social and cognitive foundations* (pp. 39–70). Mahwah, NJ: Lawrence Erlbaum Associates.

Oliver, M. B. 1993. Exploring the paradox of the enjoyment of sad films. *Human Communication Research* 19(3):315–42. doi: 10.1111/j.1468-2958.1993.tb00304.x.

———. 2003. Mood management and selective exposure. In J. Bryant, D. Roskos-Ewoldsen, and J. Cantor (Eds.), *Communication and emotion* (pp. 85–106). Mahway, NJ: Lawrence Erlbaum Associates.

Panksepp, J. 2011. Empathy and the laws of affect. *Science* 334(6061):1358–59. doi: 10.1126/science.1216480.

Pechmann, C., and E. T. Reibling. 2006. Antismoking advertisements for youths: An independent evaluation of health, counter-industry, and industry approaches. *American Journal of Public Health* 96(5):906–13. doi: 10.2105/ajph.2004.057273.

Raghunathan, R., and K. Corfman. 2004. Sadness as pleasure-seeking prime and anxiety as attentiveness prime: The "different affect–different effect" (DADE) model. *Motivation and Emotion* 28(1):23–41. doi: 10.1023/B:MOEM.0000027276.32709.30.

Raghunathan, R., and Y. Trope. 2002. Walking the tightrope between feeling good and being accurate: Mood as a resource in processing persuasive messages. *Journal of Personality and Social Psychology* 83(3):510–25. doi: 10.1037/0022-3514.83.3.510.

Rizzolatti, G. 2008. *Mirrors in the brain: How our minds share actions, emotions.* Oxford; New York: Oxford University Press.

Salovey, P., and J. D. Mayer. 1988. Emotional intelligence. *Imagination, Cognition and Personality* 9(3):185–211. doi: 10.2190/DUGG-P24E-52WK-6CDG.

Schwarz, N., and Clore, G. L. 1983. Mood, misattribution, and judgments of well-being: Informative and directive functions of affective states. *Journal of Personality and Social Psychology* 45(3):513–23. doi: 10.1037/0022-3514.45.3.513.

———. 1988. How do I feel about it? The informative function of mood. In K. Fiedler and J. P. Forgas (Eds.), *Affect, cognition and social behavior* (pp. 44–62). Toronto: C. J. Hogrefe.

———. 2003. Mood as Information: 20 years later. *Psychological Inquiry* 14(3–4):296–303. doi: 10.1080/1047840x.2003.9682896.

Shamay-Tsoory, S. G., J. Aharon-Peretz, and D. Perry. 2009. Two systems for empathy: A double dissociation between emotional and cognitive empathy in inferior frontal gyrus versus ventromedial prefrontal lesions. *Brain* 132(3):617–27. doi: 10.1093/brain/awn279.

Shen, L. 2010. Mitigating psychological reactance: The role of message-induced empathy in persuasion. *Human Communication Research* 36(3):397–422. doi: 10.1111/j.1468-2958.2010.01381.x.

———. 2011. The effectiveness of empathy- versus fear-arousing antismoking PSAs. *Health Communication* 26(5):404–15. doi: 10.1080/10410236.2011.552480.

Slater, M. D., and D. Rouner. 2002. Entertainment-education and elaboration likelihood: Understanding the processing of narrative persuasion. *Communication Theory* 12(2):173–91. doi: 10.1111/j.1468-2885.2002.tb00265.x.

Slovic, P., M. L. Finucane, E. Peters, and D. G. MacGregor. 2004. Risk as analysis and risk as feelings: Some thoughts about affect, reason, risk, and rationality. *Risk Analysis* 24(2):311–22. doi: 10.1111/j.0272-4332.2004.00433.x.

Slovic, P., and E. Peters. 2006. Risk perception and affect. *Current Directions in Psychological Science* 15(6):322–25. doi: 10.1111/j.1467-8721.2006.00461.x.

Slovic, P., E. Peters, M. L. Finucane, and D. G. Macgregor. 2005. Affect, risk, and decision making. *Health Psychology* 24(4):S35–S40.

Stiff, J. B., J. P. Dillard, L. Somera, H. Kim, and C. Sleight. 1988. Empathy, communication, and prosocial behavior. *Communication Monographs* 55(2):198–213. doi: 10.1080/03637758809376166.

Tal-Or, N., and J. Cohen. 2010. Understanding audience involvement: Conceptualizing and manipulating identification and transportation. *Poetics* 38(4):402–18. doi: http://dx.doi.org/10.1016/j.poetic.2010.05.004.

Tian, Y., and J. H. Yoo. 2014. Connecting with *The Biggest Loser*: An extended model of parasocial interaction and identification in health-related reality TV shows. *Health Communication*, 1–7. doi: 10.1080/10410236.2013.836733.

Trope, Y., and E. Neter. 1994. Reconciling competing motives in self-evaluation: The role of self-control in feedback seeking. *Journal of Personality and Social Psychology* 66(4):646–57. doi: 10.1037/0022-3514.66.4.646.

Trope, Y., and E. M. Pomerantz. 1998. Resolving conflicts among self-evaluative motives: Positive experiences as a resource for overcoming defensiveness. *Motivation and Emotion* 22(1):53–72. doi: 10.1023/a:1023044625309.

Tugade, M. M., and B. L. Fredrickson. 2004. Resilient individuals use positive emotions to bounce back from negative emotional experiences. *Journal of Personality and Social Psychology* 86(2):320–33.

White, M., and S. M. Dorman. 2001. Receiving social support online: Implications for health education. *Health Education Research* 16(6):693–707. doi: 10.1093/her/16.6.693.

Williams, W. W., P. J. Lu, M. C. Lindley, E. D. Kennedy, and J. A. Singleton. 2012. Influenza vaccination coverage among adults—National Health Interview Survey, United States, 2008–09 influenza season. *Morbidity and Mortality Weekly Report* 61 Suppl:65–72.

Zillmann, D. 1971. Excitation transfer in communication-mediated aggressive behavior. *Journal of Experimental Social Psychology* 7(4):419–34. doi: 10.1016/0022-1031(71)90075-8.

———. 1988. Mood management through communication choices. *American Behavioral Scientist* 31(3):327–40. doi: 10.1177/000276488031003005.

———. 2006. Exemplification effects in the promotion of safety and health. *Journal of Communication* 56:S221–S237. doi: 10.1111/j.1460-2466.2006.00291.x.

Zillmann, D., and H.-B. Brosius. 2000. *Exemplification in communication: The influence of case reports on the perception of issues.* Mahwah, NJ: Lawrence Erlbaum Associates.

Zillmann, D., and J. Bryant. 1985. *Selective exposure to communication.* Hillsdale, NJ: Erlbaum Associates.

Zillmann, D., J. W. Perkins, and S. S. Sundar. 1992. Impression-formation effects of printed news varying in descriptive precision and exemplifications. *Zeitschrift für Medienpsychologie* 4(3):168–85.

Index

action tendencies: in health campaigns, 173; in health information seeking, 202–203, 205–206, 208–209; in interactive experiences, 225, 226, 227; in health journalism, 193–194; of anger and sadness, 46, 51–52, 53–54, 57, 58, 72; of elevation, 147, 148, 149, 152, 156–157; of fear and guilt, 13, 14, 18, 23, 31, 39; of happiness and pride, 87, 94, 104, 108; of hope, 132, 134; of interest, 123, 127; themes of, 243–244, 249, 257, 273; theoretical foundations, xvii, 3, 7–8

advertising, 42, 89, 172

affect-as-information, 255, 256, 257

Affordable Care Act, xii, 28, 96

alcohol, xii, 38, 45, 55, 64, 92, 94, 108, 112, 164, 178, 226

anger: as an emotion, 2, 3, 5; definition of and applications in media messaging, 51–65; discrete emotions, xiii, xv; in Anger Activism Model (AAM), 56; in appraisal theory, 5, 6–7, 8; in emotion regulation and mood management, 203, 209, 211, 212, 213; in the Extended Parallel Process Model, 18; in framing, xvii; in guilt communication, 41, 42, 44, 47; in health campaigns, 165, 169–170, 171, 173, 175, 176; in health journalism, 187, 188, 189, 190, 193–194, 195; in hope and prevention

messages, 135, 139; in message design, 247, 249, 257; in video games, 230; negative emotions, xx, xxii, 72; reduced through laughter, 88

anticipated emotions, xv, 232

anxiety, xv, xx, 3, 14, 17, 20, 26, 27, 29, 62, 77, 93, 97, 106, 114, 149, 155, 175, 183, 186, 188, 190, 199–202, 205, 206, 210, 215, 227, 229, 230, 246, 248, 256, 257, 268, 270

appraisal, xvii, xx, 2; in health journalism, 187, 193, 194; in health seeking information, 205, 206, 211; in mobile health, 225; in relation to meta-emotions, 268; of anger, 52, 53, 54, 61, 64; of fear appeals, 13, 14, 15–17, 19, 23, 24, 29, 31; of guilt appeals, 42, 43; of hope, 132, 133–134, 135, 137, 138, 141; of humor, 86; of interest, 120, 121–122, 124, 126; of pride, 111; of sadness, 71, 74; patterns of, 243, 247, 257

Appraisal Tendency Framework, 209

appraisal theory, xviii, xx, 1, 5–9, 18, 79, 111, 202, 205, 208–209, 244, 249, 257

arousal, 2, 4, 5, 8, 17, 23, 29, 87, 121, 152, 155, 163, 166, 169, 175, 194, 203, 211, 222, 223, 226, 230, 233, 236, 243, 250, 256, 260, 263, 271, 273